WORLD REPORT ON **AGEING AND HEALTH**

WHO Library Cataloguing-in-Publication Data

World report on ageing and health.

1.Aging. 2.Life Expectancy. 3.Aged. 4.Health Services for the Aged. 5.Global Health.
6.Population Dynamics. 7.Delivery of Health Care. I.World Health Organization.

ISBN 978 92 4 156504 2   (NLM classification: WT 104)
ISBN 978 92 4 069479 8 (ePub)
ISBN 978 92 4 069480 4 (Daisy)
ISBN 978 92 4 069481 1 (PDF)

Cover: The painting on the cover of the Report is Rose Wiley's 'PV Windows and Floorboards'. At 81 years old Rose Wiley's style is fresh, unpredictable and cutting edge. This painting won the John Moores Painting Prize in 2014 from more than 2,500 entries. At double the age of previous winners, Rose Wiley shows that older age need not be a barrier to success. The John Moores Painting Prize unlike other prestigious art prizes does not restrict submissions for contemporary works by age. The copyright for this painting is held by the artist.

Printed in Luxembourg

Contents

Preface

At a time of unpredictable challenges for health, whether from a changing climate, emerging infectious diseases, or the next microbe that develops drug resistance, one trend is certain: the ageing of populations is rapidly accelerating worldwide. For the first time in history, most people can expect to live into their 60s and beyond. The consequences for health, health systems, their workforce and budgets are profound.

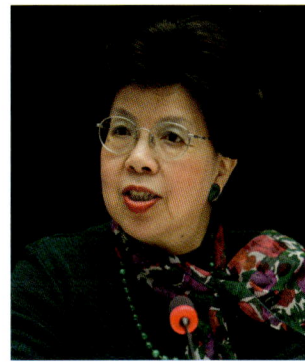

The *World report on ageing and health* responds to these challenges by recommending equally profound changes in the way health policies for ageing populations are formulated and services are provided. As the foundation for its recommendations, the report looks at what the latest evidence has to say about the ageing process, noting that many common perceptions and assumptions about older people are based on outdated stereotypes.

As the evidence shows, the loss of ability typically associated with ageing is only loosely related to a person's chronological age. There is no "typical" older person. The resulting diversity in the capacities and health needs of older people is not random, but rooted in events throughout the life course that can often be modified, underscoring the importance of a life-course approach. Though most older people will eventually experience multiple health problems, older age does not imply dependence. Moreover, contrary to common assumptions, ageing has far less influence on health care expenditures than other factors, including the high costs of new medical technologies.

Guided by this evidence, the report aims to move the debate about the most appropriate public health response to population ageing into new – and much broader – territory. The overarching message is optimistic: with the right policies and services in place, population ageing can be viewed as a rich new opportunity for both individuals and societies. The resulting framework for taking public health action offers a menu of concrete steps that can be adapted for use in countries at all levels of economic development.

In setting out this framework, the report emphasizes that healthy ageing is more than just the absence of disease. For most older people, the maintenance of functional ability has the highest importance. The greatest costs to society are not the expenditures made to foster this functional ability, but the benefits that might be missed if we fail to make the appropriate adaptations and investments. The recommended societal approach to population ageing, which includes the goal of building an age-friendly world, requires a transformation of health systems away from disease-based curative models and towards the provision of integrated care that is centred on the needs of older people.

The report's recommendations are anchored in the evidence, comprehensive, and forward-looking, yet eminently practical. Throughout, examples of experiences from different countries are used to illustrate how specific problems can be addressed through innovation solutions. Topics explored range from strategies to deliver comprehensive and person-centred services to older populations, to policies that enable older people to live in comfort and safety, to ways to correct the problems and injustices inherent in current systems for long-term care.

In my view, the *World report on ageing and health* has the potential to transform the way policy-makers and service-providers perceive population ageing – and plan to make the most of it.

Dr Margaret Chan
Director-General
World Health Organization

Acknowlededgments

The report was prepared by an editorial team comprising John Beard, Alana Officer and Andrew Cassels, under the overall guidance of Flavia Bustreo, Assistant Director-General Women and Children's Health; Anne Marie Worning; and Anarfi Asamoa-Baah, Deputy Director-General. Many other WHO staff from the regional offices and a range of departments contributed both to specific sections relevant to their areas of work and to the development of the overall conceptual framework. Without their dedication, support and expertise this report would not have been possible.

A core group responsible for developing the conceptual framework and writing the report included Islene Araujo de Carvalho, John Beard, Somnath Chatterji, JoAnne Epping Jordan, Alison Harvey, Norah Keating, Aki Kuroda, Wahyu Retno Mahanani, Jean-Pierre Michel, Alana Officer, Anne Margriet Pot, Ritu Sadana, Jotheeswaran Amuthavalli Thiyagarajan and Lisa Warth. Chapter development was led by John Beard and Ritu Sadana (Chapter 1), John Beard and Jean-Pierre Michel (Chapter 2), John Beard and Somnath Chatterji (Chapter 3), Islene Araujo de Carvalho and JoAnne Epping Jordan (Chapter 4), Anne Margriet Pot and Peter Lloyd-Sherlock (Chapter 5) and Alana Officer and John Beard (Chapter 6).

General research support was provided by Meredith Newlin, Jannis Pähler vor der Holte and Harleen Rai, and data analysis was provided by Colin Mathers, Nirmala Naidoo, Gretchen Stevens and Emese Verdes. Data on volunteering was obtained from the Gallup World Poll, provided by Gallup, Inc. Photos were provided by HelpAge International.

The report benefited from the rich inputs of a number of experts and academics. It was also informed by many individuals from various institutions who provided background papers, which were coordinated by Catherine d'Arcangues. Their names are listed as contributors.

The report also benefited from the efforts of many other people, in particular Miriam Pinchuk, who edited the final text of the report.

Thanks are also due to the following: Christopher Black, Alison Brunier, Anna Gruending, Giles Reboux, Sarah Russell, Marta Seoane Aguilo and Sari Setiogi for media and communication; Amanda Milligan for proofreading, and Laurence Errington for indexing; Eddie Hill and Sue Hobbs for graphic design; Christelle Cazabat and Melanie Lauckner for producing the report in alternative formats;

Mira Schneiders for coordinating the translation and printing; and Charlotte Wristberg for her administrative support.

The World Health Organization also wishes to thank the governments of Japan and the Netherlands for their generous financial support for the development, translation and publication of the report. The development of the report was supported through Core Voluntary Contributions.

Contributors

Additional contributors

Sharon Anderson, Yumiko Arai, Alanna Armitage, Marie-Charlotte Bouesseau, Francesco Branca, Mathias Braubach, David Burnes, Esteban Calvo, James Campbell, Matteo Cesari, Shelly Chadha, Hannie Comijs, Catherine d'Arcangues, Adrian Davis, Jens Deerberg, Joan Dzenowagis, Robert Enderbeek, Laura Ferguson, Ruth Finkelstein, Kelly Fitzgerald, Pascale Fritsch, Loic Garçon, Francisco Javier Gomez Batiste-Alentorn, Mike Hodin, Manfred Huber, Elif Islek, Josephine Jackisch, Matthew Jowett, Rania Kawar, Ed Kelley, Silvio Mariotti, Mike Martin, Hernan Montenegro, John Morris, Wendy Moyle, Karl Pillemer, Bill Reichman, Alex Ross, Martin Smalbrugge, Nuria Toro Polanco, Kelly Tremblay, Bruno Vellas, Armin Von Gunten, Robert Wallace, Huali Wang, Martin Webber.

Peer reviewers

Isabella Aboderin, Maysoon Al-Amoud, George Alleyne, Yumiko Arai, Alanna Armitage, Said Arnaout, Senarath Attanayake, Julie Byles, Matteo Cesari, Heung Cha, Shelly Chadha, Sung Choi, Alexandre Cote, June Crown, Joan Dzenowagis, Robert Eendebak, Ruth Finkelstein, Loic Garçon, Emmanuel Gonzalez-Bautista, Gustavo Gonzalez-Canali, Sally Greengross, Luis Miguel Gutierrez Robledo, Anna Howe, Manfred Huber, Alexandre Kalache, Rania Kawar, Rajat Khosla, Michael Kidd, Hyo Jeong Kim, Tom Kirkwood, Hans-Horst Konkolewsky, Nabil Kronfol, Ritchard Ledgerd, Bengt Lindstom, Stephen Lungaro-Mifsud, John McCallum, Roar Maagaard, Melissa Medich, Verena Menec, Juan Mezzich, Tim Muir, Leendert Nederveen, Triphonie Nkurunziza, S.Jay Olshansky, Desmond O'Neill, Paul Ong, Du Peng, Silvia Perel-Levin, Poul Erik Petersen, Toby Porter, Vinayak Mohan Prasad, Thomas Prohaska, Parminder Raina, Glenn Rees, William Reichman, Andreas Alois Reis, Nathalie Roebbel, Perminder Sachdev, Xenia Scheil-Adlung, Dorothea Schmidt, Shoji Shinkai, Alan Sinclair, Martin Smalbrugge, Mike Splaine, Victor Tabbush, Virpi Timonen, Andreas Ullrich, Enrique Vega, Adriana Velazquez Berumen, Armin von Gunten, Huali Wang, Ruth Warick, Jennifer Wenborn, Anthony Woolf, Tom Wright, Tuohong Zhang.

Box authors

John Beard and Laura Ferguson (1.1); Michael Marmot (1.2); Paul Nash (1.3); David Phillips (1.4); Ursula Staudinger (3.1); Tarun Dua and Shekhar Saxena (3.2, 3.3); Hiroshi Ogawa and Poul Erik Petersen (3.4); Ebtisam Alhuwaidi (4.1); Islene Araujo de Carvalho (4.2); Kiran Iyer, Nandita Kshetrimayum and Ganesh Shenoy Panchmal (4.3); Islene Araujo de Carvalho (4.4, 4.5); Silvia Costa, Alexandre Kalache, and Ina Voelcker (4.6); Islene Araujo de Carvalho (4.7); Islene Araujo de Carvalho, Luc Besançon and Alison Roberts (4.8); Eduardo Augusto Duque Bezerra (4.9); ; Loic Garçon (5.1); Amit Dias (5.2); Anne Margriet Pot (5.3); John Beard (5.4); Anne Margriet Pot (5.5); Dawn Brooker (5.6); Hussain Jafri and Theresa Lee (5.7); Marie-Charlotte Bouesseau, Xavier Gomez and Nuria Toro (5.8); Elif Islek (5.9); Fred Lafeber (5.10); Anne Margriet Pot (5.11); Jim Pearson (5.12); Lindsey Goldman and Lisa Warth (6.1); Laura Fergusen (6.2); HelpAge International (6.3); Lindy Clemson, Monica R Perracini, Vicky Scott, Catherine Sherrington, Anne Tiedemann and Sebastiana Zimba Kalula (6.4); Frances Heywood (6.5); Bobby Grewal (6.6); Jannis Pahler vor der Holte (6.7); David Hutton (6.8); Alana Officer (6.9); Thuy Bich Tran and Quyen Ngoc Tran (6.10); Adrian Bauman, David Buchner, Fiona Bull, Maria Fiatarone Singh, Alison Harvey and Dafna Merom (6.11); Jaclyn Kelly, Anne Berit Rafoss and Lisa Warth (6.12); Senarath Attanayake (6.13); Alana Officer and Lisa Warth (6.14); Lisa Warth (6.15); Jaclyn Kelly and Lisa Warth (6.16); Alana Officer and Lisa Warth (6.17); Stéphane Birchmeier (6.18); Islene Araujo de Carvalho and JoAnne Epping Jordan (7.1); Mitch Besser and Sarah Rohde (7.2); Jaclyn Kelly and Lisa Warth (7.3); Suzanne Garon (7.4); Tine Buffel (7.5).

Authors of background papers

- *Age-associated skin conditions and diseases: current perspectives and future options.* Ulrike Blume-Peytavi, Jan Kottner, Wolfram Sterry, Michael W Hodin, Tamara W Griffiths, Rachel EB Watson, Roderick J Hay, Christopher EM Griffiths.
- *Ageing and hearing health.* Adrian Davis, Catherine McMahon, Kathleen Pichora-Fuller, Shirley Russ, Frank Lin, Bolajoko Olusanya, Shelly Chadha, Kelly Tremblay.
- *Ageing, work, and health.* Ursula Staudinger, Ruth Finkelstein, Esteban Calvo, Kavita Sivaramakrishnan.
- *Developmental aspects of a life course approach to healthy ageing.* Mark Hanson, Cyrus Cooper, Avan Aihie-Sayer, John Beard.
- *Elder abuse.* Karl Pillemer, David Burnes, Catherine Riffin Mark S Lachs.
- *Ethics and older people.* Julian C Hughes.
- *Falls in older adults: current evidence gaps and priority challenges.* Monica Perracini, Lindy Clemson, Anne Tiedemann, Sebastiana Zimba Kalula, Vicky Scott, Catherine Sherrington.

- *Frailty: an emerging public health priority.* Matteo Cesari, Martin Prince, Roberto Bernabei, Piu Chan, Luis Miguel Gutierrez-Robledo, Jean-Pierre Michel, John E Morley, Paul Ong, Leocadio Rodriguez Manas, Alan Sinclair, Chang Won Won, Bruno Vellas.
- *Gender and ageing.* Julie Byles, Cate D'Este, Paul Kowal, Cassie Curryer, Louise Thomas, Adam Yates, Britta Baer, Anjana Bhushan, Joanna Vogel, Lilia Jara.
- *Genetic influences on functional capacities in ageing.* Andrea D Foebel, Nancy L Pedersen.
- *Healthy ageing: raising awareness of inequalities, determinants, and what could be done to improve health equity.* Ritu Sadana, Erik Blas, Suman Budhwani, Theadora Koller, Guillermo Paraje.
- *Investing in health to create a third demographic dividend.* Linda P Fried.
- *Medical and assistive health technologies: meeting the needs of ageing populations in low- and middle-income countries.* Chapal Khasnabis, Loic Garçon, Lloyd Walker, Yukiko Nakatani, Jostacio Lapitan, Alex Ross, Adriana Velazquez Berumen, Johan Borg.
- *Musculoskeletal (MSK) health and the impact of MSK disorders in the elderly.* Anthony Woolf, Lyn March, Alana Officer, Marita J Cross, Andrew M Briggs, Damian Hoy, Lidia Sanchez Riera, Fiona Blyth.
- *Older people as a resource for their own health.* Paul Ong.
- *Older people in humanitarian contexts: the impact of disaster on older people and the means of addressing their needs.* Hyo-Jeong Kim, Pascale Fritsch.
- *Physical activity in older adults.* Adrian Bauman, Maria Fiatarone Singh, David Buchner, Dafna Merom, Fiona Bull.
- *The right to health of older people.* Britta Baer, Anjana Bhushan, Hala Abou Taleb, Javier Vasquez, Rebekah Thomas.
- *What does rehabilitation offer to an ageing population?* Alarcos Cieza Moreno, Marta Imamura.

Conflicts of interest

None of the experts involved in the development of this report declared any conflicts of interest.

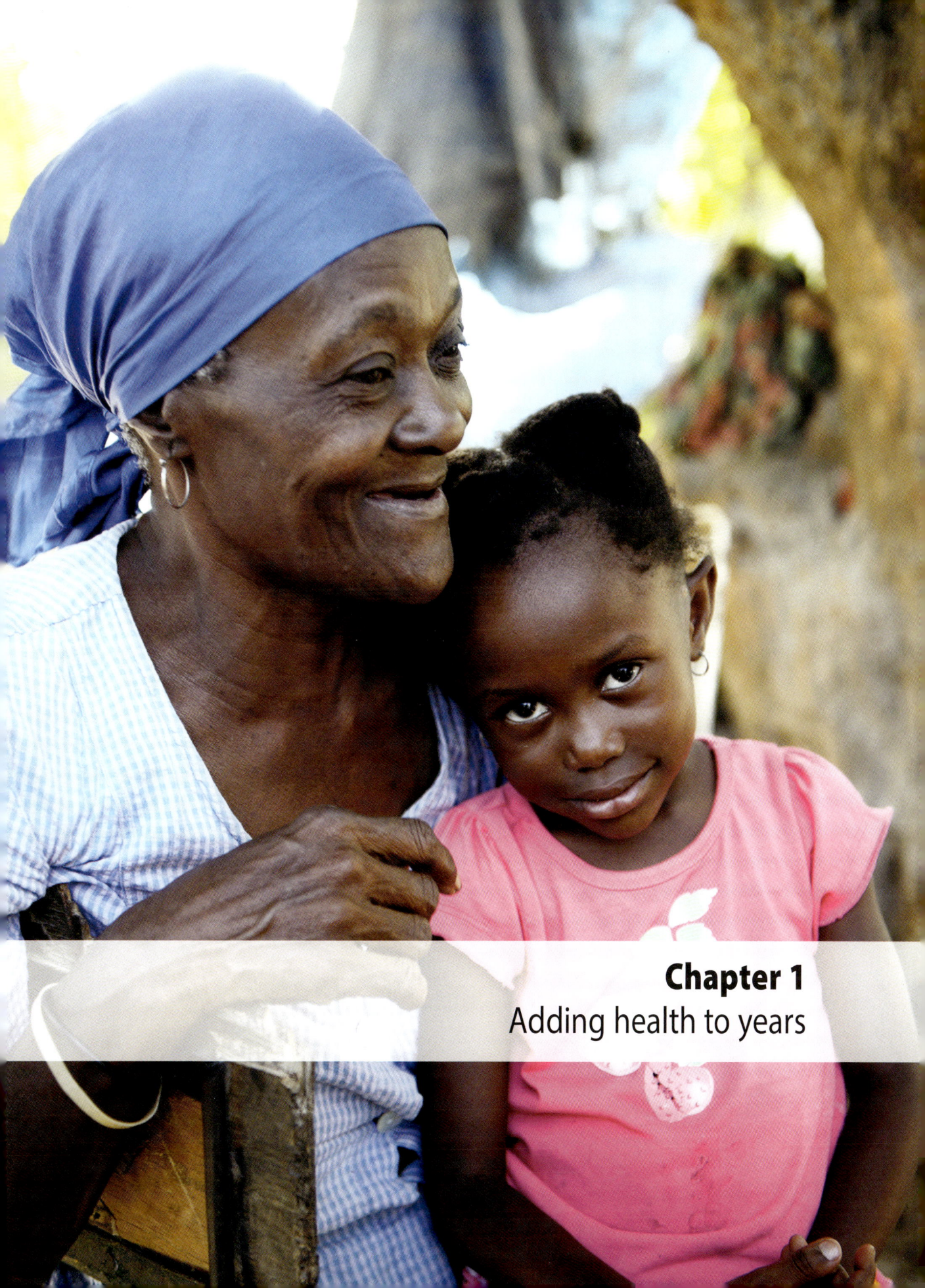

Chapter 1
Adding health to years

Yolande, 56, Haiti

Yolande is the sole provider for her children, two grandchildren and a little boy who she took in because he needed care. Yolande lost her home in the 2011 earthquake in Port-au-Prince and lives in temporary housing on the same site. She sells sweets and other produce from a street stall she established using a low interest loan.

"One of my dreams for the children would be that I could afford to send them to school."

1

Adding health to years

Introduction

Today, for the first time in history most people can expect to live into their 60s and beyond (*1*). In low- and middle-income countries, this is largely the result of large reductions in mortality at younger ages, particularly during childhood and childbirth, and from infectious diseases (*2*). In high-income countries, continuing increases in life expectancy are now mainly due to declining mortality among those who are older (*3*).

These changes are dramatic. A child born in Brazil or Myanmar in 2015 can expect to live 20 years longer than one born in those countries just 50 years ago. When combined with the marked falls in fertility occurring in almost every country, these trends are having equally significant impacts on the structure of populations. In the Islamic Republic of Iran in 2015, around 10% of the population is older than 60 years. In just 35 years' time, this will have increased to around 33% of the population.

These extra years of life and demographic shifts have profound implications for each of us, as well as for the societies we live in. They offer unprecedented opportunities, and are likely to have a fundamental impact on the way we live our lives, the things we aspire to and the ways we relate to each other (*4*). And, unlike most of the changes that societies will experience during the next 50 years, these underlying trends are largely predictable. We know that the demographic transition to older populations will occur, and we can plan to make the most of it.

Older people contribute to society in many ways – whether it be within their family, to their local community or to society more broadly. However, the extent of these human and social resources, and the opportunities available to each of us as we age, will be heavily dependent on one key characteristic: our health. If people are experiencing these extra years in good health, their ability to do the things they value will have few limits. If these added years are dominated by declines in physical and mental capacities, the implications for older people and for society may be much more negative.

Although it is often assumed that increasing longevity is being accompanied by an extended period of good health, the evidence that older people today are experiencing better health than their parents is less encouraging (Chapter 3).

Some longitudinal research has suggested that the prevalence of severe disability may have declined in wealthy countries, but this trend does not appear to extend to less severe disability, and may even have stalled (5–9). The picture from low- and middle-income countries is even less clear (10).

But poor health does not have to be the dominant and limiting feature of older populations. Most of the health problems of older age are the result of chronic diseases. Many of these can be prevented or delayed by engaging in healthy behaviours. Indeed, even in very advanced years, physical activity and good nutrition can have powerful benefits for health and well-being. Other health problems can be effectively managed, particularly if they are detected early enough. Even for people experiencing declines in capacity, supportive environments can ensure that they can still get where they need to go and do what they need to do. Long-term care and support can ensure that they live dignified lives with opportunities for continued personal growth. Yet unhealthy behaviours remain prevalent among older people, health systems are poorly aligned with the needs of the older populations they now serve, in many parts of the world it is unsafe and impractical for an older person to leave their home, caregivers are often untrained, and at least 1 in 10 older people is a victim of some form of elder abuse (Chapter 3).

The ageing of populations thus demands a comprehensive public-health response. However, debate about just what this might comprise has been limited (11). In many areas the evidence for what works is thin (12).

The context for action

The international legal and policy frameworks

Two international policy instruments have guided action on ageing since 2002: the *Politi-cal declaration and Madrid international plan of action on ageing* (13) and the World Health Organization's *Active ageing: a policy framework* (14) (Box 1.1). These documents sit within the context of an international legal framework afforded by human rights law. They celebrate rising life expectancy and the potential of older populations to act as powerful resources for future development (Box 1.1). They highlight the skills, experience and wisdom of older people, and the contributions they make. They map a broad range of areas where policies can enable these contributions and ensure security in older age. Each document identifies the importance of health in older age, both in its own right and for the instrumental benefits of enabling the participation of older people (and the benefits that this, in turn, may have on health) (14). However, little detail is given on the systemic changes necessary to achieve these goals.

Yet a recent review of the progress made globally since 2002, covering more than 130 countries, noted that "there is low priority within health policy to the challenge of the demographic transition"; "there are low levels of training in geriatrics and gerontology within the health professions, despite increasing numbers of older persons"; and "care and support for caregivers… is not a priority focus of government action on ageing" (17).

This lack of progress, occurring despite clear opportunities for action, is doubly important because population ageing is inextricably linked with many other global public-health agendas, particularly in relation to universal health coverage, noncommunicable diseases and disability, as well as the post-2015 development agenda and specifically the Sustainable Development Goals (18). Without considering the health and well-being of older adults, many of these agendas do not make sense or will simply be unachievable.

Box 1.1.   International legal and policy frameworks on ageing

International human rights law

Human rights are the universal freedoms and entitlements of individuals and groups that are protected by law. These include civil and political rights, such as the right to life, as well as social, economic and cultural rights, which include rights to health, social security and housing. All rights are interrelated, interdependent and inalienable. Human rights cannot be taken away due to a person's age or health status. Article 1 of the *International Covenant on Economic, Social and Cultural Rights* proscribes discrimination based on an individual's status, and this proscription encompasses age (*15*). By definition, human rights apply to all people, including older people, even when there is no specific reference in the text to older age groups or ageing.

During the past two decades, major strides have been made in efforts to advance human rights, including those of older people. Several international human rights treaties and instruments refer to ageing or older persons, enshrining the freedom from discrimination of older women, older migrants and older people with disabilities; discussing health, social security and an adequate standard of living; and upholding the right to be free from exploitation, violence and abuse.

The Madrid international plan of action on ageing

In 2002, the United Nations General Assembly endorsed the *Political declaration and Madrid international plan of action on ageing* (*13*). Three priorities for action were identified in their recommendations: "older persons and development; advancing health and well-being into old age; and ensuring that older people benefit from enabling and supportive environments".

Several key issues were flagged in the plan. These remain relevant in 2015 and are emphasized in this report. They include: promoting health and well-being throughout life; ensuring universal and equal access to health-care services; providing appropriate services for older persons with HIV or AIDS; training care providers and health professionals; meeting the mental health needs of older persons; providing appropriate services for older persons with disability (addressed in the health priority); providing care and support for caregivers; and preventing neglect and abuse of, and violence against, older people (addressed in the environments priority). The plan also emphasizes the importance of ageing in place.

Active ageing

The idea of active ageing emerged as an attempt to bring together strongly compartmentalized policy domains in a coherent way (*16*). In 2002, the World Health Organization (WHO) released *Active ageing: a policy framework* (*14*). This framework defined active ageing as "the process of optimizing opportunities for health, participation and security to enhance quality of life as people age". It emphasizes the need for action across multiple sectors and has the goal of ensuring that "older persons remain a resource to their families, communities and economies".

The WHO policy framework identifies six key determinants of active ageing: economic, behavioural, personal, social, health and social services, and the physical environment. It recommends four components necessary for a health-policy response:

- prevent and reduce the burden of excess disabilities, chronic disease and premature mortality;
- reduce risk factors associated with major diseases and increase factors that protect health throughout the life course;
- develop a continuum of affordable, accessible, high-quality and age-friendly health and social services that address the needs and rights of people as they age;
- provide training and education to caregivers.

Current public-health response – more of the same will not be enough

Achieving the goals outlined in the *Political declaration and Madrid international plan of action on ageing* and *Active ageing: a policy framework* is not simply a case of doing more of what is already being done or doing it better. Systemic change is needed. In high-income countries, health systems are often better designed to cure acute conditions than to manage and minimize the consequences of the chronic states prevalent in older age (*19–21*). Moreover, these systems are often developed in professional silos and so address each of these issues separately. This can lead to polypharmacy, unnecessary interventions and care that is less than adequate (*22, 23*).

For example, in 2015 it was estimated that in one of France's biggest hospitals, 20% of all patients older than 70 were significantly less able to perform the basic tasks necessary for daily living at the time of discharge than they were when they entered the hospital. Yet the presenting condition accounted for this fall in ability in less than half of these cases. In the others, the decline in functional ability related to limitations in the care that patients had received. In 80%, the problem was preventable, usually through the use of easy and affordable alternative care models, such as encouraging mobilization or by better managing incontinence (*24*).

Nor are health services in high-income countries adequately integrated with long-term care systems. This can lead to costly acute services being used to meet chronic care needs and a failure to fully foster the functioning of older people receiving long-term care (*23, 25*).

In lower-income countries or in resource-poor settings around the world, access to health services is often limited. Health workers may have little training in how to deal with issues common in older age, such as dementia or frailty, and opportunities for the early diagnosis and management of conditions, such as high blood pressure (a key risk factor for the biggest killers of older people – heart disease and stroke), may be missed.

This can be seen in findings from the WHO Study on global AGEing and adult health (SAGE), which draws on nationally representative samples of older people from China, Ghana, India, Mexico, the Russian Federation and South Africa (*26*). Across the countries included in SAGE, effective health coverage has been estimated to range from 21% of patients in Mexico to 48% in South Africa. This indicates that vast numbers of older adults either forgo or underuse health services, or end up impoverished due to the need to pay for health services which may, or may not, be able to provide the care they need (*27*). Thus, while around 53% of older adults included in SAGE have been found to have high blood pressure, only 4–14% of them were receiving effective treatment (*28*). Spending on catastrophic health care is also very high, ranging from about 8% of income to 46%, even among older people with insurance (*27*).

These gaps in health care in low- and middle-income countries result in high rates of older people who have limitations in functioning (Chapter 3). Because these settings often have limited or non-existent infrastructure for long-term care, this responsibility is passed on to families who generally lack the training or support to provide the care needed. This may require another family member, usually a woman, to forgo work.

A comprehensive, global public-health response to population ageing will therefore need to transform systems that are fundamentally misaligned with the populations they increasingly serve. Achieving such alignment will require a clear understanding of health in older age and a focused conceptualization of what can be done to improve it. This will need to be framed in a way that speaks to all sectors because the health of older people is influenced not only by the systems providing health and long-term care but also by the environments they live in and have lived in throughout their lives.

As a step towards meeting this aspiration, this report seeks to bring together what is currently known about ageing and health, and to outline a public-health framework for action relevant to countries at all levels of development. Thus, the report can be considered to be giving substance to the health priorities identified more than 10 years ago by the *Political declaration and Madrid international plan of action on ageing* and *Active ageing: a policy framework*. However, given the significance of this task, the lack of action to date and the need to stimulate a global public-health response, we suggest a twin-track approach to policy that emphasizes the need for both healthy and active ageing. This emphasis is consistent with recent initiatives undertaken within the European Union (*29*). Because the determinants of health in older age are being established even before we are born, this report applies a life-course approach (*30*, *31*), but the focus of the report is on the second half of life.

The challenges for policy development

Four key challenges will need to be overcome if a comprehensive public-health response to population ageing is to be successful.

Diversity in older age

One major challenge arises from the sheer diversity of health and functional states experienced by older people. These reflect subtle physiological changes that occur over time but are only loosely associated with chronological age.

For example, Fig. 1.1 illustrates trajectories of physical capacity across the life course using data from the large Australian Longitudinal Study on Women's Health (*32*). The range of physical functioning (denoted by the dark lines at the top and bottom of Fig. 1.1) is far greater in older age than in younger ages. This diversity is a hallmark of older age. It means that some

Fig. 1.1.   Physical capacity across the life course stratified by ability to manage on current income

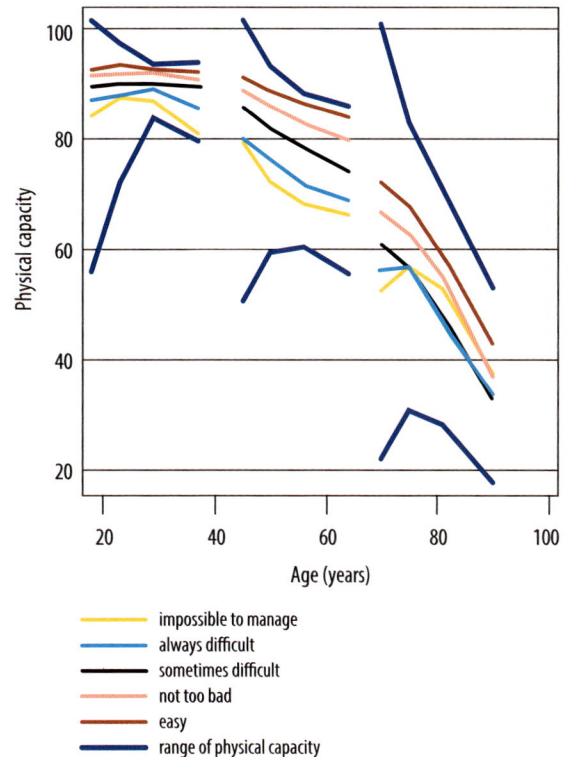

Source: G Peeters, J Beard, D Deeg, L Tooth, WJ Brown, A Dobson; unpublished analysis from the Australian Longitudinal Study on Women's Health.

80-year-olds will have levels of both physical and mental capacities similar to that of many 20-year-olds. Public-health policy must be framed to maximize the number of people who experience these positive trajectories of ageing. And it must serve to break down the many barriers that limit their ongoing social participation and contributions. But Fig. 1.1 also highlights the fact that many other people will experience significant declines in capacity at much younger ages. Some 60- or 70-year-olds will require help from others to undertake basic activities. A comprehensive public-health response to population ageing must address their needs too.

These diverse needs of older people are best viewed as a continuum of functioning. Yet policy responses often appear disjointed, focusing on one end of the continuum or the other. This reflects a broader public discourse that is often polarized between two very different perspectives on ageing.

On the one hand, deficit conceptualizations cast old age as a period of vulnerability and disengagement (33). From this perspective, decline and increasing irrelevance appear inevitable, and decision-makers focus on the "care of the elderly" and fret over what is portrayed as dependence and increasing demands for health care, pensions and social services.

On the other hand are models that emphasize the importance of social engagement in older age, the contribution that older people can make to all levels of society and the potential to make this the norm rather than an exception (16, 33–37). From this viewpoint, 70 becomes the new 60 and decision-makers look to overcome outdated stereotypes and foster active or successful ageing to create a society where the contribution of older people generally outweighs social investments (38).

The debate over these models can become quite heated. For example, while the more optimistic perspective can be seen as an "attempt to set something positive against the negative societal stereotypes of ageing", it has also been criticized as a "new orthodoxy" with fundamental flaws that are likely to have negative consequences for more vulnerable members of older populations (39). Others have suggested that these approaches may have helped shift public and political perceptions of older people from a homogenous "group of 'deserving poor' unable to work" to an even "more negative image of 'greedy geezers' who are unwilling to work" (40).

In 1961, Robert J. Havighurst, one of the fathers of modern gerontology, suggested that each position in this polarized debate was "an affirmation of certain values" (35). To some extent, this remains true today. Furthermore, the great diversity in the experience of older age suggests that there is some truth in each perspective.

Although many people continue to experience personal growth in older age, some disengage. Some experience good health, but others experience a significant loss of capacity and require substantial care. Policies cannot just focus on one end of this spectrum.

Therefore, one of the goals of this report is to build a public-health framework for action on ageing that is relevant to all older people.

The impact of inequity

The diversity seen in older age is not random. Although some diversity reflects genetic inheritance (41) or choices made by individuals during their lives, much is driven by influences that are often beyond an individual's control or outside the options available to them. These arise from the physical and social environments that people inhabit that can affect health directly, or through barriers or incentives that affect opportunities, decisions and behaviour (Chapter 6).

Moreover, the relationship we have with our environments varies according to many personal characteristics including the family we were born into, our sex and our ethnicity. The impact of these environments is often fundamentally skewed by these characteristics, leading to inequalities in health, and where unfair and avoidable, to health inequities (42). Indeed, a significant proportion of the vast diversity of capacity and circumstances that we see in older age is likely to be underpinned by the cumulative impact of these health inequities across the life course. This is sometimes referred to as cumulative advantage/disadvantage (43).

Thus, in Fig. 1.2, the lines between the darker boundaries of physical functioning show the cohort divided into quintiles of income adequacy. Those with the lowest income adequacy at baseline have a lower peak of physical functioning, and this disparity tends to persist across the whole life course. As most people would agree that differences in physical functioning should not be correlated with income, this report would consider that such differences and their persistence are inequitable.

These influences are important for policymakers for two reasons. First, they need to be aware that the people with the greatest health need at any time may also be those with the fewest resources to address it. Second, public-health policies need to be crafted in ways that overcome, rather than reinforce, these inequities (Box 1.2). These themes cut across much of this report.

Box 1.2.   Inequities in health and pensions

A review of health inequalities since 2010 in the United Kingdom found that while, on average, people could expect to live to age 77, 15 of these years would be spent with some form of disability. Moreover, both life expectancy and disability-free life expectancy varied depending on where someone lived. On average, people living in wealthier neighbourhoods in England die approximately 6 years later than those living in poorer neighbourhoods. The difference in disability-free life expectancy was even greater: 13 years. So people living in poorer areas not only die sooner, but they also spend more of their shorter lives with limitations of capacity (44). And poorer areas often lack the infrastructure and resources that might enable someone with restricted capacity to do what they need to do.

Fig. 1.2.   Life expectancy and disability-free life expectancy at birth, by neighbourhood income level, England, 1999–2003

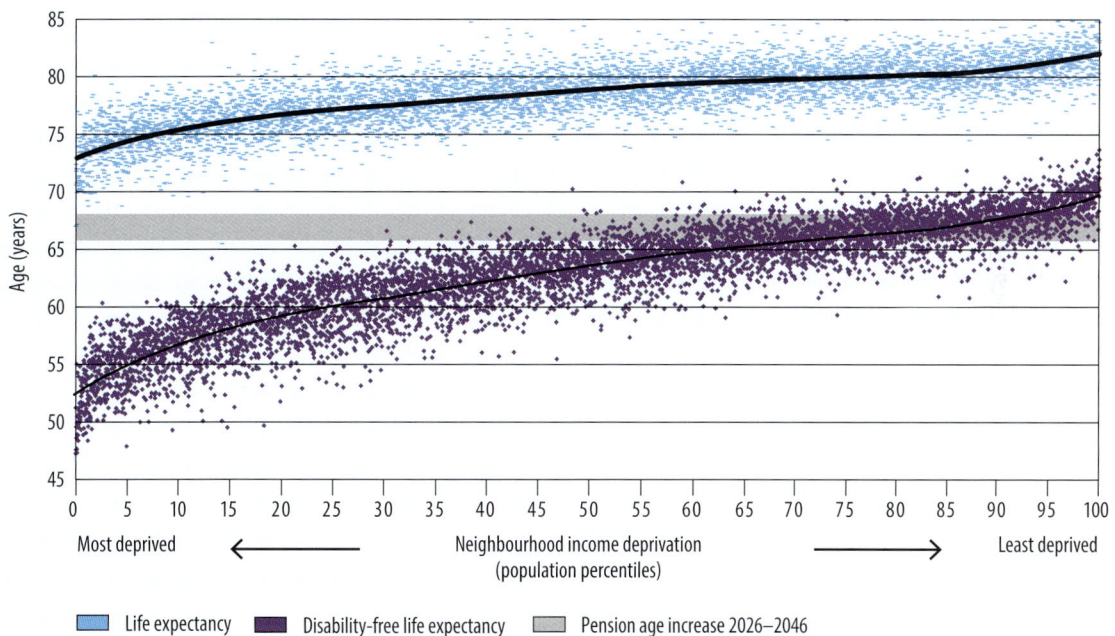

The analysis also compared disability-free life expectancy with the planned age for pension eligibility in the United Kingdom, which is 68 years. More than three quarters of people had experienced some form of disability by age 68, most of whom lived in poorer neighbourhoods. Moreover, the length of time someone with a disability might expect to live beyond 68 (and thus benefit from a pension) is likely to be significantly less than for someone in good health. Thus, policies that limit the availability of resources strictly on the basis of chronological age can reinforce and extend inequity because they can deny resources to those who need them most and, at the same time, provide them for longer to those who need them less.

Outdated stereotypes, new expectations

Some of the most important barriers to developing good public-health policy on ageing are pervasive misconceptions, attitudes and assumptions about older people (45, 46). Although there is substantial evidence that older people contribute to society in many ways, they are instead often stereotyped as frail, out of touch, burdensome or dependent (47). These ageist attitudes (Box 1.3) limit the way problems are conceptualized, the questions that are asked, and the capacity to seize innovative opportunities (46). As a starting point for policy-making, they often lead to great emphasis on cost containment.

These outdated stereotypes extend to the way we often frame the life course, assuming it is inevitably categorized into fixed stages. In high-income settings, these are typically early childhood, studenthood, a defined period of working age, and then retirement. Yet these are social constructs that have little physiological basis. The notion of retirement is relatively new, and for many people in low- and middle-income countries it remains abstract. The idea that learning is something that should occur only during the early stages of life reflects outdated employment patterns in which a person trained for a role and, with luck, worked at it for life, sometimes with a single employer (52).

One consequence of this rigid framing of the life course is that the extra years that accrue from longevity are often considered as simply extending the period of retirement. However, if these extra years can be experienced in good health, then this approach to how they might be used is very limiting. For example, the anticipation of living longer might allow people to raise children and then start a career at age 40 or even 60, to change career paths at any stage in life, or perhaps to choose to retire for a while at 35 and then re-enter the workforce. Retirement itself may evolve into choices that are less stark.

Thus, if policies permit, the combination of greater longevity and good health can allow endless variations on the traditional categories of the life course. Such shifts may benefit not only the individual but also society more broadly, by offering expanded opportunities for older people to contribute through participation in the workforce and other social activities.

Research suggests that at least in some high-income countries, older people are looking for innovative alternatives to the traditional life frame (53). Surveys in the United States, for example, have found that the majority of people approaching traditional retirement age do not actually want to retire (53). For some, this may reflect the impact of poverty and a need to continue to work, but for most it appears that there is a broader interest in remaining active participants in society. However, what respondents reported they were looking for was not more of the same. What they wanted was flexibility and the opportunity to shift careers, work part-time or start a business. Indeed, there is some evidence that older people are acting on these ambitions and are good at these transitions. In the United States, 23% of new entrepreneurs during 2011–2012 were aged 55–64 (54), and twice as many successful entrepreneurs were older than 50 years of age than were under 25 (55).

In low- and middle-income countries, the life course may be less clearly demarcated. This is true particularly for the poor, who may have had limited educational opportunities in their youth and who are likely to have to work to support themselves into advanced old age unless they have family who can help them (56).

Yet it would be wrong to stereotype the situation in low- and middle-income countries. For example, socioeconomic development is allowing many to introduce tax-funded minimum pensions. This is vital for the financial security of older populations (57), and particularly important for people who have worked in the informal workforce (for example, women who have played a caregiving role throughout their life or

Box 1.3. **Ageism**

Ageism is the stereotyping of and discrimination against individuals or groups based on their age. Ageism can take many forms, including prejudicial attitudes, discriminatory practices, or institutional policies and practices that perpetuate stereotypical beliefs (46).

Negative ageist attitudes are widely held across societies and not confined to one social or ethnic group. Research suggests that ageism may now be even more pervasive than sexism and racism (48, 49). This has serious consequences both for older people and society at large. It can be a major barrier to developing good policies because it steers policy options in limited directions. It may also seriously impact the quality of health and social care that older people receive.

These negative stereotypes are so pervasive that even those who outwardly express the best of intentions may have difficulty avoiding engaging in negative actions and expressions. Furthermore, negative ageist attitudes are often seen as humorous and based in some degree of fact; thus, the humour is often mistakenly assumed to counteract any negative effects on the older person. Yet ageism has been shown to cause lowered levels of self-efficacy, decreased productivity, and cardiovascular stress (50). And these stereotypes can become a self-fulfilling prophecy, reinforcing the inaction and deficits that result from their internalization. These negative attitudes are also widely present even within the health and social-care settings where older adults are at their most vulnerable.

Some of this prejudice arises from observable biological declines. This so-called objective starting point for the stereotype of older age may be distorted by awareness of disorders such as dementia, which may be mistakenly thought to reflect normal ageing. Furthermore, because ageism is assumed to be based on these presumed physiological and psychological facts, little or no account is taken of the less obvious adaptations made by older people to minimize the effects of age-related loss, nor the positive aspects of ageing, the personal growth that can occur during this period of life and the contributions made by older people.

This socially ingrained ageism can become self-fulfilling by promoting in older people stereotypes of social isolation, physical and cognitive decline, lack of physical activity and economic burden (51).

agricultural workers) and who have not had the opportunity to accrue benefits such as pensions or health insurance.

However, some of the life-course attitudes and limitations in high-income countries are also apparent in low- and middle-income countries. For example, privileged subsections of the population, such as public sector workers, may have access to generous pensions that are similar to, and sometimes even more restrictive than, those seen in high-income countries (58). Attaining these benefits may become an aspiration for other sections of the community, and the assumptions within these goals can influence broader policy development.

Developing policies that can ensure the financial security essential for well-being in older age while providing the flexibility for innovative approaches to the life course and,

at the same time, being financially sustainable and fair will be major challenges for all governments in the 21st century. Resolving how these might be achieved is beyond the scope of this report. Yet ensuring the health of older populations, and that this benefit is equitably spread, is a prerequisite for effective policy-making in this area.

To achieve these goals, public-health policy will need to take account of the significant rethinking that is underway about what older age is and what it could be. However, although policy responses cannot be based on outdated stereotypes, predicting how attitudes and behaviours will change in the future is perilous. Rather than steering older people towards predetermined social purposes, public-health policy would be better aimed at empowering older people to achieve things previous generations could never imagine.

The world is changing too

Not only can an older person today expect to live much longer than previously, but the world around them has changed (*59*). For example, the past 50 years have seen a massive demographic shift from rural to urban living. Now, for the first time, the majority of the world's population lives in cities (*60*). The world has also become much wealthier through almost global socioeconomic development, although in many places this has been associated with increasing disparity, much of which is avoidable. Advances in transportation and communications have seen rapid globalization of economic and cultural activities, with increased migration, the deregulation of labour markets and the shifting of jobs from those traditionally filled by many now-ageing people to new sectors of the economy (*61, 62*).

For some older people, particularly those with desirable knowledge, skills and financial flexibility, these changes create new opportunities. For others, they can remove social safety nets that might otherwise have been available. For example, while globalization and global connectivity may make it easier for younger generations to migrate to areas of growth, this may result in older family members being left in poor rural areas without the traditional family structures they could have otherwise turned to for support.

Other changes are happening within families too. Some of these reflect local cultural norms, responses to external events or factors specific to the family (*63*). In Zambia, for example, due to internal migration and the impact of AIDS, 30% of older women are at the head of skipped-generation households in which they have responsibility for at least one grandchild without the presence of middle-generation family members (*64*).

But broader trends are also underway. As life expectancy increases, so do the odds of different generations within a family being alive at the same time. However, although the number of surviving generations in a family may have increased, today these generations are more

likely than in the past to live separately. Indeed, in many countries the proportion of older people living alone is rising dramatically. For example, in some European countries, more than 40% of women aged 65 and older now live alone (*65*).

In societies with strong traditions of older parents living with children, such as in Japan, traditional, multigenerational living arrangements are also becoming less common (*66*). Even in India, a country where strong family ties have often been assumed to continue, only 20% of households include people living in joint or extended families (*67*).

Falling family size may be associated with less opportunity to enjoy reciprocal care arrangements or to share the goods that may typically be available in a larger household, and this may also increase the risk of poverty (*68*). Older people living alone may be at increased risk of isolation and suicide (*69*). However, as is explored in later chapters of this report, many older people still prefer to live in their own home and community for as long as possible (*70*).

These changes in family structure are reinforced by two other significant trends. Dramatic falls in fertility in many parts of the world mean that the relative number of younger people in a family is much lower than it used to be (Fig. 3.8). At the same time, there have been major changes in gender norms and opportunities for women. In the past, one key role for women was often that of caregiver, both for children and for older relatives. This restricted women's participation in the paid workforce, which had many negative consequences for them in later life, including a greater risk of poverty, less access to quality health and social-care services, a higher risk of abuse, poor health and reduced access to pensions. Today, women are increasingly filling other roles, which provides them with greater security in older age. But these shifts also limit the capacity of women and families to provide care for older people who need it. Former models of family care are unlikely to be sustainable.

Other social changes will further influence what it means to be old in the 21st century. For example, in many parts of the world, the traditional position of being respected as an older person within a family or society may be weakening or at least transforming (Box 1.4). However, new assistive devices and supportive environments may improve the ability of older people to do the things that are important to them despite significant limitations in their capacity; for example, the Internet can provide video access to distant family and online learning opportunities, and workforce shortages, government encouragement and changing attitudes mean that employment opportunities in some areas are increasing.

It is within this dynamic world that more and more people are living into older age.

Box 1.4.   Social change, filial piety and ageing in the Asia-Pacific region

The Asia-Pacific area is leading in many global demographic trends. Many countries have undergone enormous economic and industrial development and urbanization. At the same time, the region has experienced, and will continue to experience, huge changes in family size and composition. This has been accompanied by shifts in intergenerational relations in almost all countries, but particularly in China, Japan, the Republic of Korea, Singapore and Thailand (71).

Across the region, many feel that traditional attributes, such as filial piety, have been weakened or are changing. Filial piety (孝, xiào) involves a complex set of reciprocal emotional and practical relations and duties between a parent and a child. Respect, obedience, loyalty and practical support are important components and may extend beyond immediate generations to encompass reverence for ancestors (for example, through ancestor worship and grave cleaning) (71, 72).

Tensions are rising in many countries as younger generations feel either less reason to, or have a reduced ability to, fulfil filial duties. The rise of smaller families and the increase in migration for work often mean that fewer children are at home to share physical, emotional and financial responsibilities for ageing parents and grandparents. This has the potential to lead to social exclusion, isolation, poverty and even abuse of older people, as well as to an increasing mismatch in intergenerational expectations (72).

In response, some countries have introduced or expanded legislation to force children to support, visit or care for elderly parents, although this raises challenges of fairness and enforceability. For example, certain groups – such as older people with no children, those whose children have emigrated and lost contact, or in families with divorces and remarriages – effectively have no filial supporters and risk being neglected (72).

Yet filial norms appear to remain strong, although practical expressions of filial piety are becoming much more varied than the provision of direct personal care. Older people, children and, in many places, the state are increasingly accepting this reality. These shifts can be seen in direct contact being substituted by telephone calls and messaging. For many, sending financial remittances and paying for care, the cost of which is sometimes shared among children with different resources, have become major modern expressions of filial duty.

Furthermore, trends seen elsewhere are increasing, including the reliance on institutional care for older people, and the delegation of personal, social and health care to public and private sources. In China, for example, some parents feel it is a mark of success if their children can pay for an expensive care home or a live-in domestic care worker (73, 74).

Debates will be needed about future reliance on families, the state or private sectors in caring for older persons. In many places, family care has been assumed to be the norm, but many societies now recognize that an overreliance on family care may be detrimental to older people's well-being, as well as placing a particular burden on women as traditional caregivers. Moreover, many older people will want to work or take care of themselves, or both. Some older people undoubtedly feel they may be a burden to their children and thus choose to live apart from them. A better understanding of the impact of these shifts and the social isolation that may accompany them will be crucial for policy development.

Why act on ageing and health?

The rights of older people

There are many justifications for devoting public resources to improving the health of older populations (*4*). The first is the human right that older people have to the highest attainable standard of health (*75*). This right is enshrined in international law. Yet people often experience stigma and discrimination, and violations of their rights at individual, community and institutional levels simply as a result of their age. A rights-based approach to healthy ageing can help address the legal, social and structural barriers to good health for older people, and clarify the legal obligations of state and non-state actors to respect, protect and fulfil these rights (*76, 77*).

A human rights-based approach to health states that the right to health "embraces a wide range of socioeconomic factors that promote conditions in which people can lead a healthy life, and extends to the underlying determinants of health, such as food and nutrition, housing, access to safe and potable water and adequate sanitation, safe and healthy working conditions, and a healthy environment" (*78*). A wide range of laws, policies and actions is therefore required to help create the appropriate conditions to ensure that older people can enjoy the highest attainable standard of health. Indeed, under the right to health, states are obligated to deliver, without discrimination of any kind, health facilities, goods and services that are available, accessible, acceptable and of good quality. State parties must move forward in line with the principle of progressive realization, which requires that they take steps to the maximum of their available resources to move towards the full realization of the right to health and other related human rights of older people.

Availability refers to having a sufficient quantity of effective public-health and health-care facilities, goods and services, as well as pro-grammes. In the context of ageing, availability implies considering the extent to which health facilities, goods and services meet the specific health needs of older people. This report will make clear that these services are quite different from the services often offered by health systems.

The accessibility of health facilities, goods and services has four subdimensions: nondiscrimination, physical accessibility, economic accessibility (or affordability), and the accessibility of information. All are particularly relevant to older people who may face aged-based rationing of services, physical limitations that make access particularly difficult, financial insecurity as a result of their age, and information barriers ranging from literacy to the ability to use web-based material, a form with which they may not be familiar or have access to.

Older people's right to health also upholds the element of the acceptability of health facilities, goods and services, in keeping with the standards of medical ethics and the use of gender-responsive and culturally appropriate approaches. For example, assessing acceptability includes considering whether services are age-friendly or responsive to older people's needs and taking into account the diversity of older people, who are not a homogeneous group but face varying health risks and circumstances. In some low-income countries, services may be available but require queuing for many hours, which may be difficult for some older people due to physical limitations or the need to frequently use the toilet. Some countries have taken steps to address these needs by setting aside certain times to see only older people, providing chairs to sit on and ensuring that older people can use the toilet without losing their place in a queue.

The fourth element of the right to health underlines the importance of good-quality facilities, goods and services. When services are restructured to better meet older people's needs, systems must ensure these improvements continue to be delivered. Furthermore, a human rights focus demands that states monitor access to services for older people against these crite-ria, underscoring again the importance of robust and routine evidence.

More broadly, the right to non-discrimina-tion encompasses the right not to be discrimi-nated against on the basis of age. Not only does this mean that older people have the same rights as everyone else but also that states have an obli-gation to make particular efforts to reach any groups of older people who are disadvantaged or vulnerable, and to target resources towards these groups in an effort to promote equality.

Central to a human rights-based approach is the idea that older people participate actively and make informed decisions about their health and well-being; this is also a core element of the person-centred public-health approach. Poli-cies and programmes should empower older people to contribute to, and remain active mem-bers of, their communities for as long as pos-sible, according to their capacity (79). However, ensuring meaningful participation and contin-uing community leadership require adequate financial and technical support. Ensuring that attention is paid to human rights also adds value to efforts to improve ageing and health by recognizing the importance of accountability. Accountability empowers individuals to claim their rights. Accountability for health can be enhanced through the use of multiple mecha-nisms, including human rights mechanisms at the international, regional and national levels, as well as by developing national committees on ageing, or other monitoring, complaint and redress processes. These may help to unearth hidden issues, such as violence against older people. For example, the Asia Pacific Forum of National Human Rights Institutions has helped call attention to the vulnerability of older people in institutional care to discrimination and abuse, emphasizing its "systemic rather than individ-ual nature", which requires action across sectors and domains, including by advocates for human rights, public health and older people (80).

Ageing, health and development

The second key justification for taking action on ageing and health is to foster sustainable devel-opment (81). Today most people will live into older age, and an increasingly significant pro-portion of the population will be older people. If we are to build societies that are cohesive, peace-ful, equitable and secure, development will need to take account of this demographic transition and actions will need to both harness the contri-butions that older people make to development and ensure that they are not left behind (13).

Older people contribute to development in numerous ways, for example through food pro-duction or the raising of future generations (82). Including them in development processes not only helps build a more equitable society but is likely to reinforce development by support-ing these contributions. Excluding older people from these processes, not only undermines their well-being and contributions but can heavily impact on the well-being and productivity of other generations. For example, a lack of acces-sible or affordable health care may mean that an older person's high blood pressure is left untreated and this may result in a stroke. Not only could this endanger their future contribu-tion to family security, but it may require other family members (usually women and girls) to provide supportive care and then themselves be unable to pursue work or schooling. Neglecting the needs of older people has ramifications for development that extend far beyond individuals.

Because older people are often stereotyped as part of the past, they can be overlooked in the surge towards the future. Sustainable develop-ment requires that we address the unacceptable number of older people who live in poverty, lack adequate income security, experience threats to personal safety (through elder abuse or unmet needs in disasters, for example) and have lim-ited access to health care and social care (81). Ensuring "development for all" will require that the root causes of inequity are tackled and all generations gain equal access to health care and social care, lifelong learning and opportunities to contribute. Specific consideration will need to be given to the needs of older people to ensure that environments are accessible, including homes, public spaces and buildings, workplaces and transportation.

Closely evaluating the impact of policies on older adults in different age, sex, socioeconomic, geographical and ethnic groups can help identify which policies might enhance equity and which might make older people worse off. For example, several higher-income countries have considered increasing the out-of-pocket payments made for health-care services as a way to reduce spending on health and decrease the overutilization of services. However, an investigation in Germany of older adults' out-of-pocket expenses on health care found that this placed a significantly lower financial burden on the wealthiest quintile of the population compared with the poorest one (83). Whether the objectives of development policies aim to contain costs or expand coverage, such information is crucial when thinking through options to enhance equity within and across age groups. Involving older people in making decisions about issues that concern them and their families can ensure that responses are more relevant.

The economic imperative

A third reason for taking action is the economic imperative to adapt to shifts in the age structure in ways that minimize the expenditures associated with population ageing while maximizing the many contributions that older people make. These contributions may be made by direct participation in the formal or informal workforce, through taxes and consumption, through transfers of cash and property to younger generations and through a myriad of less tangible benefits that accrue to their families and communities.

However, economic analyses of the implications of population ageing are evolving, and

the models that are often used today may lead to inappropriate responses. For example, one commonly used economic indicator is what is known as the old-age dependency ratio, which has been defined as the ratio of older dependents (people aged 65 or older) to the working-age population (those aged 15–64) (84). As a starting point for policy development, this leads to a focus on the costs that may arise from supporting what are presumed to be dependent populations.

Moreover, there are many flaws in this measure, particularly in the assumption that chronological age is a valid marker of behaviour. One of the hallmarks of older age is diversity, and chronological age is only loosely associated with levels of functioning. Yet the dependency ratio assumes that everyone between the ages of 15 and 65 works (although in 2009, more than one third of what was considered to be the working-age population in the European Union was not actually working), and everyone older than 64 is considered to be dependent (when many people over the age of 64 are active participants in the formal workforce) (85). It also ignores the influence that policies and other external factors may have on the proportion of older people participating in the formal workforce.

Furthermore, this widespread use of the word dependency is based on ageist assumptions. Many older people may no longer be in the workforce but may be independently financially secure through the assets they have accumulated during their lives or contributions made to their pension funds. Detailed analyses within families show that, contrary to the expectation of dependency, in many countries cash flows run from older family members to younger members until people are well into their eighties (86). Furthermore, older people make strong economic contributions to society through consumption. In the United States, those who are older than 55 will control 70% of all disposable income by 2017 (87). In France, those older than 55 will be responsible for two thirds of all increased consumption between 2015 and 2030 (88).

Research from 2010 in the United Kingdom highlights how different the economic picture concerning older populations might appear if these diverse contributions were taken into account. This suggests that public expenditure on older people (through the provision of pensions, other welfare and health care) totalled £136 billion. However, in return, older people made contributions through taxation totalling £45 billion and other direct financial contributions worth £10 billion. They also added a further £76 billion to the national economy through their spending, and £44 billion through economically tangible benefits such as providing social care and volunteering. Indeed, when both the costs and contributions of older people were taken into account, older people were estimated to make a net contribution to society of nearly £40 billion, and this was expected to grow to £77 billion by 2030 (47).

Research from lower-income countries is more limited but highlights the contributions that older people make in sometimes surprising ways. For example, the average age of farmers in Kenya is 60 years (82), making them crucial for ensuring food security. Many other older people in lower-income countries have significant roles in raising the next generation.

This report, therefore, takes a different approach to the economic implications of population ageing. Rather than portraying expenditures on older people as a cost, these are considered as investments that enable the well-being and various contributions of older people (Fig. 1.3). These investments include expenditures on health systems, long-term care and on enabling environments more broadly. The return on some of these investments is obvious (for example, better health from appropriate investment in health systems leads to increased participation in society). Others may be less direct and less obvious but require equal consideration: for example, investment in long-term care will not only benefit older people who have significant losses of capacity but can also allow women to remain in the workforce instead of at home caring for older relatives; the availability of

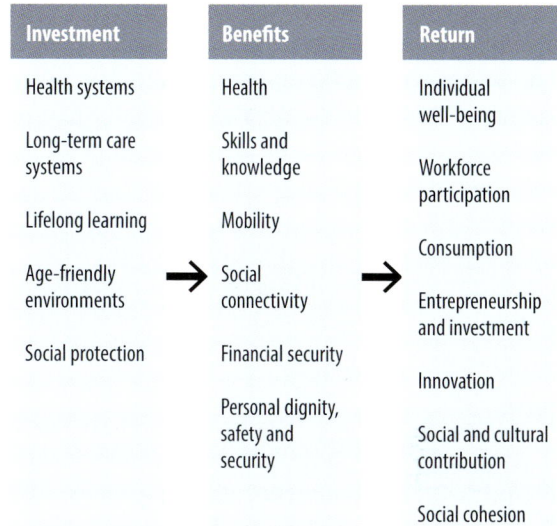

Fig. 1.3.   **Investment in and return on investment in ageing populations**

Source: adapted from unpublished information from the World Economic Forum's Global Agenda Council on Ageing, 2013.

long-term care may also foster social cohesion by sharing risk across the community. Fully quantifying and considering the extent of these dividends on the investment in ageing will be crucial if decision-makers are to shape truly informed policies.

Moreover, this report considers investments from a life-course perspective and with the goal of ensuring a fair distribution of society's resources. This does not require people in each age group to be treated exactly the same (given their different needs), but instead that they be treated fairly throughout their life (89).

Reframing the economic questions in this way shifts debate from a singular focus on minimizing the costs of population ageing to an analysis that considers the benefits that might be missed if society fails to make the appropriate adaptations and investments. Subsequent sections of this report will suggest how some of these investments can be prioritized.

Conclusion

Current public-health approaches to population ageing have clearly been ineffective. The health of older people is not keeping up with increasing longevity (5, 9); marked health inequities are apparent in the health status of older people; current health systems are poorly aligned to the care that older populations require even in high-income countries (17–21); long-term care models are both inadequate and unsustainable (Chapter 5); and physical and social environments present multiple barriers and disincentives to both health and participation (Chapter 6) (90).

A new framework for global action is required. It will need to encompass the great diversity of older populations and address the inequities that lie beneath it. It must drive the development of new systems for health care and long-term care that are more in tune with the needs of older people, and it must ensure that all sectors focus on common goals so that action can be coordinated and balanced. Above all, it will need to transcend outdated ways of think-ing about ageing, foster a major shift in how we understand ageing and health, and inspire the development of transformative approaches. Because social change is ongoing and unpredictable, these cannot be prescriptive but, instead, should look to strengthen the ability of older people to thrive in the turbulent environment they are likely to live in.

This report offers a framework for this response. Chapter 2 explores what health might mean to an older person and how a public-health strategy might be framed to foster it. Chapter 3 uses this model as the basis for assessing health trends and priorities in older age. The final chapters explore in detail actions that might be taken in key sectors: Chapter 4 examines health systems, Chapter 5 examines long-term care systems, and Chapter 6 looks at the role of other sectors. However, throughout this report it is emphasized that all these aspects of an older person's environment need to work together in an integrated way if healthy ageing is to be achieved. Chapter 7, the final chapter, identifies the key steps that need to be taken next.

References

1. World Economic and Social Survey 2007: development in an ageing world. New York: United Nations Department of Social and Economic Affairs; 2007 (Report No. E/2007/50/Rev.1 ST/ESA/314; http://www.un.org/en/development/desa/policy/wess/wess_archive/2007wess.pdf, accessed 4 June 2015).

2. Bloom DE. 7 billion and counting. Science. 2011 Jul 29;333(6042):562–9.doi: http://dx.doi.org/10.1126/science.1209290 PMID: 21798935

3. Christensen K, Doblhammer G, Rau R, Vaupel JW. Ageing populations: the challenges ahead. Lancet. 2009 Oct 3;374(9696):1196–208.doi: http://dx.doi.org/10.1016/S0140-6736(09)61460-4 PMID: 19801098

4. Beard JR, Biggs S, Bloom DE, Fried LP, Hogan P, Kalache A, et al. Introduction. In: Beard JR, Biggs S, Bloom DE, Fried LP, Hogan P, Kalache A, et al., editors. Global population ageing: peril or promise? Geneva: World Economic Forum; 2012:4–13. (http://www3.weforum.org/docs/WEF_GAC_GlobalPopulationAgeing_Report_2012.pdf, accessed 24 July 2015).

5. Crimmins EM, Beltrán-Sánchez H. Mortality and morbidity trends: is there compression of morbidity? J Gerontol B Psychol Sci Soc Sci. 2011 Jan;66(1):75–86.doi: http://dx.doi.org/10.1093/geronb/gbq088 PMID: 21135070

6. Manton KG, Gu X, Lamb VL. Change in chronic disability from 1982 to 2004/2005 as measured by long-term changes in function and health in the U.S. elderly population. Proc Natl Acad Sci U S A. 2006 Nov 28;103(48):18374–9.doi: http://dx.doi.org/10.1073/pnas.0608483103 PMID: 17101963

7. Lin S-F, Beck AN, Finch BK, Hummer RA, Masters RK. Trends in US older adult disability: exploring age, period, and cohort effects. Am J Public Health. 2012 Nov;102(11):2157–63.doi: http://dx.doi.org/10.2105/AJPH.2011.300602 PMID: 22994192

8. Jagger C, Gillies C, Moscone F, Cambois E, Van Oyen H, Nusselder W, et al.; EHLEIS team. Inequalities in healthy life years in the 25 countries of the European Union in 2005: a cross-national meta-regression analysis. Lancet. 2008 Dec 20;372(9656):2124–31.doi: http://dx.doi.org/10.1016/S0140-6736(08)61594-9 PMID: 19010526

9. Chatterji S, Byles J, Cutler D, Seeman T, Verdes E. Health, functioning, and disability in older adults–present status and future implications. Lancet. 2015 Feb 7;385(9967):563–75.doi: http://dx.doi.org/10.1016/S0140-6736(14)61462-8 PMID: 25468158

10. Zheng X, Chen G, Song X, Liu J, Yan L, Du W, et al. Twenty-year trends in the prevalence of disability in China. Bull World Health Organ. 2011 Nov 1;89(11):788–97. PMID: 22084524

11. Lloyd-Sherlock P, McKee M, Ebrahim S, Gorman M, Greengross S, Prince M, et al. Population ageing and health. Lancet. 2012 Apr 7;379(9823):1295–6.doi: http://dx.doi.org/10.1016/S0140-6736(12)60519-4 PMID: 22480756

12. Smith A. Grand challenges of our aging society. Washington DC: National Academies Press; 2010.

13. Political declaration and Madrid international plan of action on ageing. New York: United Nations; 2002 (http://www.un.org/en/events/pastevents/pdfs/Madrid_plan.pdf, accessed 4 June 2015).

14. Active ageing: a policy framework. Geneva: World Health Organization; 2002 (WHO/NMH/NPH/02.8; http://whqlibdoc.who.int/hq/2002/who_nmh_nph_02.8.pdf, accessed 4 June 2015).

15. International Covenant on Economic, Social and Cultural Rights. New York: United Nations; 1966 (http://www.ohchr.org/Documents/ProfessionalInterest/cescr.pdf, accessed 7 June 2015).

16. Walker A. A strategy for active ageing. Int Soc Secur Rev. 2002;55(1):121–39. doi: http://dx.doi.org/10.1111/1468-246X.00118

17. Overview of available policies and legislation, data and research, and institutional arrangements relating to older persons – progress since Madrid. New York: United Nations Population Fund, Help Age International; 2011 (http://www.ctc-health.org.cn/file/Older_Persons_Report.pdf, accessed 4 June 2015).

18. Sustainable development. In: United Nations Department of Economic and Social Affairs, Sustainable Development Knowledge Platform [website]. New York: United Nations; 2015 (https://sustainabledevelopment.un.org/index.html, accessed 17 June 2015).

19. Goodwin N, Sonola L, Thiel V, Kodner DL. Co-ordinated care for people with complex chronic conditions: key lessons and markers for success. London: The King's Fund; 2013 (http://www.kingsfund.org.uk/sites/files/kf/field/field_publication_file/co-ordinated-care-for-people-with-complex-chronic-conditions-kingsfund-oct13.pdf, accessed 4 June 2015).

20. Patterson L. Making our health and care systems fit for an ageing population: David Oliver, Catherine Foot, Richard Humphries. King's Fund March 2014. Age Ageing. 2014 Sep;43(5):731.doi: http://dx.doi.org/10.1093/ageing/afu105 PMID: 25074536

21. Smith SM, Soubhi H, Fortin M, Hudon C, O'Dowd T. Managing patients with multimorbidity: systematic review of interventions in primary care and community settings. BMJ. 2012;345:e5205.doi: http://dx.doi.org/10.1136/bmj.e5205 PMID: 22945950

22. Peron EP, Gray SL, Hanlon JT. Medication use and functional status decline in older adults: a narrative review. Am J Geriatr Pharmacother. 2011 Dec;9(6):378–91.doi: http://dx.doi.org/10.1016/j.amjopharm.2011.10.002 PMID: 22057096

23. Low LF, Yap M, Brodaty H. A systematic review of different models of home and community care services for older persons. BMC Health Serv Res. 2011;11(1):93.doi: http://dx.doi.org/10.1186/1472-6963-11-93 PMID: 21549010

24. Sourdet S, Lafont C, Rolland Y, Nourhashemi F, Andrieu S, Vellas B. Preventable iatrogenic disability in elderly patients during hospitalization. J Am Med Dir Assoc. 2015 Aug 1;16(8):674–81. PMID: 25922117

25. Eklund K, Wilhelmson K. Outcomes of coordinated and integrated interventions targeting frail elderly people: a systematic review of randomised controlled trials. Health Soc Care Community. 2009 Sep;17(5):447–58.doi: http://dx.doi.org/10.1111/j.1365-2524.2009.00844.x PMID: 19245421

26. Kowal P, Chatterji S, Naidoo N, Biritwum R, Fan W, Lopez Ridaura R, et al.; SAGE Collaborators. Data resource profile: the World Health Organization Study on global AGEing and adult health (SAGE). Int J Epidemiol. 2012 Dec;41(6):1639–49.doi: http://dx.doi.org/10.1093/ije/dys210 PMID: 23283715

27. Goeppel C, Frenz P, Tinnemann P, Grabenhenrich L. Universal health coverage for elderly people with non-communicable diseases in low-income and middle-income countries: a cross-sectional analysis. Lancet. 2014 Oct;384:S6. doi: http://dx.doi.org/10.1016/S0140-6736(14)61869-9

28. Lloyd-Sherlock P, Beard J, Minicuci N, Ebrahim S, Chatterji S. Hypertension among older adults in low- and middle-income countries: prevalence, awareness and control. Int J Epidemiol. 2014 Feb;43(1):116–28.doi: http://dx.doi.org/10.1093/ije/dyt215 PMID: 24505082

29. Stegeman I, Otte-Trojel T, Costongs C, Considine J. Healthy and active ageing. Brussels: EuroHealthNet and Bundeszentrale für gesundheitliche Aufklaerung (BZgA); 2012 (http://www.healthyageing.eu/sites/www.healthyageing.eu/files/featured/Healthy%20and%20Active%20Ageing.pdf, accessed 4 June 2015).

30. Alwin DF. Integrating varieties of life course concepts. J Gerontol B Psychol Sci Soc Sci. 2012 Mar;67(2):206–20.doi: http://dx.doi.org/10.1093/geronb/gbr146 PMID: 22399576

31. Liu S, Jones RN, Glymour MM. Implications of lifecourse epidemiology for research on determinants of adult disease. Public Health Rev. 2010 Nov;32(2):489–511. PMID: 24639598

32. Lee C, Dobson AJ, Brown WJ, Bryson L, Byles J, Warner-Smith P, et al. Cohort Profile: the Australian Longitudinal Study on Women's Health. Int J Epidemiol. 2005 Oct;34(5):987–91.doi: http://dx.doi.org/10.1093/ije/dyi098 PMID: 15894591

33. Cumming E, Henry W. Growing old, the process of disengagement. New York: Arno; 1979.

34. Lemon BW, Bengtson VL, Peterson JA. An exploration of the activity theory of aging: activity types and life satisfaction among in-movers to a retirement community. J Gerontol. 1972 Oct;27(4):511–23.doi: http://dx.doi.org/10.1093/geronj/27.4.511 PMID: 5075497

35. Havighurst RJ. Successful aging. Gerontologist. 1961;1(1):8–13. doi: http://dx.doi.org/10.1093/geront/1.1.8

36. Butler RN. The study of productive aging. J Gerontol B Psychol Sci Soc Sci. 2002 Nov;57(6):S323.doi: http://dx.doi.org/10.1093/geronb/57.6.S323 PMID: 12426440

37. Knapp MR. The activity theory of aging: an examination in the English context. Gerontologist. 1977 Dec;17(6):553–9.doi: http://dx.doi.org/10.1093/geront/17.6.553 PMID: 924178

38. Steverink N. Successful development and ageing: theory and intervention. In: Pachana N, Laidlaw K, editors. Oxford handbook of geropsychology. Oxford: Oxford University Press; 2014:84–103.

39. Schroeter KR. [The Doxa of the social-gerontological field: successful and productive aging-orthodoxy, heterodoxy or allodoxy?]. Z Gerontol Geriatr. 2004 Feb;37(1):51–5.doi: http://dx.doi.org/10.1007/s00391-004-0163-z PMID: 14991297

40. Dillaway HE, Byrnes M. Reconsidering successful aging: a call for renewed and expanded academic critiques and conceptualizations. J Appl Gerontol. 2009;28(6):702–22. doi: http://dx.doi.org/10.1177/0733464809333882

41. Steves CJ, Spector TD, Jackson SH. Ageing, genes, environment and epigenetics: what twin studies tell us now, and in the future. Age Ageing. 2012 Sep;41(5):581–6.doi: http://dx.doi.org/10.1093/ageing/afs097 PMID: 22826292

42. Commission on Social Determinants of Health. Closing the gap in a generation: health equity through action on social determinants of health. Final report of the Commission on Social Determinants of Health. Geneva: World Health Organization; 2008 (http://whqlibdoc.who.int/publications/2008/9789241563703_eng.pdf, accessed 5 June 2015).

43. Dannefer D. Cumulative advantage/disadvantage and the life course: cross-fertilizing age and social science theory. J Gerontol B Psychol Sci Soc Sci. 2003 Nov;58(6):S327–37.doi: http://dx.doi.org/10.1093/geronb/58.6.S327 PMID: 14614120

44. Fair society. Healthy lives. Strategic review of health inequalities in England post-2010. London: UCL Institute of Health Equity; 2010 (The Marmot Review; http://www.instituteofhealthequity.org/projects/fair-society-healthy-lives-the-marmot-review, accessed 4 June 2015).

45. Tam T, Hewstone M, Harwood J, Voci A, Kenworthy J. Intergroup contact and grandparent–grandchild communication: the effects of self-disclosure on implicit and explicit biases against older people. Group Process Intergroup Relat. 2006;9(3):413–29. doi: http://dx.doi.org/10.1177/1368430206064642

46. Butler RN. Ageism: a foreword. J Soc Issues. 1980;36(2):8–11. doi: http://dx.doi.org/10.1111/j.1540-4560.1980.tb02018.x

47. Cook J. The socioeconomic contribution of older people in the UK. Working Older People. 2011;15(4):141–6 doi: http://dx.doi.org/10.1108/13663661111191257

48. Levy B, Banaji M. Implicit ageism. In: Nelson TD, editor. Ageism: stereotyping and prejudice against older persons. Cambridge (MA): MIT Press; 2002:127–8.

49. Kite M, Wagner L. Attitudes toward older and younger adults. In: Nelson TD, editor. Ageism: stereotyping and prejudice against older persons. Cambridge (MA): MIT Press; 2002:129–61.

50. Levy B, Ashman O, Dror I. To be or not to be: the effects of aging stereotypes on the will to live. Omega (Westport). 1999-2000;40(3):409–20.doi: http://dx.doi.org/10.2190/Y2GE-BVYQ-NF0E-83VR PMID: 12557880

51. Angus J, Reeve P. Ageism: a threat to "aging well" in the 21st century. J Appl Gerontol. 2006;25(2):137–52. doi: http://dx.doi.org/10.1177/0733464805285745

52. Guillemard A-M. The advent of a flexible life course and the reconfigurations of welfare. In: Goul Andersen J, Guillemard A-M, Jensen PH, Pfau-Effinger B, editors. The changing face of welfare: consequences and outcomes from a citizenship perspective. Bristol: Policy Press Scholarship Online; 2005:55–73. doi: http://dx.doi.org/10.1332/policypress/9781861345929.003.0004

53. The SunAmerica Retirement Re-Set Study: redefining retirement post recession. Los Angeles: SunAmerica Financial Group; 2011 (http://www.agewave.com/research/retirementresetreport.pdf, accessed 4 June 2015).

54. Lin LP, Hsia YC, Hsu SW, Loh CH, Wu CL, Lin JD. Caregivers' reported functional limitations in activities of daily living among middle-aged adults with intellectual disabilities. Res Dev Disabil. 2013 Dec;34(12):4559–64.doi: http://dx.doi.org/10.1016/j.ridd.2013.09.038 PMID: 24139711

55. Holly K. Why great entrepreneurs are older than you think. In: Forbes Tech [website]. 2014 (http://www.forbes.com/sites/krisztinaholly/2014/01/15/why-great-entrepreneurs-are-older-than-you-think/, accessed 4 June 2015).

56. Lloyd-Sherlock P. Population ageing and international development: from generalisation to evidence. Bristol: Policy Press; 2010.

57. Palacios R, Knox-Vydmanov C. The growing role of social pensions: history, taxonomy and key performance indicators. Public Adm Dev. 2014;34(4):251–64. doi: http://dx.doi.org/10.1002/pad.1682

58. Palacios R, Whitehouse E. Civil-service pension schemes around the world. Washington (DC): World Bank; 2006.

59. Beard JR, Biggs S, Bloom DE, Fried LP, Hogan P, Kalache A, et al., editors. Global population ageing: peril or promise? Geneva: World Economic Forum; 2012. (http://www3.weforum.org/docs/WEF_GAC_GlobalPopulationAgeing_Report_2012.pdf, accessed 4 June 2015).

60. Hidden cities: unmasking and overcoming health inequities in urban settings. Kobe: World Health Organization, WHO Centre for Health Development, United Nations Human Settlements Programme; 2010 (http://www.who.int/kobe_centre/publications/hiddencities_media/who_un_habitat_hidden_cities_web.pdf, accessed 4 June 2015).

61. Polivka L. Globalization, population, aging, and ethics. J Aging Identity. 2001;6(3):147–63. doi: http://dx.doi.org/10.1023/A:1011312300122

62. Arxer SL, Murphy JW. The symbolism of globalization, development, and aging. Dordrecht: Springer; 2012. (http://www.springer.com/us/book/9781461445074, accessed 17 June 2015).

63. Suzman R, Beard J. Global health and ageing. Bethesda, MD: U.S. Department of Health and Human Services, World Health Organization; 2011 (NIH Publication no. 11-7737; http://www.who.int/ageing/publications/global_health.pdf, accessed 4 June 2015).

64. Living arrangements of older persons around the world. New York: United Nations; 2005 (http://www.un.org/esa/population/publications/livingarrangement/report.htm, accessed 4 June 2015).

65. Ageing in Ireland. 2007. Dublin: Central Statistics Office; 2007. (http://www.cso.ie/en/media/csoie/releasespublications/documents/otherreleases/2007/ageinginireland.pdf, accessed 17 June 2015).

66. Household projections for Japan 2010–2035. Tokyo: National Institute of Population and Social Security Research; 2013 (http://www.ipss.go.jp/pp-ajsetai/e/hhprj2013/t-page_e.asp, accessed 4 June 2015).

67. National Family Health Survey Mumbai. India: International Institute of Population Sciences and ORC Macro; 2007.

68. Casey B, Yamada A. Getting older, getting poorer? A study of the earnings, pensions, assets and living arrangements of older people in nine countries. Paris: OECD Publishing; 2002 (OECD Labour Market and Social Policy Occasional Papers, No. 60; http://www.oecd-ilibrary.org/social-issues-migration-health/getting-older-getting-poorer_345816633534, accessed 4 June 2015).

69. Poudel-Tandukar K, Nanri A, Mizoue T, Matsushita Y, Takahashi Y, Noda M, et al.; Japan Public Health Center-based Prospective Study Group. Differences in suicide risk according to living arrangements in Japanese men and women–the Japan Public Health Center-based (JPHC) prospective study. J Affect Disord. 2011 Jun;131(1-3):113–9.doi: http://dx.doi.org/10.1016/j.jad.2010.11.027 PMID: 21168916

70. Healthy aging & the built environment. In: Centers for Disease Control and Prevention [website]. Atlanta, GA: Centers for Disease Control and Prevention; 2015 (http://www.cdc.gov/healthyplaces/healthtopics/healthyaging.htm, accessed 17 June 2015).

71. Phillips DR. Overview of health and ageing issues in the Asia-Pacific region. In: Chan W, editor. Singapore's ageing population: managing healthcare and end of life decisions. Abingdon, Oxford: Routledge; 2011:13–39.

72. Phillips DR, Cheng KHC. The impact of changing value systems on social inclusion: an Asia-Pacific perspective. In: Scharf T, Keating NC, editors. From exclusion to inclusion in old age. Bristol: Policy Press; 2012:109–24. doi: http://dx.doi.org/10.1332/policypress/9781847427731.003.0007

73. Phillips DR, Cheng KHC. Challenges for the ageing family in the People's Republic of China. Can J Aging. 2015;34(3):1–15. http://www.ncbi.nlm.nih.gov/entrez/query.fcgi?cmd=Retrieve&db=PubMed&list_uids=25511315&dopt=Abstractdoi: http://dx.doi.org/10.1017/S0714980815000203 PMID: 25511315

74. Yeh KH, Yi CC, Tsao WC, Wan PS. Filial piety in contemporary Chinese societies: a comparative study of Taiwan, Hong Kong, and China. Int Sociol. 2013;28(3):277–96. doi: http://dx.doi.org/10.1177/0268580913484345

75. Baera B, Bhushan A, Abou Taleb H, Vasquez J, Thomas R, Fergusen L. The right to health of older people. Gerontologist. 2016 (In press).

76. Doron I, Apter I. The debate around the need for an international convention on the rights of older persons. Gerontologist. 2010 Oct;50(5):586–93.doi: http://dx.doi.org/10.1093/geront/gnq016 PMID: 20185521

77. Kalache A. Human rights in older age. In: Beard JS, Bloom DE, Fried LP, Hogan P, Kalache A, et al., editors. Global population ageing: peril or promise? Geneva: World Economic Forum; 2012: 89–92. (http://www3.weforum.org/docs/WEF_GAC_GlobalPopulationAgeing_Report_2012.pdf, accessed 4 June 2015).

78. The right to the highest attainable standard of health. New York: United Nations; 2000 (E/C.12/2000/4, General Comments; http://www.nesri.org/sites/default/files/Right_to_health_Comment_14.pdf, accessed 4 June 2015).

79. Kornfeld-Matte R, editor. United Nations Office of the High Commisioner for Human Rights. [website]. New York: United Nations; 2014. (http://www.ohchr.org/EN/NewsEvents/Pages/DisplayNews.aspx?NewsID=15148&LangID=E, accessed 4 June 2015).

80. Open-ended working group on ageing for the purpose of strengthening the protection of the human rights of older persons: General Assembly resolution 65/182. New York: United Nations; 2011 (http://social.un.org/ageing-working-group/documents/Chair_summary_2nd_session_OEWG_final.pdf, accessed 4 June 2015).

81. Ageing in the twenty-first century: a celebration and a challenge. New York, London: United Nations Population Fund; HelpAge International; 2012 (http://www.unfpa.org/sites/default/files/pub-pdf/Ageing%20report.pdf, accessed 20 July 2015).

82. Aboderin IA, Beard JR. Older people's health in sub-Saharan Africa. Lancet. 2015 Feb 14;385(9968):e9–11.doi: http://dx.doi.org/10.1016/S0140-6736(14)61602-0 PMID: 25468150

83. Bock J-O, Matschinger H, Brenner H, Wild B, Haefeli WE, Quinzler R, et al. Inequalities in out-of-pocket payments for health care services among elderly Germans–results of a population-based cross-sectional study. Int J Equity Health. 2014;13(1):3. doi: http://dx.doi.org/10.1186/1475-9276-13-3 PMID: 24397544

84. World population prospects: the 2012 revision. Methodology of the United Nations population estimates and projections. New York: United Nations Department of Economic and Social Affairs, Population Division; 2014. (http://esa.un.org/wpp/Documentation/pdf/WPP2012_Methodology.pdf, accessed 4 June 2015).

85. Wöss J, Türk E. Dependency ratios and demographic change. The labour market as a key element. Brussels: European Trade Union Institute; 2011.

86. Lee R, Mason A. Population aging and the generational economy. a global perspective. Cheltenham: Edward Elgar; 2011. doi: http://dx.doi.org/10.4337/9780857930583

87. Introducing boomers: marketing's most valuable generation. New York: Nielsen; 2012 (http://www.nielsen.com/us/en/reports/2012/introducing-boomers--marketing-s-most-valuable-generation.html, accessed 4 June 2015).

88. Desvaux G, Regout B. Older, smarter, more value conscious: the French consumer transformation. McKinsey Quarterly. 2010 Jun; (http://www.mckinsey.com/insights/consumer_and_retail/older_smarter_more_value_conscious_the_french_consumer_transformation, accessed 4 June 2015).

89. Daniels N. Just health: meeting health needs fairly. New York: Cambridge University Press; 2007. doi: http://dx.doi.org/10.1017/CBO9780511809514

90. Beard JR, Petitot C. Aging and urbanization: can cities be designed to foster active aging? Public Health Rev. 2011;32(2):427–50.

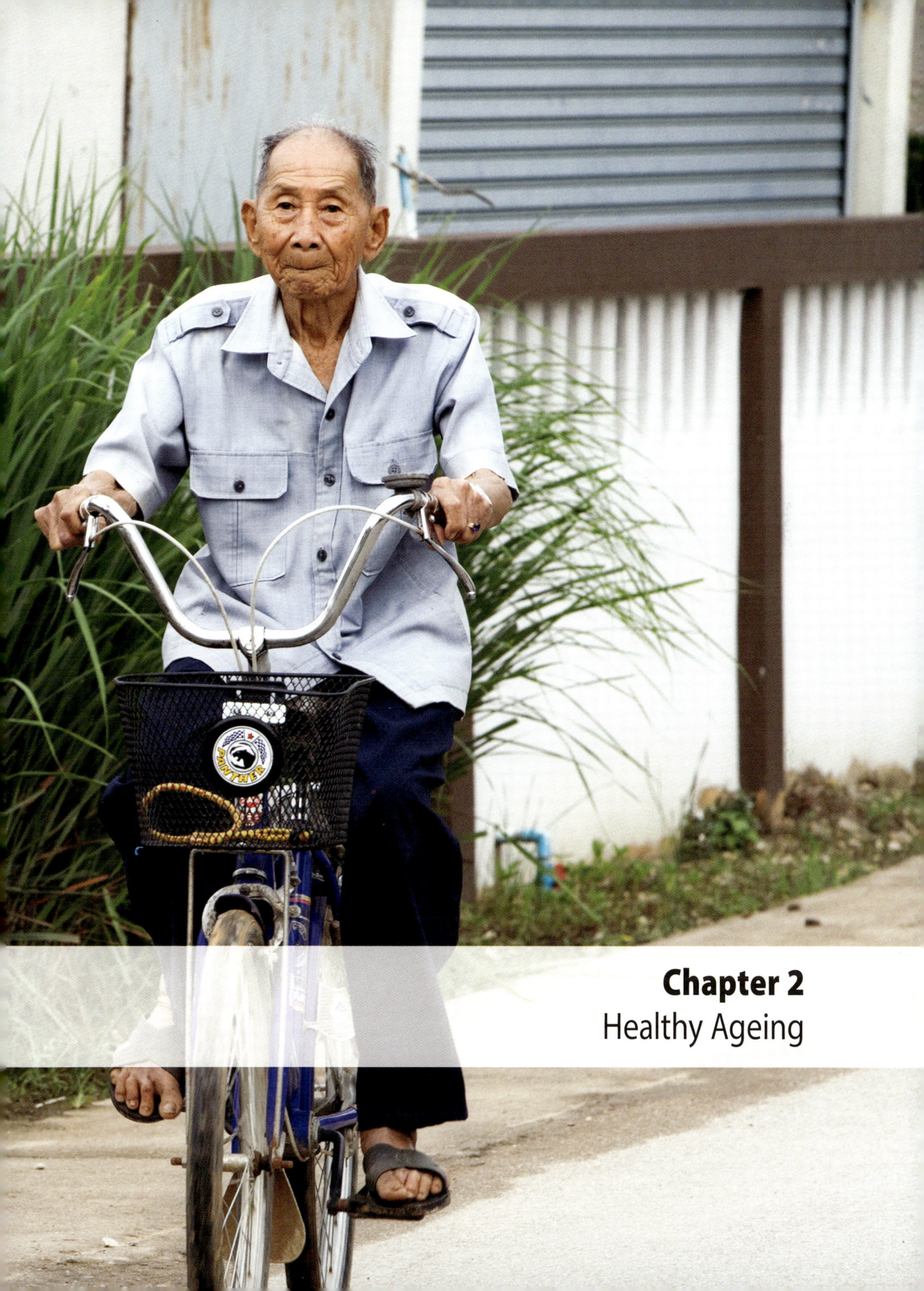

Chapter 2
Healthy Ageing

Moon, 88, Thailand

Moon leads an active life. Joyful and energetic,
he enjoys helping his community.
"I like to stay active, and get around by riding my bicycle",
he explains, adding, "sadness is not a good thing".
He hopes to continue investing his energy into doing what
he can for his community.

2

Healthy Ageing

What is ageing?

The changes that constitute and influence ageing are complex (*1*). At a biological level, ageing is associated with the gradual accumulation of a wide variety of molecular and cellular damage (*2*, *3*). Over time, this damage leads to a gradual decrease in physiological reserves, an increased risk of many diseases, and a general decline in the capacity of the individual. Ultimately, it will result in death.

But these changes are neither linear nor consistent, and they are only loosely associated with age in years (*2*). Thus, while some 70-year-olds may enjoy good physical and mental functioning, others may be frail or require significant support to meet their basic needs. In part, this is because many of the mechanisms of ageing are random. But it is also because these changes are strongly influenced by the environment and behaviours of the individual (Chapter 1).

Beyond these biological losses, older age frequently involves other significant changes. These include shifts in roles and social positions, and the need to deal with the loss of close relationships. In response, older adults tend to select fewer and more meaningful goals and activities, optimize their existing abilities through practise and the use of new technologies, and compensate for the losses of some abilities by finding other ways to accomplish tasks (*4*). Goals, motivational priorities and preferences also appear to change (*5*), with some suggesting that older age may even be the stimulus for a shift from materialistic perspectives to more transcendent ones (*6*, *7*). Although some of these changes may be driven by adaptations to loss, others reflect ongoing psychological development in older age that may be associated with "the development of new roles, viewpoints and many interrelated social contexts" (*4*, *8*). These psychosocial changes may explain why in many settings older age can be a period of heightened subjective well-being (*9*).

In developing a public-health response to ageing, it is thus important not just to consider approaches that ameliorate the losses associated with older age but also those that may reinforce recovery, adaptation and psychosocial growth. These strengths may be particularly important in helping people navigate the systems and marshal the resources that will enable them to deal with the health issues that often arise in older age (*10*).

Ageing, health and functioning

The dynamics of health in older age are complex and are more fully described in the following chapter. How these play out is ultimately expressed in the older person's physical and mental capacities and functioning.

With increasing age, numerous underlying physiological changes occur, and the risk of chronic disease rises. By age 60, the major burdens of disability and death arise from age-related losses in hearing, seeing and moving, and noncommunicable diseases, including heart disease, stroke, chronic respiratory disorders, cancer and dementia (Chapter 3). These are not just problems for higher-income countries. In fact, the burden associated with these conditions in older people is generally far higher in low- and middle-income countries.

Yet the presence of these health conditions says nothing about the impact they may have on an older person's life (11). High blood pressure in one older person may be easily controlled with medication, while in another it may require multiple treatments which lead to significant side-effects. Similarly, older people with age-related visual impairment may retain full functioning with the aid of glasses, but without them they may be unable to perform simple tasks, such as reading or preparing food.

Moreover, since ageing is also associated with an increased risk of experiencing more than one chronic condition at the same time (known as multimorbidity), it is simplistic to consider the burden from each of these conditions independently. For example, in Germany, it has been estimated that 24% of people aged 70–85 years, experience five or more diseases concurrently (12) (Chapter 3). The impact of multimorbidity on an older person's capacity, health-care utilization and their costs of care is often significantly greater than might be expected from the summed effects of each condition (13).

Furthermore, the multifaceted dynamics among underlying physiological change, disease and multimorbidity can result in health states in older age that are not captured by traditional disease classifications. These states can be chronic (for example, frailty, which may have a prevalence of around 10% in people older than 65 years) (14) or acute (for example, delirium, which can result from multiple determinants as diverse as the side-effects of medication or surgery) (15).

Nor are these complex health states static. Older people with congestive heart failure, for example, may follow several different typical trajectories of illness, and their needs, and those of their caregivers, may vary predictably, according to which path they are on (16).

In assessing the health needs of an older person, it is therefore important to consider not just the specific diseases they may be experiencing but how these interact and impact on trajectories of functioning. Such comprehensive functional assessments of health in older age are significantly better predictors of survival and other outcomes than the presence of individual diseases or even the extent of comorbidities (17). Moreover, health care that considers and manages the complex needs of older age in an integrated way has been shown to be more effective than services that simply react to specific diseases individually (18–20). Approaches based on functioning can also be useful in framing a public-health response to population ageing.

However, functioning is determined not just by assessing physical and mental capacities but also by the interactions each of us has with the environments we inhabit across our lives (21). These environmental influences on health in older age may take many forms, including the broad policies that affect us, the economic situation, a community's attitudes or norms, the physical characteristics of the natural and built environments, the social networks that we can draw on, and even the assistive devices that may be available to us. These shape both the physical and mental capacities we have at any time (for example, by influencing our available options and our choice about health behaviours), and whether for any given level of capacity we can do the things we want to do (for example, if we want to go somewhere, is there transport available to get us where we need to go?) (*22*). An understanding of the role of these wide-ranging contextual factors must be central to any strategy aimed at fostering health in older age.

A framework for action on ageing and health

As described in Chapter 1, in developing the public-health framework for action on ageing outlined in this report, WHO has looked to build on the platform provided by the *Political declaration and Madrid international plan of action on ageing* (*23*), WHO's *Active ageing: a policy framework* (*24*), and international human rights norms and standards. The report has also sought to draw on, and hopes to inform, ongoing work on multiple other frameworks in related domains, including the *International classification of functioning, disability and health* (*21*); the *United Nations Convention on the rights of persons with disabilities* (*25*); the *Global action plan for the prevention and control of noncommunicable diseases 2013–2020* (*26*); the *Beijing declaration and platform for action* for advancing women's rights (*27*); and the final report of the WHO Commission on Social Determinants of Health (*28*). Particular attention has been paid to key issues that emerged in the previous chapter. These include the need to:

- consider the heterogeneity of experiences in older age and be relevant to all older people, regardless of their health status;
- address the inequities that underlie this diversity;
- avoid ageist stereotypes and preconceptions;
- empower older people to adapt to and shape the challenges they face and the social change that accompanies population ageing;
- consider the environments an older person inhabits;

- consider health from the perspective of an older person's trajectory of functioning rather than the disease or comorbidity they are experiencing at a single point in time.

Furthermore, this report has attempted to avoid the negative attitudes and norms that often underpin conceptualizations of the issues arising from population ageing and society's responses to them. Instead, it starts from an assumption that ageing is a valuable if often challenging process and that older people make multiple crucial contributions to society. This report considers that it is good to get old, and that societies are better off for having these older people. At the same time, it acknowledges that many older people will experience significant losses, whether in their physical or cognitive capacities, or through the loss of family, friends and the roles they had earlier in life. Some of these losses can be avoided, and efforts should be made by individuals and society to prevent them. But other losses will be inevitable. Societal responses to ageing should not deny these challenges but look to foster recovery and adaptation.

These are complex considerations that cannot be addressed by a narrow conceptualization of health in older age as a state defined by the absence of disease. Instead, this report considers health as a fundamental and holistic attribute that enables older people to achieve the things that are important to them. This is consistent with work undertaken in other spheres on capabilities (*29–38*). Moreover, rather than considering health in older age in a static sense, the report views it in terms of dynamic change, where subtle shifts in capacity or environment can have significant long-term consequences.

Finally, in framing a public-health response that might strengthen an older person's ability to navigate and adapt to these dynamics and the losses they are likely to experience, we have drawn on the concept of resilience. Originally conceptualized in gerontology as a psychological trait inherent to the individual, this has more recently been explored as "a dynamic process of positive adaptation in the face of adversity" (*39*) or a process enabled by both "internal traits, such as hardiness or high self-efficacy" as well as "external factors, such as social support, that promote coping" (*40*). This ability to adapt is a crucial resource for older people and allows differentiation between individuals who may otherwise have similar levels of other characteristics. Further, there is mounting evidence to suggest that resilience is not static, but varies across an individual's life course, making it a potential target for public-health policy (*41*).

Healthy Ageing

The term healthy ageing is widely used in academic and policy circles, yet there is surprisingly little consensus on what this might comprise or how it might be defined or measured (*42–46*). Furthermore, it is often used to identify a positive disease-free state that distinguishes between healthy and unhealthy individuals. This is prob-

lematic in older age because many individuals may have one or more health conditions that are well controlled and have little influence on their ability to function. Therefore, in framing the goal for a public-health strategy on ageing, WHO considers *Healthy Ageing* in a more holistic sense, one that is based on life-course and functional perspectives.

This report defines **Healthy Ageing** as **the process of developing and maintaining the functional ability that enables well-being in older age** (Fig. 2.1).

Functional ability comprises the health-related attributes that enable people to be and to do what they have reason to value. It is made up of the intrinsic capacity of the individual, relevant environmental characteristics and the interactions between the individual and these characteristics.

Intrinsic capacity is the composite of all the physical and mental capacities of an individual.

Environments comprise all the factors in the extrinsic world that form the context of an individual's life. These include – from the micro-

Fig. 2.1. *Healthy Ageing*

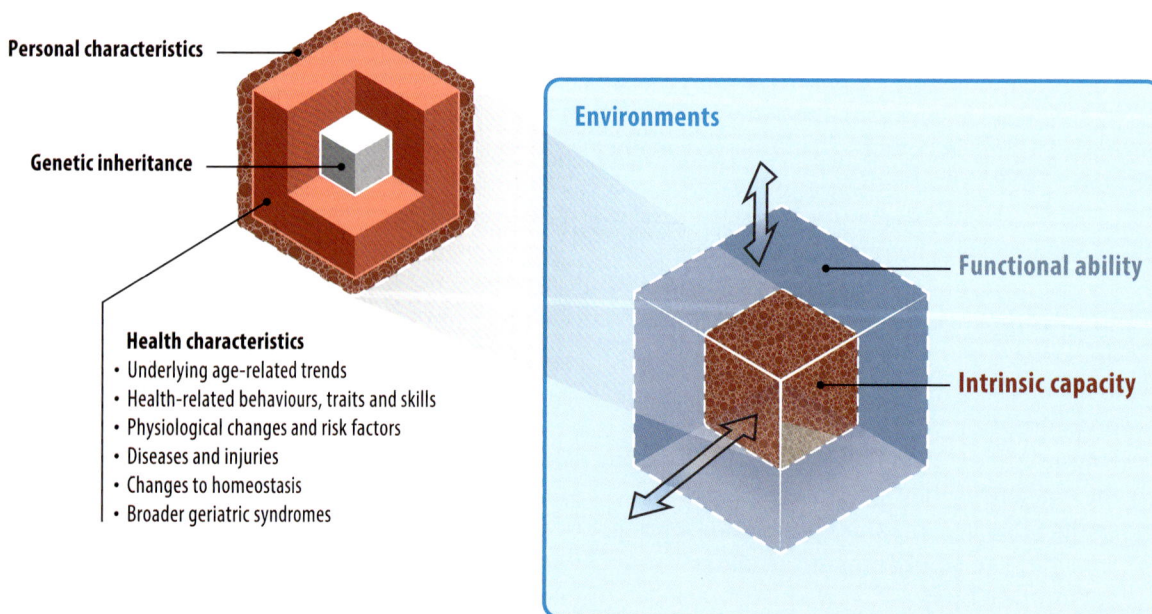

Personal characteristics

Genetic inheritance

Health characteristics
- Underlying age-related trends
- Health-related behaviours, traits and skills
- Physiological changes and risk factors
- Diseases and injuries
- Changes to homeostasis
- Broader geriatric syndromes

Environments

Functional ability

Intrinsic capacity

level to the macro-level – home, communities and the broader society. Within these environments are a range of factors, including the built environment, people and their relationships, attitudes and values, health and social policies, the systems that support them, and the services that they implement (*21*).

Well-being is considered in the broadest sense and includes domains such as happiness, satisfaction and fulfilment.

The process of *Healthy Ageing* is outlined in Fig. 2.1. *Healthy Ageing* starts at birth with our **genetic inheritance**. The expression of these genes can be influenced by experiences in the womb, and by subsequent environmental exposures and behaviours.

But each of us is also born into a social milieu. **Personal characteristics** include those that are usually fixed, such as our sex and ethnicity, as well as those that have some mobility or reflect social norms, such as our occupation, educational attainment, gender or wealth. These contribute to our social position within a particular context and time, which shapes the exposures, opportunities and barriers we face, as well as our access to resources. These interactions can be unfair or inequitable, as our share of opportunities and resources may not be based on need or right, but on our social or economic position (*28*).

As people age, they experience a gradual accumulation of molecular and cellular damage that results in a general decrease in physiological reserves. These broad physiological and homeostatic changes are largely inevitable, although their extent will vary significantly among individuals at any particular chronological age. On top of these underlying changes, exposures to a range of positive and negative environmental influences across the life course can influence the development of other **health characteristics**, such as physiological risk factors (for example, high blood pressure), diseases, injuries and broader geriatric syndromes.

The interaction among these health characteristics will ultimately determine the **intrinsic capacity** of the individual – that is, the composite of all the physical and mental capacities that an individual can draw on.

However, whether older people can achieve the things that they have reason to value will be determined not just by this capacity but also by further interactions with the environments they inhabit at a particular point in time. For example, older people with limitations in their physical capacity may still have the mobility they need if they use an assistive device and live close to public transport that provides access for people with disabilities. Another person with the same physical limitation but who lives in less enabling environments may find it much more difficult. This final combination of the individual and their environments, and the interaction between them, is the individual's **functional ability**.

At any point in time, an individual may have reserves of functional ability that they are not drawing on. These reserves contribute to an older person's **resilience**. Although this is not shown in Fig. 2.1, the *Healthy Ageing* model conceptualizes resilience as the ability to maintain or improve a level of functional ability in the face of adversity (either through resistance, recovery or adaptation). This ability comprises both components intrinsic to each individual (for example, psychological traits that help an individual frame problems in a way that can lead to a positive outcome, or physiological reserves that allow an older person to recover quickly after a fall) and environmental components that can mitigate deficits (for example, strong social networks that can be called on in times of need, or good access to health and social care).

The beings and doings that people have reason to value differ among individuals, and change over the course of people's lives (*5*). Although research is limited, some of the things that older people identify as important include having (*46–49*):

- **a role or identity;**
- **relationships;**
- **the possibility of enjoyment;**

- **autonomy** (being independent and being able to make their own decisions);
- **security**;
- **the potential for personal growth**.

Several domains of functional ability appear crucial to allowing people to achieve these ends. These will be discussed later in this report, particularly in Chapter 6, which looks at the broader impact of the environments an older person inhabits. These are the abilities to:

- move around;
- build and maintain relationships;
- meet their own basic needs;
- learn, grow and make decisions;
- contribute.

Most of the variability we see in both life span and intrinsic capacity in older age can be explained by our interaction with the environments we have experienced across our lives (50, 51). These experiences can take many forms. For example, safe and walkable environments may encourage physical activity and have multiple health benefits for people at almost all stages in life. Access to preventive services may lead to the diagnosis and management of hypertension and the prevention of ischaemic heart disease. If older people have a stroke, their ability to recover their intrinsic capacity will be significantly influenced by their access to rehabilitation.

The environment may be an even stronger influence on functional ability because it determines whether at any given level of intrinsic capacity we can ultimately do the things that are important to us.

One way of assessing the interaction between individuals and their environment is through the notion of **person–environment fit**. This reflects the dynamic and reciprocal relationship between individuals and their environments (Chapter 6) (52). Where the fit between people and their environments is good, they will enjoy the greatest opportunities to build and maintain both their intrinsic capacity and functional ability. The concept of person–environment fit considers:

- individuals and their health characteristics and capacity;
- societal needs and resources;
- the dynamic and interactive nature of the relationship between older people and the environments they inhabit;
- the changes that occur in people and places over time.

However, an environment is not neutral in its relationship with different individuals. Indeed, the same environment may affect different individuals in very different ways, influenced strongly by the range of personal characteristics that help determine a person's social position. These characteristics influence not only the nature of the environments around us (for example, whether we live in a poor or rich community) but also our relationship with an environment (for example, a man may feel safe in an environment where a woman may not). The result can be a systematic and unequal distribution of access to resources or exposure to negative environmental characteristics, or both.

When these interactions are unfair they result in health inequities. The cumulative impact of these inequities across our life course is a powerful influence on *Healthy Ageing*. For example, being poor may have many impacts across a lifetime including limiting access to healthy food or information that is important for making decisions about health. This may result in an older person experiencing atherosclerosis and diminished intrinsic capacity. Moreover, if the individual remains poor in older age, he or she may also only be able to afford to live in a disadvantaged neighbourhood where there is less access to the community and personal resources that might be available to a more financially secure person of the same age and with the same capacity. The functional ability and resilience of the poorer person is thus also likely to be comparatively lower.

Trajectories of *Healthy Ageing*

Healthy Ageing reflects the ongoing interaction between individuals and the environments they inhabit. This interaction results in trajectories of both intrinsic capacity and functional ability. To illustrate how these might be conceptualized and used, Fig. 2.2 shows three hypothetical trajectories of physical capacity for individuals beginning from the same starting point in midlife.

In Fig. 2.2, individual A can be considered as having the optimal trajectory, in which intrinsic capacity remains high until the end of life. Individual B has a similar trajectory until a point when an event causes a sudden fall in capacity, followed by some amount of recovery and then a gradual deterioration. Individual C has a steady decline in function. Each trajectory sees the person die at around the same age, but the levels of physical capacity they have enjoyed in the interim are very different.

From the original starting point in Fig. 2.2, the goal would be for each individual to experience the same trajectory as individual A. Experience in monitoring trajectories of intrinsic capacity suggests that already it is possible to assess individuals and predict their likely future trajectories given information on behaviours, health characteristics, genes and personal factors. Such predictive models are likely to be increasingly accurate and useful as more data are collected. These models could provide the opportunity to intervene in specific ways to help achieve this ideal goal.

Fig. 2.2 also shows alternative trajectories for individuals B and C. For individual B, a more positive trajectory might, for example, result from access to rehabilitation, and a negative trajectory might result from a lack of access to care (perhaps through rationing in a poor community or within a socially excluded subgroup of the population). For individual C, a more positive trajectory might result from a change in a health-related behaviour or having access to medication. Measuring functioning over time,

Fig. 2.2.   Three hypothetical trajectories of physical capacity

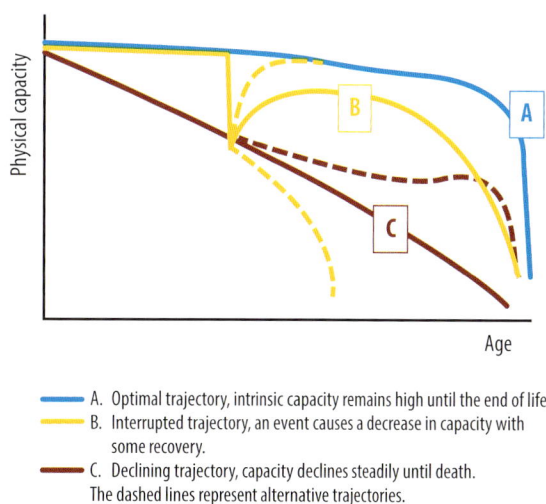

—— A. Optimal trajectory, intrinsic capacity remains high until the end of life.
—— B. Interrupted trajectory, an event causes a decrease in capacity with some recovery.
—— C. Declining trajectory, capacity declines steadily until death.
The dashed lines represent alternative trajectories.

understanding the plausible pathways that have led to it, and evaluating the influence of events at different points in time can thus help identify the interventions that have the most significant impacts during a person's life.

These hypothetical curves are an example of the diversity of older age and reflect the weak link at an individual level between intrinsic capacity and chronological age. However, at a population level, more general trends can be observed, with the average capacity at age 65 being very different from that at 80. These population averages can be seen in Fig. 3.16. It is worth noting, however, that even at a population level, there are significant differences in these average trajectories of intrinsic capacity. In developing a country-specific response to population ageing, a first step might be to identify these differences and why they exist.

Even if an individual's intrinsic capacity has fallen below its peak, the person may still be able to do the things that matter to them if they live in a supportive environment. This reflects the concept of functional ability: the ultimate goal of *Healthy Ageing*. Here, too, the concept of trajectories can be applied. Thus, Fig. 2.3 shows average trends from midlife in intrinsic capacity and functional ability. The additional functioning associated with functional ability reflects the net benefits accrued from the environment that a person lives in. This may become increasingly important as decrements in a person's capacity increase. Of course, the environment has also contributed to the level of capacity that an individual has achieved at any point in time.

In Fig. 2.3 it is assumed that the environment always enables functional ability to be greater than might be possible through intrinsic capacity alone. Even in a poor country, for example, a road and a bicycle add to mobility, and the opportunity to have a role can enhance well-being. However, it is possible that in some settings the barriers that the environment puts in the way of older people may be greater than the benefits it provides. Examples of environmental barriers might include barriers to education that result in illiteracy, or laws that prevent segments of the population from participating in certain fundamental activities (for example, by imposing mandatory retirement ages or sex-based exclusion from key roles).

Fig. 2.3.   Trajectories of functional ability and intrinsic capacity

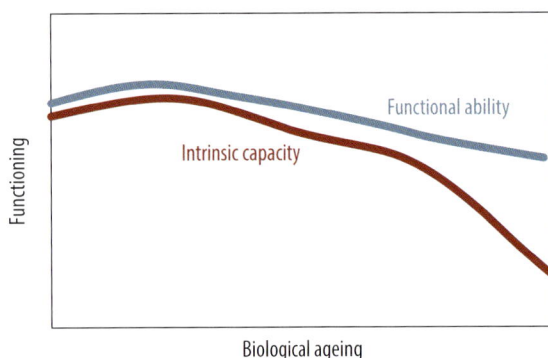

A public-health framework for *Healthy Ageing*

Numerous entry points can be identified for actions to promote *Healthy Ageing*, but all will have one goal: to foster functional ability (Fig. 2.4). This can be achieved in two ways: by supporting the building and maintenance of intrinsic capacity, and by enabling those with a decrement in their functional capacity to do the things that are important to them.

Fig. 2.3 and Fig. 2.4 show how, when considering the population as a whole, functional ability and intrinsic capacity can vary across the second half of the life course. These general trajectories can be divided into three common periods: a period of relatively high and stable capacity, a period of declining capacity, and a period of significant loss of capacity. It is important to note that these periods are not defined by chronological age, are not necessarily monotonic (that is, continually decreasing) and that trajectories will differ markedly among individuals (and may be disrupted entirely by an unexpected event such as an accident). Some people may, for example, die suddenly from any of a variety of causes while still in the period of high and stable capacity.

However, a random sample of older people at any particular age is likely to include people in each of these phases, thus reflecting much of the observed heterogeneity of older age. Furthermore, the needs of people in these different phases of the life course are quite distinct (Chapter 4). Therefore, they are used here to help frame public-health actions that might be applied across the second half of life.

The focus of public-health strategies targeting people with high and stable levels of intrinsic capacity should be on building and maintaining this for as long as possible. Health systems will need to detect and control disease and risk factors early. Environmental strategies will be crucial in encouraging healthy behaviours, both by building personal skills and knowledge, and

Fig. 2.4.   A public-health framework for *Healthy Ageing:* opportunities for public-health action across the life course

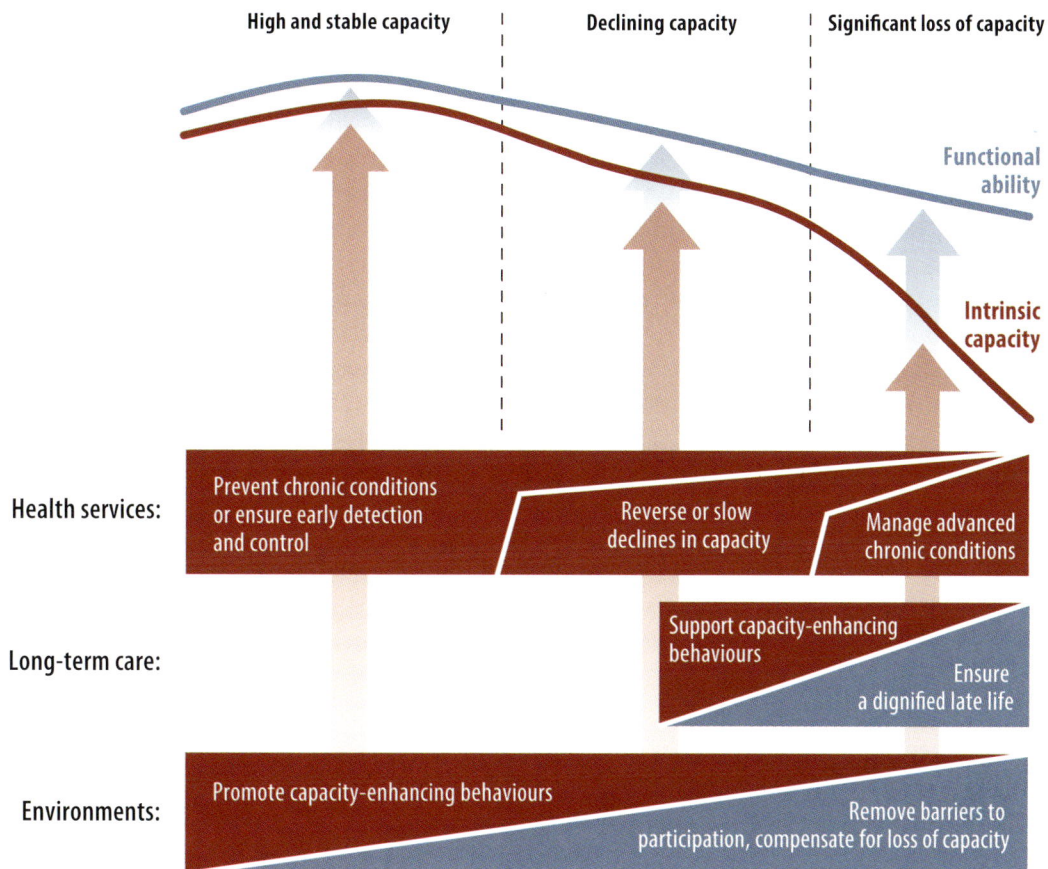

through the implementation of broader environmental strategies, such as taxing tobacco or providing safe and pleasant environments for physical activity. Environments will also have a role in enabling functional ability during this period, with particular emphasis on removing barriers to the expression of this capacity.

Public-health interventions targeting the segment of the population with declining capacities need a different emphasis. During this stage, diseases may have become established, and the emphasis of health systems will generally shift from prevention or cure to minimizing the impacts of these conditions on a person's overall capacity. Therefore, services are needed to help stop, slow or reverse declines in capacity. Furthermore, the role of the environment in enabling functional ability will broaden as capacity falls, with strategies that help people overcome these decrements becoming increasingly important. For example, if physical capacity becomes limited public seating may make shopping more achievable by providing a place for an older person to rest, or good street lighting may allow an older person with slight visual impairment to get home in the evening. The role of the environment in enabling healthy behaviours will continue to be important for this segment of the older population, but the emphasis may change. For example, physical activity may be promoted as much for building and maintaining muscle mass and balance as for reducing the risk of disease.

The focus of a public-health response to the needs of older people who have, or are at high risk of, significant losses in capacity will be the provision of long-term care (Chapter 5). The role of long-term care systems is to enable an older person to maintain a level of functional ability consistent with their basic rights, fundamental freedoms, and human dignity. This requires both ensuring the optimal trajectory of intrinsic capacity and enabling older people to perform with dignity the basic tasks that are necessary for their well-being. This can take many forms. For example, early care to reduce declines in capacities might include family members encouraging older people to become more active and assisting them with this as well as encouraging them to eat well. Later care may include support for basic tasks, such as washing and cooking, but will also need to be fully integrated with health systems to ensure that trajectories of capacity are optimized. These tasks will be made easier if the older person lives in an enabling environment (for example, in a home that is fully wheelchair accessible, or a dementia-friendly community for someone with cognitive decline).

Although public-health strategies will need to be framed to meet the specific needs of these typical subpopulations, and tailored to the structure and needs of the population as a whole, *Healthy Ageing* considers these phases of older age as part of a continuous trajectory of ability and capacity. Public-health interventions should similarly be seamless to remain relevant for older people as they transition from one phase to another.

Key issues for public-health action

Dealing with diversity

Shaping policy to foster *Healthy Ageing* will require active efforts to better understand the diverse needs of older populations. This could start with the collection of data that are more disaggregated and nuanced to help identify older people's needs and gaps in services, to better describe the process of *Healthy Ageing*, and to better understand the diverse pathways from determinants to intrinsic capacity and functional ability. Another approach that is increasingly used is the concept of being **person-centred**. This approach evolved in the practice of psychotherapy, but has been extended to health and long-term care settings and is central to the *WHO global strategy on people-centred and integrated health services* (53). This strategy is designed to encourage a fundamental paradigm shift in the way health services are funded, managed and delivered so that all people have access to health services that respond to their preferences, are coordinated around their needs, and are safe, effective, timely, efficient and of an acceptable quality.

This strategy can equally be applied in long-term care. For example, in 2003 the Japanese government introduced the concept of the unit-care model, which shifted emphasis from standardized care practices to the structure and staffing needed for care. It has been shown that this model facilitates flexibility in care, for example by providing choices for meals and activities for patients' spare time (54). Similarly, the provision of care in small-scale home-like facilities for people with dementia in the Netherlands has been shown to be related to a higher involvement of residents in overall activities and their preferred activities (55). In fact, the principles of person-centred care can be applied to every interaction in a care home, whether helping someone use the toilet or when asking a person's opinion.

A person-centred approach can also be useful in helping other sectors tailor and prioritize their responses to population ageing. For example, the WHO Global Network of Age-friendly Cities and Communities brings together municipal authorities from across the world who have committed to making their jurisdictions better places for older people to live. One of the core elements of this initiative is to involve older people in helping frame both the key issues and the responses to them. This has been done even in megacities such as New York, which have diverse populations in terms of personal characteristics and socioeconomic gradients (56).

Reducing inequity

If the inequities that often underpin the diversity observed in older age are to be addressed, strategies must look not just to improve conditions for the best-off or the average older person. Attention must also be given to levelling-up capacity and functional ability across social gradients and to narrowing the gaps in the total inequalities observed among older individuals, particularly by giving assistance to those at the bottom of the range. This type of action reflects the human rights principles of equality and nondiscrimination, specifically because they require governments to make disproportionate efforts to reach groups that are particularly disadvantaged.

Several steps can help ensure that policy choices enhance equity (57, 58). These include:
- making a commitment that all older people will have equal opportunities to improve or maintain their health;
- assessing health policies and programmes in relation to inequalities, from inputs to outcomes, and gauging to what extent these are fair or unfair. For example, when only the poorest people do not have access to a service, policies may need to focus on expanding the provision of that service to the particular groups that are excluded or marginalized. When almost no one has access to

a service, more wide-ranging strategies are usually required. In many settings a combination of strategies will be needed (52);
- involving older people and other stakeholders in identifying interventions that draw on the evidence for what works locally and elsewhere.

Policies aiming to level-up social gradients are not only fair but can also produce significant health benefits for older adults. For example, around 1 in 5 cases of Alzheimer's disease worldwide is estimated to be to some extent attributable to low educational attainment (population attributable risk, 19.1%), with almost 6.5 million attributable cases occurring globally in 2010 alone (59). It has been suggested that incidence might be significantly reduced through improved access to education and use of effective methods targeted at reducing the prevalence of vascular risk factors and depression (60).

Enabling choice

Older people are not passive in their relationship with their environments. Rather, this interaction is shaped to varying degrees by the choices they make to respond to, or change, their situation. Retaining the ability and right to choose is closely linked to notions of agency and autonomy (61, 62), which have been shown to have a powerful influence on an older person's dignity, integrity, freedom and independence (63, 64). This is true whether they live in the community, in an assisted living facility or in an institution (65, 66).

Our ability to make the best choices at different stages in our lives is influenced by a range of environmental and personal resources. As with intrinsic capacity more broadly, financially secure, better educated and more socially connected older people are likely to have the greatest access to these resources. Understanding this association is crucial because it means that older people with the lowest intrinsic capacity and functional ability at any given age are not only less likely to be financially secure and well educated, but are also less likely to have had the opportunity to develop the skills and knowledge that allows them to make the choices that are in their best interest. Therefore, fostering the abilities to choose and to self-manage in this group may be a useful strategy for overcoming some of the inequities experienced in older age.

Public-health strategies that might empower older people to retain control of their lives and make the choices that are in their best interest are discussed in particular detail in Chapter 6 as being in the domain of the functional ability to learn, grow and make decisions.

Ageing in place

Declines in capacity often require older people to make transitions in their living environments, either by adapting their current residence or by relocating to a more supportive environment (67). In deciding where to live, older people often view their existing home or community as having the advantages of maintaining a sense of connection, security and familiarity, and as being related to their sense of identity and autonomy (68). Indeed, the right for all people with some form of functional limitation to live and be included in their community is a central focus of the *United Nations convention on the rights of persons with disabilities* (25). Furthermore, institutional settings are sometimes seen as dehumanizing and as posing structural and cultural barriers that impede social interactions (69).

One common policy response to population ageing has therefore been to encourage what is known as ageing in place – that is, the ability of older people to live in their own home and community safely, independently, and comfortably, regardless of age, income or level of intrinsic capacity (70). This is generally viewed as better for the older person and may also hold significant financial advantages in terms of health-care expenditure (71).

Emerging technologies, particularly those used to foster communication and engagement, provide opportunities to learn, and monitor the safety and ensure the security of an older person, may make this goal more achievable in the future. Ageing in place can be further enhanced by creating age-friendly environments that enable mobility and allow older people to engage in basic activities, such as shopping.

However, as with other policies on ageing, putting too rigid an emphasis on one-size-fits-all solutions can present problems. For example, ageing in place may not be the prime goal for isolated older people, for those with high unmet needs for care and inappropriate housing, or for those living in unsafe or less than supportive neighbourhoods (72). Furthermore, ageing in place should not be viewed as a policy that allows governments to simply minimize costs by failing to provide more costly alternatives. Indeed, it has been suggested that ageing in place requires a family of caregivers and appropriate medical care to allow it to occur (73).

Moreover, older people generally have a nuanced and realistic perspective on the residential decisions they face. Recent advances in developing new forms of assisted living and nursing-home care provide many alternatives to the stereotypical choice between living at home or in a home (73). These alternatives can enable an older person to thrive in ways that might not be possible in their original community.

References

1. Kirkwood TB. A systematic look at an old problem. Nature. 2008 Feb 7;451(7179):644–7.doi: http://dx.doi.org/10.1038/451644a PMID: 18256658
2. Steves CJ, Spector TD, Jackson SH. Ageing, genes, environment and epigenetics: what twin studies tell us now, and in the future. Age Ageing. 2012 Sep;41(5):581–6.doi: http://dx.doi.org/10.1093/ageing/afs097 PMID: 22826292
3. Vasto S, Scapagnini G, Bulati M, Candore G, Castiglia L, Colonna-Romano G, et al. Biomarkes of aging. Front Biosci (Schol Ed). 2010;2(1):392–402.doi: http://dx.doi.org/http://dx.doi.org/ PMID: 20036955
4. Baltes P, Freund A, Li S-C. The psychological science of human ageing. In: Johnson ML, Bengtson VL, Coleman PG, Kirkwood TBL, editors. The Cambridge handbook of age and ageing. Cambridge: Cambridge University Press; 2005:47–71.
5. Carstensen LL. The influence of a sense of time on human development. Science. 2006 Jun 30;312(5782):1913–5.doi: http://dx.doi.org/10.1126/science.1127488 PMID: 16809530
6. Adams KB. Changing investment in activities and interests in elders' lives: theory and measurement. Int J Aging Hum Dev. 2004;58(2):87–108.doi: http://dx.doi.org/10.2190/0UQ0-7D8X-XVVU-TF7X PMID: 15259878
7. Hicks JA, Trent J, Davis WE, King LA. Positive affect, meaning in life, and future time perspective: an application of socioemotional selectivity theory. Psychol Aging. 2012 Mar;27(1):181–9.doi: http://dx.doi.org/10.1037/a0023965 PMID: 21707177
8. Dillaway HE, Byrnes M. Reconsidering successful aging: a call for renewed and expanded academic critiques and conceptualizations. J Appl Gerontol. 2009;28(6):702–22. doi: http://dx.doi.org/10.1177/0733464809333882
9. Steptoe A, Deaton A, Stone AA. Subjective wellbeing, health, and ageing. Lancet. 2015 Feb 14;385(9968):640–8. PMID: 25468152
10. Huber M, Knottnerus JA, Green L, van der Horst H, Jadad AR, Kromhout D, et al. How should we define health? BMJ. 2011;343:d4163.doi: http://dx.doi.org/10.1136/bmj.d4163 PMID: 21791490
11. Young Y, Frick KD, Phelan EA. Can successful aging and chronic illness coexist in the same individual? A multidimensional concept of successful aging. J Am Med Dir Assoc. 2009 Feb;10(2):87–92.doi: http://dx.doi.org/10.1016/j.jamda.2008.11.003 PMID: 19187875
12. Saß A-C, Wurm S, Ziese T. [Somatic and Psychological Health]. In: Tesch-Römer C, Böhm K, Ziese T, editors. [Somatic and Psychological Health]. Berlin: Robert Koch-Institut; 2009 (in German).
13. Marengoni A, Angleman S, Melis R, Mangialasche F, Karp A, Garmen A, et al. Aging with multimorbidity: a systematic review of the literature. Ageing Res Rev. 2011 Sep;10(4):430–9.doi: http://dx.doi.org/10.1016/j.arr.2011.03.003 PMID: 21402176
14. Collard RM, Boter H, Schoevers RA, Oude Voshaar RC. Prevalence of frailty in community-dwelling older persons: a systematic review. J Am Geriatr Soc. 2012 Aug;60(8):1487–92. PMID: 22881367
15. Fong TG, Tulebaev SR, Inouye SK. Delirium in elderly adults: diagnosis, prevention and treatment. Nat Rev Neurol. 2009 Apr;5(4):210–20. PMID: 19347026
16. Kheirbek RE, Alemi F, Citron BA, Afaq MA, Wu H, Fletcher RD. Trajectory of illness for patients with congestive heart failure. J Palliat Med. 2013 May;16(5):478–84.doi: http://dx.doi.org/10.1089/jpm.2012.0510 PMID: 23545095
17. Lordos EF, Herrmann FR, Robine JM, Balahoczky M, Giannelli SV, Gold G, et al. Comparative value of medical diagnosis versus physical functioning in predicting the 6-year survival of 1951 hospitalized old patients. Rejuvenation Res. 2008 Aug;11(4):829–36. PMID: 18729815
18. Ham C. The ten characteristics of the high-performing chronic care system. Health Econ Policy Law. 2010 Jan;5(Pt 1):71–90. doi: http://dx.doi.org/10.1017/S1744133109990120 PMID: 19732475
19. Low LF, Yap M, Brodaty H. A systematic review of different models of home and community care services for older persons. BMC Health Serv Res. 2011;11(1):93.doi: http://dx.doi.org/10.1186/1472-6963-11-93 PMID: 21549010
20. Eklund K, Wilhelmson K. Outcomes of coordinated and integrated interventions targeting frail elderly people: a systematic review of randomised controlled trials. Health Soc Care Community. 2009 Sep;17(5):447–58.doi: http://dx.doi.org/10.1111/j.1365-2524.2009.00844.x PMID: 19245421
21. The international classification of functioning. Disability and health. Geneva: World Health Organization; 2001.
22. Beard J, Petitot C. Aging and urbanization: can cities be designed to foster active aging? Public Health Rev. 2011;32(2):427–50.
23. Political declaration and Madrid international plan of action on ageing. New York: United Nations; 2002 (http://www.un.org/en/events/pastevents/pdfs/Madrid_plan.pdf, accessed 14 June 2015).
24. Active ageing: a policy framework. Geneva: World Health Organization; 2002 (http://whqlibdoc.who.int/hq/2002/who_nmh_nph_02.8.pdf, accessed 14 June 2015).
25. Convention on the rights of persons with disabilities and optional protocol. New York: United Nations; 2006 (http://www.un.org/disabilities/documents/convention/convoptprot-e.pdf, accessed 14 June 2015).

26. Global action plan for the prevention and control of noncommunicable diseases 2013–2020. Geneva: World Health Organization; 2013 (http://apps.who.int/iris/bitstream/10665/94384/1/9789241506236_eng.pdf, accessed 14 June 2015).

27. Beijing declaration and platform for action: Beijing+5 political declaration and outcome. New York: United Nations; 1995. (http://beijing20.unwomen.org/~/media/headquarters/attachments/sections/csw/pfa_e_final_web.pdf, accessed 14 June 2015).

28. Commission on Social Determinants of Health. Closing the gap in a generation: health equity through action on social determinants of health. Final report of the Commission on Social Determinants of Health. Geneva: World Health Organization; 2008 (http://whqlibdoc.who.int/publications/2008/9789241563703_eng.pdf, accessed 14 June, 2015).

29. Venkatapuram S. Health justice: an argument from the capabilities approach. Hoboken (NJ): Wiley; 2013. (http://USYD.eblib.com.au/patron/FullRecord.aspx?p=1174277, accessed 23 April, 2015).

30. Nussbaum M. Capabilities as fundamental entitlements: Sen and social justice. Fem Econ. 2003;9(2–3):33–59. doi: http://dx.doi.org/10.1080/1354570022000077926

31. Nussbaum MC. Creating capabilities: the human development approach. Cambridge (MA): Harvard University Press; 2011. doi: http://dx.doi.org/10.4159/harvard.9780674061200

32. Gasper D. Sen's capability approach and Nussbaum's capabilities ethic. J Int Dev. 1997;9(2):281–302. doi: http://dx.doi.org/10.1002/(SICI)1099-1328(199703)9:2<281:AID-JID438>3.0.CO;2-K

33. Nussbaum M. Capabilities and social justice. Int Stud Rev. 2003;4(2):123–35. doi: http://dx.doi.org/10.1111/1521-9488.00258

34. Sen A. Capability and wellbeing. In: Nussbaum M, Sen A, editors. The quality of life. Oxford: Oxford University Press; 1993. doi: http://dx.doi.org/10.1093/0198287976.003.0003

35. Alkire S. Why the capability approach? J Hum Dev. 2005;6(1):115–35. doi: http://dx.doi.org/10.1080/146498805200034275

36. Robeyns I. The capability approach: a theoretical survey. J Hum Dev. 2005;6(1):93–117. doi: http://dx.doi.org/10.1080/146498805200034266

37. Gasper D. What is the capability approach? Its core, rationale, partners and dangers. J Socioecon. 2007;36(3):335–59. doi: http://dx.doi.org/10.1016/j.socec.2006.12.001

38. Kimberly H, Gruhn R, Huggins S. Valuing capabilities in later life: the capability approach and the Brotherhood of St Laurence aged services. Fitzroy, VIC: Brotherhood of St Laurence; 2012 (http://www.bsl.org.au/KimberleyGruhnHuggins_Valuing_capabilities_in_later_life_2012.pdf, accessed 14 June, 2015).

39. Kuh D, Ben-Shlomo Y, Lynch J, Hallqvist J, Power C. Life course epidemiology. J Epidemiol Community Health. 2003 Oct;57(10):778–83.doi: http://dx.doi.org/10.1136/jech.57.10.778 PMID: 14573579

40. Hardy SE, Concato J, Gill TM. Resilience of community-dwelling older persons. J Am Geriatr Soc. 2004 Feb;52(2):257–62.doi: http://dx.doi.org/10.1111/j.1532-5415.2004.52065.x PMID: 14728637

41. Luthar SS, Cicchetti D, Becker B. The construct of resilience: a critical evaluation and guidelines for future work. Child Dev. 2000 May-Jun;71(3):543–62.doi: http://dx.doi.org/10.1111/1467-8624.00164 PMID: 10953923

42. Peel N, Bartlett H, McClure R. Healthy ageing: how is it defined and measured? Australas J Ageing. 2004;23(3):115–9. doi: http://dx.doi.org/10.1111/j.1741-6612.2004.00035.x

43. Fuchs J, Scheidt-Nave C, Hinrichs T, Mergenthaler A, Stein J, Riedel-Heller SG, et al. Indicators for healthy ageing–a debate. Int J Environ Res Public Health. 2013 Dec;10(12):6630–44.doi: http://dx.doi.org/10.3390/ijerph10126630 PMID: 24317381

44. Lowry KA, Vallejo AN, Studenski SA. Successful aging as a continuum of functional independence: lessons from physical disability models of aging. Aging Dis. 2012 Feb;3(1):5–15. PMID: 22500268

45. Lara J, Godfrey A, Evans E, Heaven B, Brown LJ, Barron E, et al. Towards measurement of the Healthy Ageing Phenotype in lifestyle-based intervention studies. Maturitas. 2013 Oct;76(2):189–99.doi: http://dx.doi.org/10.1016/j.maturitas.2013.07.007 PMID: 23932426

46. McLaughlin SJ, Jette AM, Connell CM. An examination of healthy aging across a conceptual continuum: prevalence estimates, demographic patterns, and validity. J Gerontol A Biol Sci Med Sci. 2012 Jun;67(7):783–9.doi: http://dx.doi.org/10.1093/gerona/glr234 PMID: 22367432

47. Grewal I, Lewis J, Flynn T, Brown J, Bond J, Coast J. Developing attributes for a generic quality of life measure for older people: preferences or capabilities? Soc Sci Med. 2006 Apr;62(8):1891–901.doi: http://dx.doi.org/10.1016/j.socscimed.2005.08.023 PMID: 16168542

48. Ward L, Barnes M, Gahagan B. Well-being in old age: findings from participatory research. Brighton: University of Brighton, Age Concern Brighton, Hove and Portslade; 2012 (https://www.brighton.ac.uk/_pdf/research/ssparc/wellbeing-in-old-age-full-report.pdf, accessed 14 June 2015).

49. Bowling A, Dieppe P. What is successful ageing and who should define it? BMJ. 2005 Dec 24;331(7531):1548–51.doi: http://dx.doi.org/10.1136/bmj.331.7531.1548 PMID: 16373748

50. Brooks-Wilson AR. Genetics of healthy aging and longevity. Hum Genet. 2013 Dec;132(12):1323–38.doi: http://dx.doi.org/10.1007/s00439-013-1342-z PMID: 23925498

51. Dato S, Montesanto A, Lagani V, Jeune B, Christensen K, Passarino G. Frailty phenotypes in the elderly based on cluster analysis: a longitudinal study of two Danish cohorts. Evidence for a genetic influence on frailty. Age (Dordr). 2012 Jun;34(3):571–82.doi: http://dx.doi.org/10.1007/s11357-011-9257-x PMID: 21567248

52. Keating N, Eales J, Phillips JE. Age-friendly rural communities: conceptualizing 'best-fit'. Can J Aging. 2013 Dec;32(4):319–32. PMID: 24128863

53. WHO global strategy on people-centred and integrated health services. Geneva: World Health Organization; 2015 (http://www.who.int/servicedeliverysafety/areas/people-centred-care/en/, accessed 14 June 2015).

54. Sawamura K, Nakashima T, Nakanishi M. Provision of individualized care and built environment of nursing homes in Japan. Arch Gerontol Geriatr. 2013 May-Jun;56(3):416–24.doi: http://dx.doi.org/10.1016/j.archger.2012.11.009 PMID: 23260333

55. Smit D, de Lange J, Willemse B, Pot AM. The relationship between small-scale care and activity involvement of residents with dementia. Int Psychogeriatr. 2012 May;24(5):722–32.doi: http://dx.doi.org/10.1017/S1041610211002377 PMID: 22221709

56. Age friendly NYC: a progress report. New York: City of New York, New York Academy of Medicine; 2011 (http://www.nyam.org/agefriendlynyc/Age-Friendly-NYC-Report-Final-High-Res2_new.pdf, accessed 14 June 2015).

57. Closing the health equity gap: policy options and opportunities for action. Geneva, World Health Organization; 2013 (http://apps.who.int/iris/handle/10665/78335, accessed 19 June 2015).

58. Sadana R, Blas E. What can public health programs do to improve health equity? Public Health Rep. 2013 Nov;128(Suppl 3) Suppl 3:12–20. PMID: 24179274

59. Lee JT, Huang Z, Basu S, Millett C. The inverse equity hypothesis: does it apply to coverage of cancer screening in middle-income countries? J Epidemiol Community Health. 2015 Feb;69(2):149–55.doi: http://dx.doi.org/10.1136/jech-2014-204355 PMID: 25311479

60. Norton S, Matthews FE, Barnes DE, Yaffe K, Brayne C. Potential for primary prevention of Alzheimer's disease: an analysis of population-based data. Lancet Neurol. 2014 Aug;13(8):788–94.doi: http://dx.doi.org/10.1016/S1474-4422(14)70136-X PMID: 25030513

61. Stephens C, Breheny M, Mansvelt J. Healthy ageing from the perspective of older people: a capability approach to resilience. Psychol Health. 2014;30(6):715–31. PMID: 24678916

62. Davies S, Laker S, Ellis L. Promoting autonomy and independence for older people within nursing practice: a literature review. J Adv Nurs. 1997 Aug;26(2):408–17.doi: http://dx.doi.org/10.1046/j.1365-2648.1997.1997026408.x PMID: 9292377

63. Welford C, Murphy K, Rodgers V, Frauenlob T. Autonomy for older people in residential care: a selective literature review. Int J Older People Nurs. 2012 Mar;7(1):65–9.doi: http://dx.doi.org/10.1111/j.1748-3743.2012.00311.x PMID: 22348264

64. Lindberg C, Fagerström C, Sivberg B, Willman A. Concept analysis: patient autonomy in a caring context. J Adv Nurs. 2014 Oct;70(10):2208–21.doi: http://dx.doi.org/10.1111/jan.12412 PMID: 25209751

65. Hillcoat-Nallétamby S. The meaning of "independence" for older people in different residential settings. J Gerontol B Psychol Sci Soc Sci. 2014 May;69(3):419–30.doi: http://dx.doi.org/10.1093/geronb/gbu008 PMID: 24578371

66. Boyle G. Facilitating choice and control for older people in long-term care. Health Soc Care Community. 2004 May;12(3):212–20.doi: http://dx.doi.org/10.1111/j.1365-2524.2004.00490.x PMID: 19777711

67. Perry TE, Andersen TC, Kaplan DB. Relocation remembered: perspectives on senior transitions in the living environment. Gerontologist. 2014 Feb;54(1):75–81.doi: http://dx.doi.org/10.1093/geront/gnt070 PMID: 23840021

68. Wiles JL, Leibing A, Guberman N, Reeve J, Allen RE. The meaning of "aging in place" to older people. Gerontologist. 2012 Jun;52(3):357–66.doi: http://dx.doi.org/10.1093/geront/gnr098 PMID: 21983126

69. Bonifas RP, Simons K, Biel B, Kramer C. Aging and place in long-term care settings: influences on social relationships. J Aging Health. 2014 Dec;26(8):1320–39.doi: http://dx.doi.org/10.1177/0898264314535632 PMID: 25502244

70. Healthy Ageing & the Built Environment [website]. Atlanta (GA): Centers for Disease Control and Prevention; 2015 (http://www.cdc.gov/healthyplaces/healthtopics/healthyaging.htm, accessed 17 June 2015).

71. Marek KD, Stetzer F, Adams SJ, Popejoy LL, Rantz M. Aging in place versus nursing home care: comparison of costs to Medicare and Medicaid. Res Gerontol Nurs. 2012 Apr;5(2):123–9.doi: http://dx.doi.org/10.3928/19404921-20110802-01 PMID: 21846081

72. Golant SM. Commentary: irrational exuberance for the aging in place of vulnerable low-income older homeowners. J Aging Soc Policy. 2008;20(4):379–97.doi: http://dx.doi.org/10.1080/08959420802131437 PMID: 19042553

73. Morley JE. Aging in place. J Am Med Dir Assoc. 2012 Jul;13(6):489–92.doi: http://dx.doi.org/10.1016/j.jamda.2012.04.011 PMID: 22682696

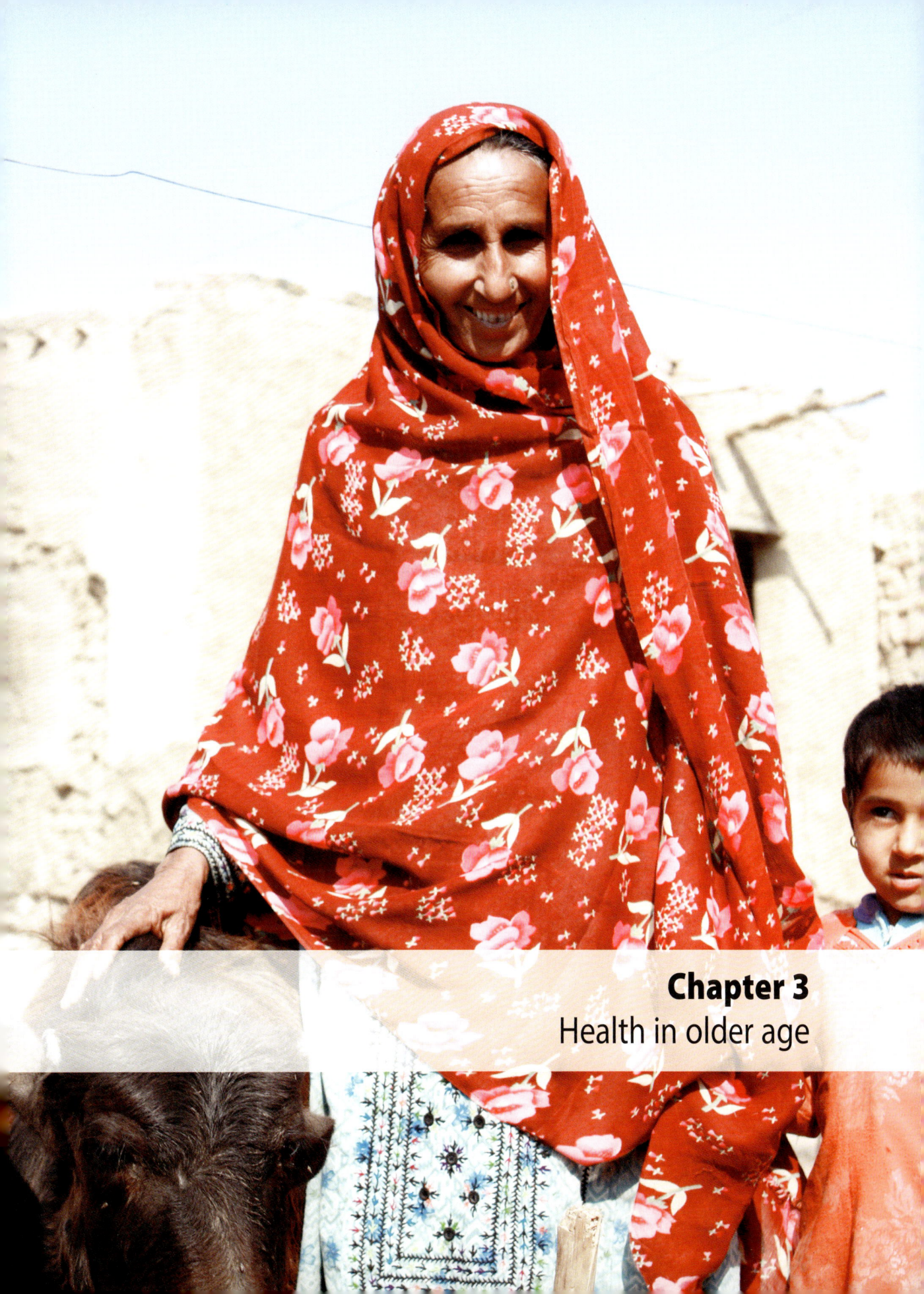

Chapter 3
Health in older age

Zenul, Age unknown, Pakistan

During the 2011 floods in Pakistan villagers lost their livestock and arable land was damaged. With a cash grant, distributed after the flood, Zenul was able to buy a calf.

"I've been a widow for at least 10 years. I have 3 sons and 1 daughter and they're all land labourers here – but now of course they cannot grow a thing. I got 15,000 rupees …. and I spent it on this calf. I'll get milk from it, some of which I'll keep for myself and the rest I can sell for 40 rupees per litre. Hopefully it'll also have calves which I'll sell.

I'm living in a tent because my house is unstable because of the floods and actually we felt an earthquake last week. Normally the mud we coat the house with protects the house - its very strong against the extreme heat and the cold in winter. But it crumbled in the floods. I'm not sure how I'll rebuild the house. If we had money we'd buy cement. Mud is free but cement is expensive. I will have to wait for the calf to grow!"

3

Health in older age

Demographic and epidemiological changes

Population ageing

One reason that ageing is emerging as a key policy issue is that both the proportion and absolute number of older people in populations around the world are increasing dramatically. Fig. 3.1 and Fig. 3.2 show the proportion of people aged 60 years or older by country in 2012 and projections for 2050. There is currently only one country where this proportion exceeds 30%: Japan. However, by the middle of the century, many countries will have a similar proportion of older people to that of Japan in 2012. These include countries in Europe and North America, but also Chile, China, the Islamic Republic of Iran, the Republic of Korea, the Russian Federation, Thailand and Viet Nam.

In Fig. 3.1 and Fig. 3.2, population ageing may appear to be less relevant to sub-Saharan Africa. Yet although the population structure in sub-Saharan Africa will stay young in relative terms, this region already has double the number of older adults than northern Europe, and this figure is expected to grow faster than anywhere else, increasing from 46 million in 2015 to 157 million by 2050 (1). Furthermore, life expectancy at age 60 in sub-Saharan Africa is 16 years for women and 14 years for men, suggesting that for those who survive the earlier perils of life, a long old age is already a reality. Older people in sub-Saharan Africa also have several roles that are critical for continued socioeconomic development (1).

The pace of population ageing in many countries is also much greater than has been the case in the past (Fig. 3.3). For example, while France had almost 150 years to adapt to a change from 10% to 20% in the proportion of the population that was older than 60 years, places such as Brazil, China and India will have slightly more than 20 years to make the same adaptation. This means that the adaptation that these countries need to go through will have to be undertaken much more quickly than was often the case in the past.

Why are populations ageing?

There are two key drivers of population ageing. The first is increasing life expectancy: on average, people around the world are living longer. Although

Fig. 3.1.   Proportion of population aged 60 years or older, by country, 2015

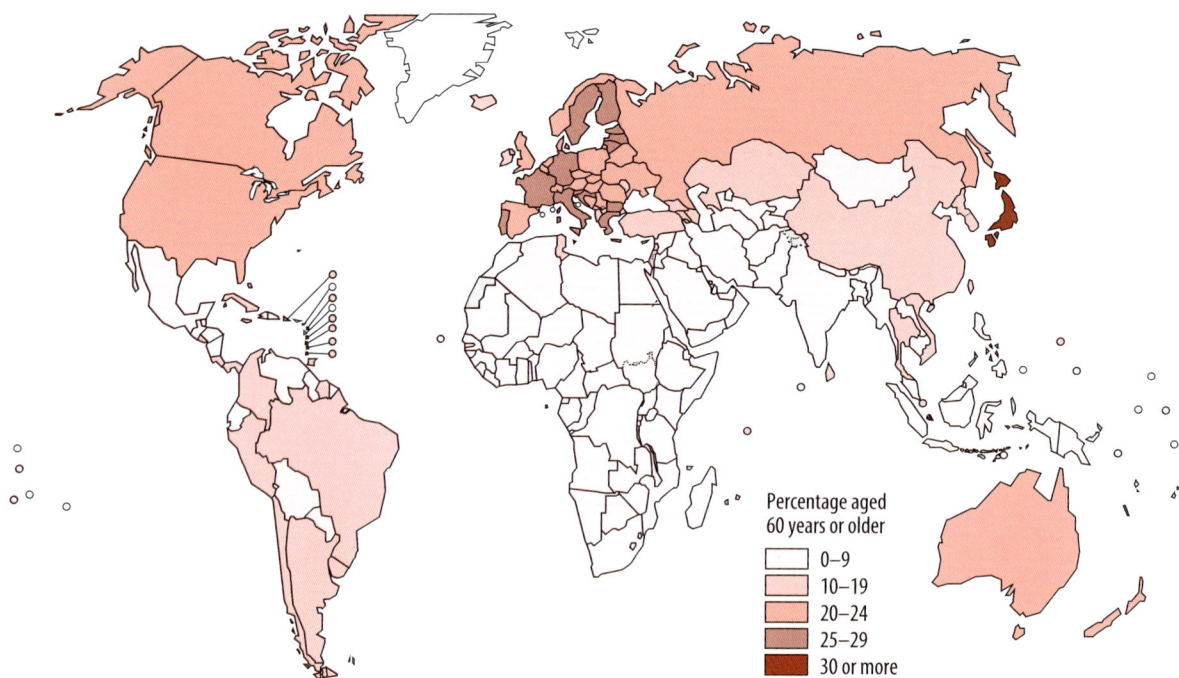

Percentage aged
60 years or older

- 0–9
- 10–19
- 20–24
- 25–29
- 30 or more

Fig. 3.2.   Proportion of population aged 60 years or older, by country, 2050 projections

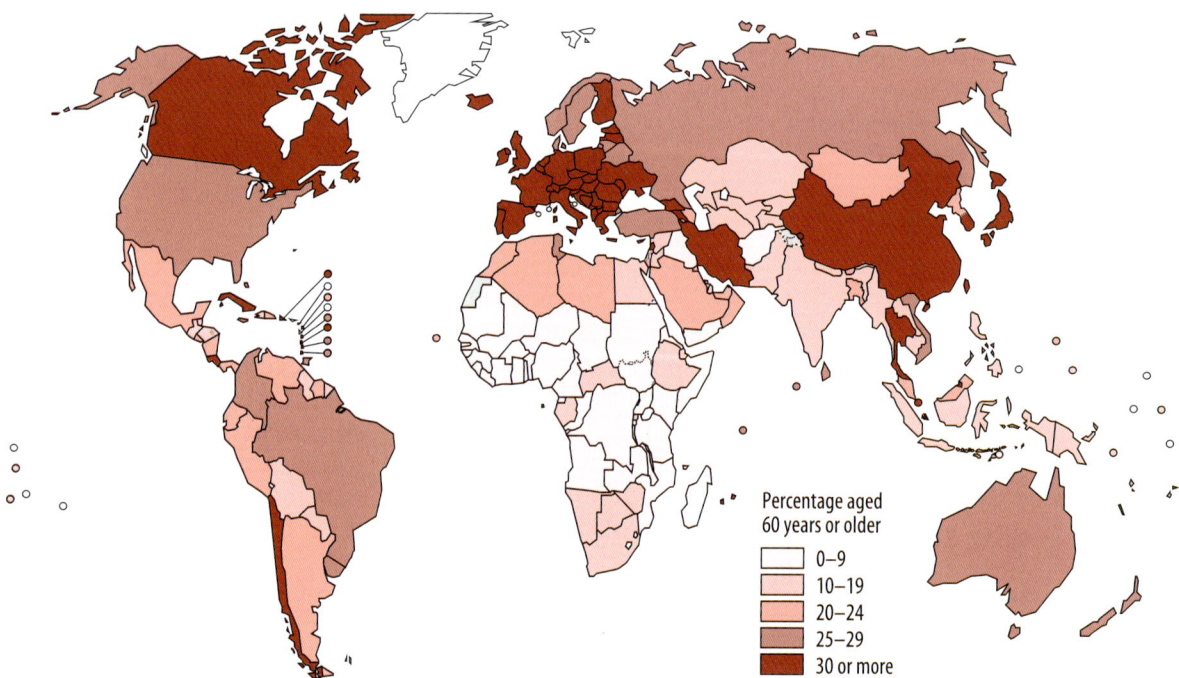

Percentage aged
60 years or older

- 0–9
- 10–19
- 20–24
- 25–29
- 30 or more

Fig. 3.3. **Period required or expected for the percentage of the population aged 60 years and older to rise from 10% to 20%**

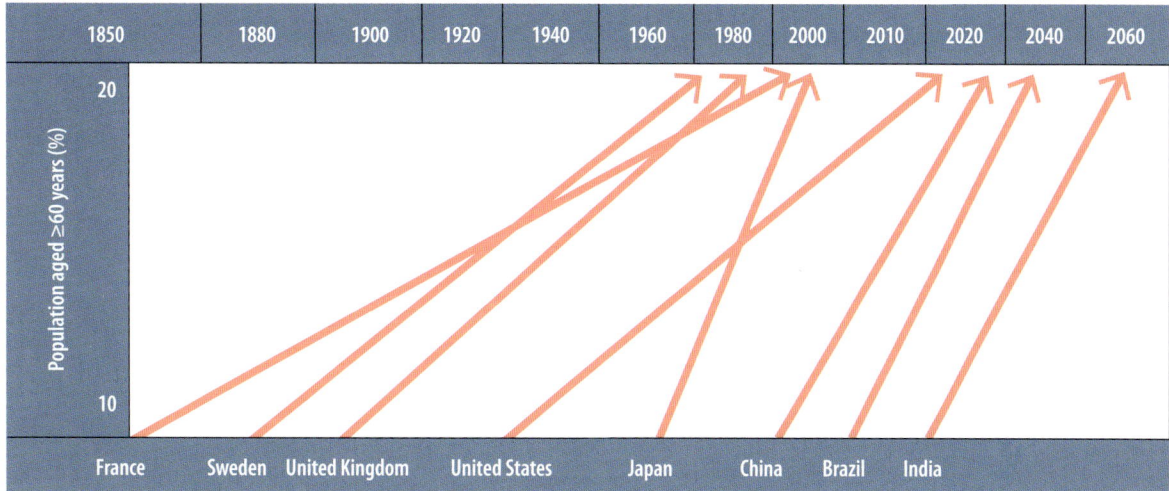

a small part of this global increase is due to the improved survival of people at older ages, most reflects improved survival at younger ages. This has accompanied the historically unprecedented socioeconomic development that has taken place globally during the past 50 years.

Fig. 3.4 and Fig. 3.5 show how strongly a country's level of socioeconomic development is associated with mortality patterns across the life course. The graphs on the right-hand side of Fig. 3.4 and Fig. 3.5 show the ages at which deaths occur in low-, middle- and high-income countries. Note that high-income countries that are members of the Organisation for Economic Co-operation and Development (OECD) are displayed separately from other high-income countries because their epidemiology is quite distinct. In lower-resource settings, death occurs most commonly in early childhood. Deaths are then evenly spread across the rest of life. As countries develop, better public health means that more people survive childhood, and the pattern of deaths changes to one in which people are more likely to die as adults. In high-income settings, the pattern of death shifts even more to old age, so that most deaths occur in people older than 70 years.

Crucially, these changes are accompanied by a change in the things that people die from (shown on the left-hand side of Fig. 3.4 and Fig. 3.5). In all settings, the dominant causes of death in older age are noncommunicable diseases, although deaths from these causes tend to occur earlier in low- and middle-income countries than in high-income countries. However, in both low- and middle-income settings, communicable diseases remain significant killers across the life course.

These shifts mean that as countries develop economically, more people live into adulthood and so life expectancy at birth increases. The majority of the increases in life expectancy seen around the world during the past 100 years (Fig. 3.6) reflect this reduced mortality at younger ages rather than older people living longer.

More recently, another trend has contributed significantly to increasing life expectancy, particularly in high-income settings: increasing survival in older age (3) (Fig. 3.7). Thus, in 1985 a 60-year-old woman in Japan could expect to live another 23 years. By 2015, this had increased to almost 30 years. This increase may reflect a mixture of better health care, public-health initia-

Fig. 3.4. Deaths among females at different ages in low-, middle- and high-income countries, 2012

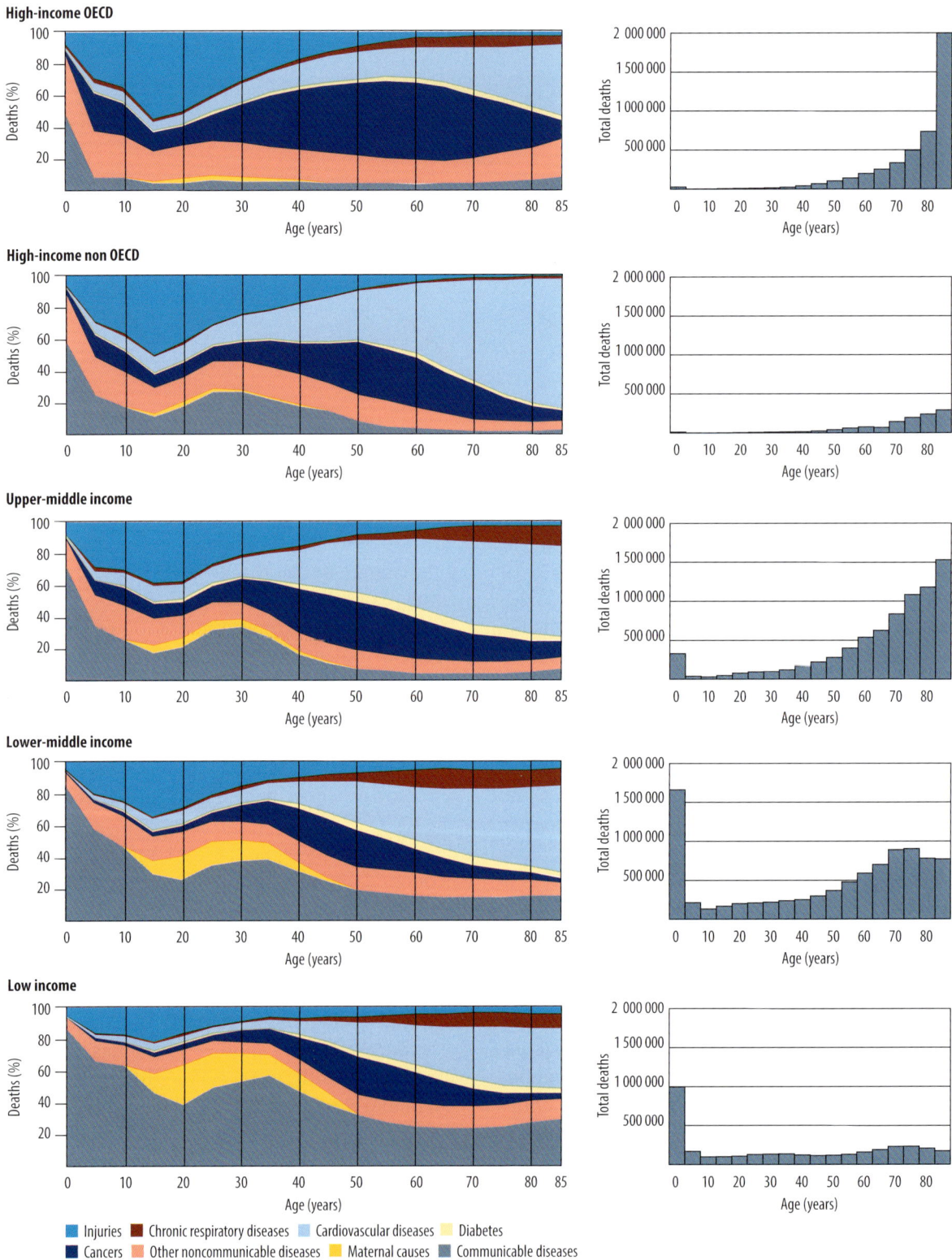

High-income OECD

High-income non OECD

Upper-middle income

Lower-middle income

Low income

Legend:
- Injuries
- Chronic respiratory diseases
- Cardiovascular diseases
- Diabetes
- Cancers
- Other noncommunicable diseases
- Maternal causes
- Communicable diseases

OECD: Organisation for Economic Co-operation and Development. *Source*: (*2*).

Fig. 3.5. **Deaths among males at different ages in low-, middle- and high-income countries, 2012**

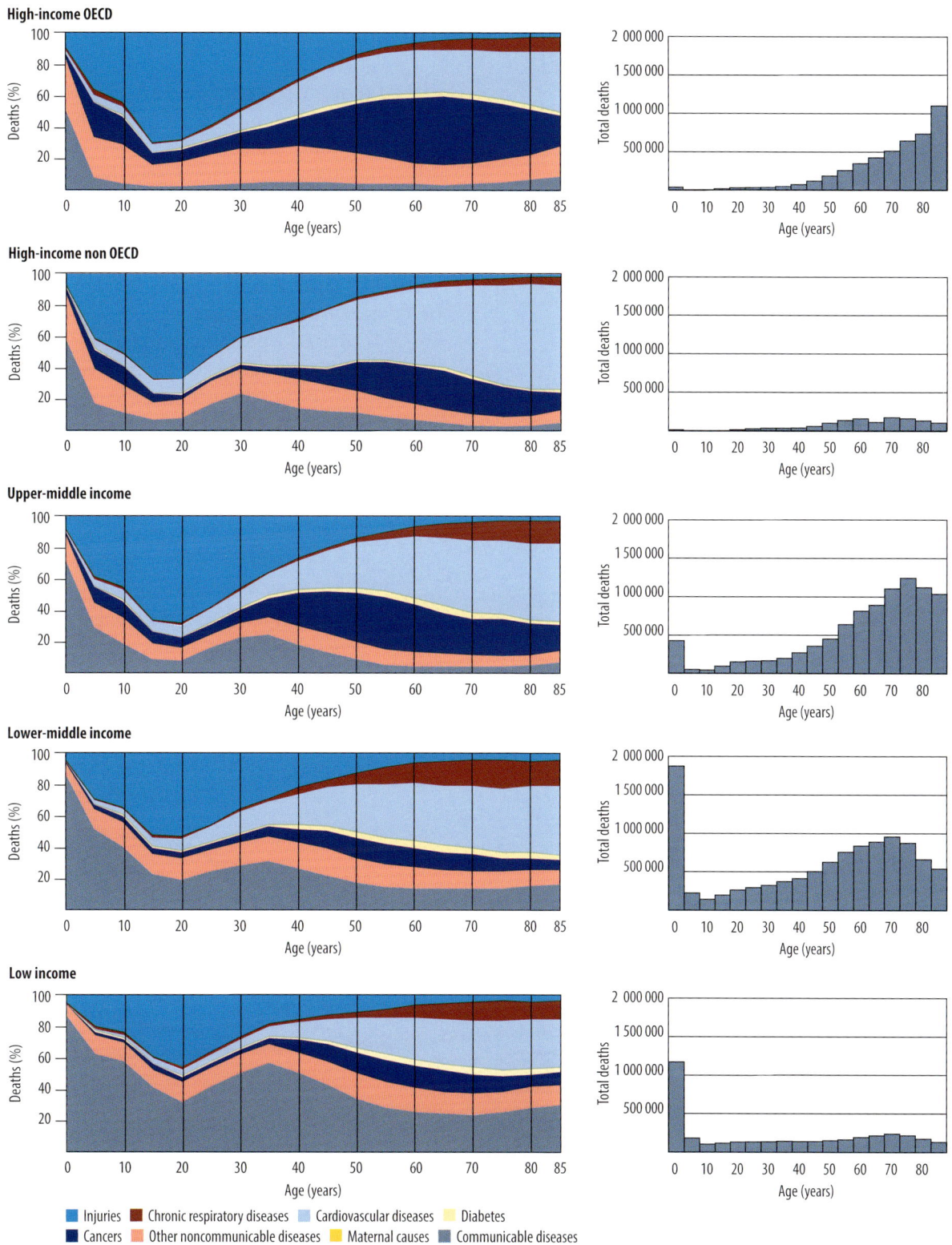

OECD: Organisation for Economic Co-operation and Development. *Source*: (*2*).

Fig. 3.6. Changes in life expectancy from 1950, with projections until 2050, by WHO Region and worldwide

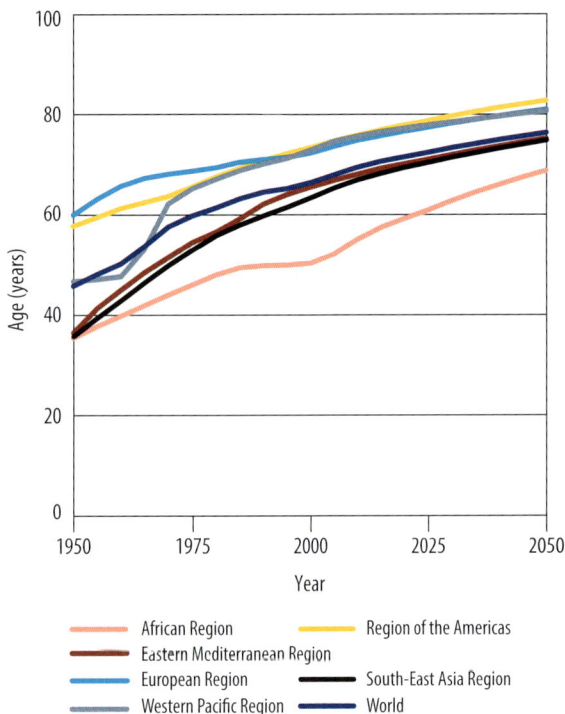

tives and the differences in the lives that people lived earlier during their life course.

However, the rate of these increases varies across the world. Life expectancy in older age is increasing at a much faster rate in high-income countries than in lower-resource settings, although this varies among specific countries and between males and females.

The second reason populations are ageing is because of falling fertility rates (Fig. 3.8). This is likely to have resulted from parents realizing their children are now more likely to survive than was the case in the past, increased access to contraception and changing gender norms. Prior to recent advances in socioeconomic development, fertility rates in many parts of the world ranged from 5 to 7 births per woman (although many of these children did not survive into adulthood). In 2015, these rates have plummeted towards, or dropped below, the level needed to maintain populations at their current size. The key exception to these dramatic falls in fertility rates is in Africa, where a slower fall has been observed and fertility rates generally remain at more than 4 births

Fig. 3.7. Male and female life expectancy at age 60 years, selected countries, 1985–2015

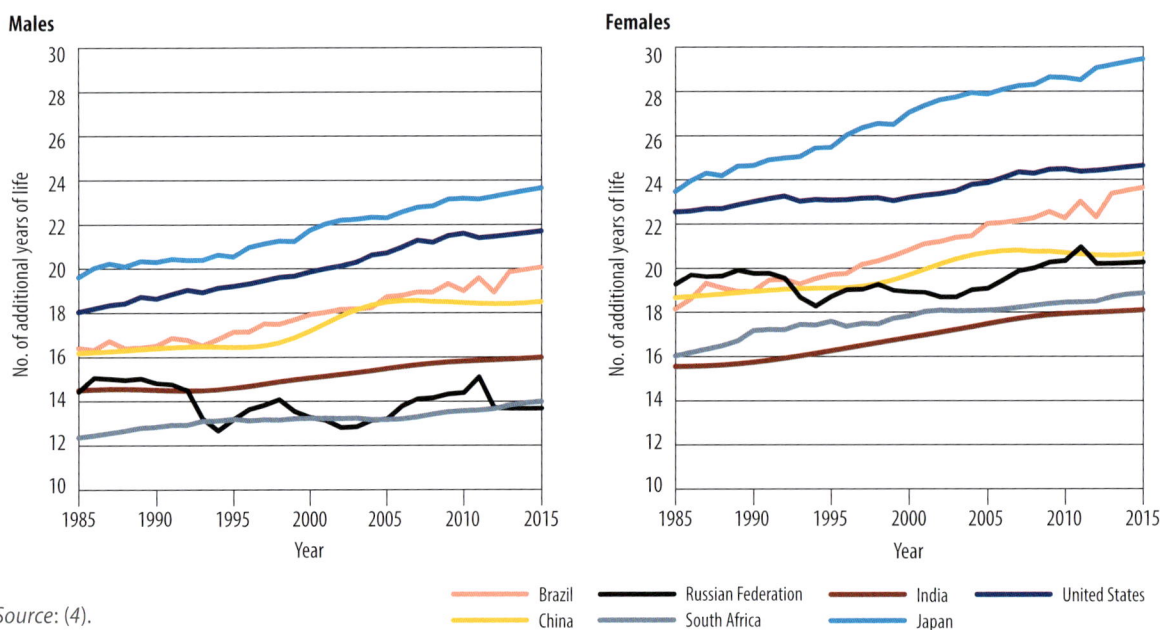

Source: (4).

Fig. 3.8. **Fertility rates in low-, middle- and high-income countries, 1960–2011**

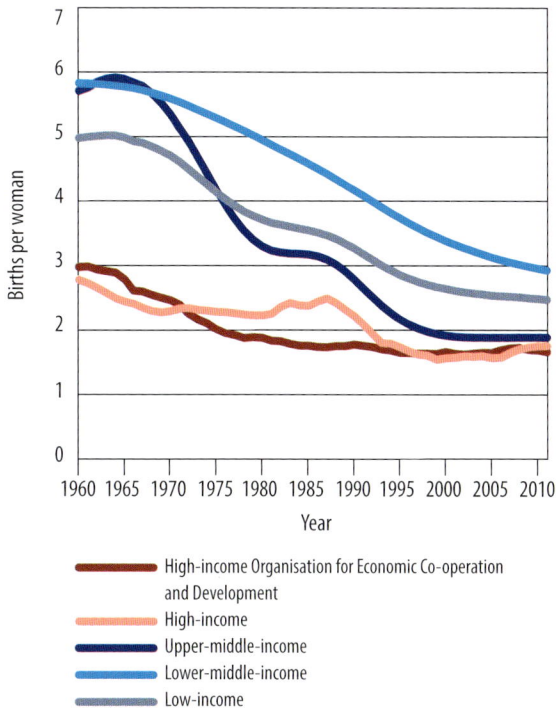

Source: (5).

per woman. The Middle East has also seen slower falls than other parts of the world. Because the fall in fertility has often lagged behind falls in child mortality, this has frequently resulted in a population bulge in younger ages. In many high-income countries, this bulge occurred shortly after the Second World War and this segment of the population is commonly referred to as baby boomers. As the members of the population bulge move into older ages, population ageing is temporarily accelerated, especially when combined with low adult mortality and continued low fertility.

Are the added years in older age being experienced in good health?

Determining whether people are living longer and healthier lives, or whether the added years of older age are lived mainly in poor health, is cru-

cial for policy development. If the added years are lived in good health, population ageing will be associated with a similarly growing human resource that might be expected to contribute to society in many ways (for example, through a longer working life). This can be summed up in the saying "70 is the new 60". However, if people are living longer but experiencing limitations in capacity at similar or higher levels to their parents at the same ages, this means demands for health care and social care will be significantly greater, and older people will be more limited in the social contributions they can make.

Understanding which of these scenarios is underway is crucial for prioritizing areas for policy action and for ensuring that any policy response is fair. For example, if everyone is living a longer and healthier life, one way of ensuring the fiscal sustainability of social-protection systems might be to increase the age at which someone is able to access a benefit such as a pension. However, if the added years are being lived in poor health, this might not be as appropriate because it may require people with significant limitations in intrinsic capacity to remain in the workforce. This may be unrealistic for the individual and less than ideal for the employer. Furthermore, if people of high socioeconomic status are living longer and healthier lives while people of low socioeconomic status are living longer but in poor health, the negative consequences of a generic policy response, such as increasing the pension age, will be shared inequitably.

Unfortunately, although there is strong evidence that older people are living longer, particularly in high-income countries, the quality of life during these extra years is quite unclear (6). This is not simply due to a lack of research in the area. Although there have been few studies in low- and middle-income countries, considerable analyses have been undertaken of data collected during the past 30 years in the United States and other high-income settings. However, the findings from this extensive research pool are inconsistent, with some studies suggesting falling levels

Fig. 3.9. **Prevalence of limitations in instrumental activities of daily living by year of birth, 1916–1958 (after controlling for age and period) (*16*)**

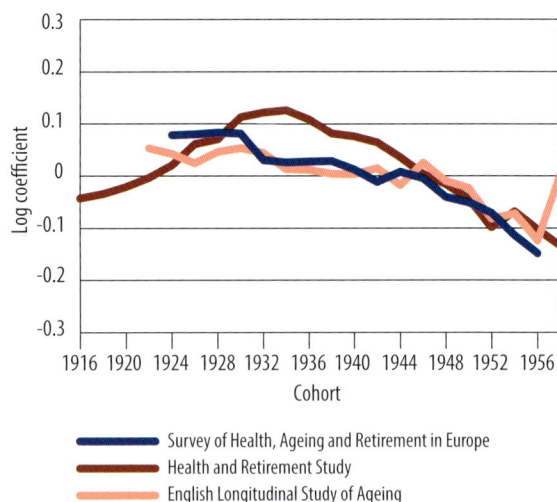

Fig. 3.10. **Prevalence of limitations in activities of daily living by year of birth, 1916–1958 (after controlling for age and period) (*16*)**

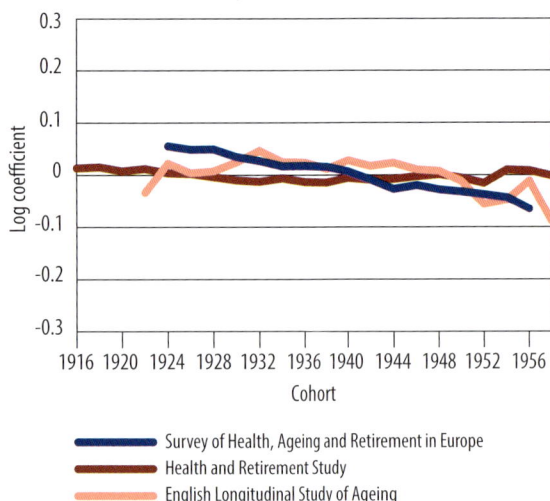

of severe disability in people older than 65 years, other studies in the same age group suggesting rising rates of chronic disease and comorbidity but steady rates of disability, and yet others suggesting an increasing prevalence of disability in 60- to 70-year-olds (*7–10*). One study that linked multiple data collections found increasing quality-adjusted life expectancy, albeit slowed down due to obesity and some decreases in capacity, while another observed that cohort-wide falls in the prevalence of disability reversed after adjustment for characteristics such as race, education, marital status, employment status, income and body mass index (*11, 12*).

These patterns may also vary geographically. Research in Europe suggests that health expectancies differ significantly among countries (*13*). For example, a multicountry assessment of patterns of milder disability in the OECD found that they had decreased in some countries, increased in others and remained the same in the rest (*14*). A pooled analysis by WHO in 2014 of large lon-

gitudinal studies conducted in high-income countries suggested that although the prevalence of severe disability (that is, a disability that requires help from another person to carry out basic activities such as eating and washing) may be declining slightly, no significant change in less severe disability has been observed during the past 30 years (*15*) (Fig. 3.9 and Fig. 3.10). Thus, the current evidence from high-income countries is confusing, but suggests there may be a small reduction in some forms of disability at a given age, although this is unlikely to be keeping up with the added years people are living.

This lack of clarity is exacerbated by several significant research limitations. First, disability is generally accepted to be a state determined by both the underlying characteristics of individuals (that is, intrinsic capacity) and the environments they live in (*17*). Unless researchers consider changes at both these levels, they will be unable to distinguish between them. For example, in the 1950s, individuals with arthritis of the hip may have found their ability to do the things that they needed to do to be compromised because there was a lack of transport options. In 2015, the same people may be able to draw on public transport that is accessible to people with disability and, thus, find that their functional ability is far better, despite the intrinsic capacity being the same. Distinguishing between trends in intrinsic capacity and environmental changes to better measure functional ability thus requires specific questions, yet the instruments commonly used generally do not make this distinction.

Furthermore, most of the data identify disability only at the severe end of the spectrum, which commonly occurs during the last years of life. Declines in intrinsic capacity generally start much earlier and are often initially very small. Although most older people are experiencing these more minor and subtle changes, information on trends in capacity during this phase of life is extremely limited.

Moreover, in high-income countries, most studies have drawn only on relatively recent data, which are largely limited to a period when the epidemiological transition outlined in Fig. 3.4 and Fig. 3.5 had already taken place. Increases in life expectancy in these settings are now largely due to increasing survival in older age, and this may be the result of prolonging the end-stage of life through medical treatments rather than of the broader public-health advances that are likely to have driven earlier epidemiological changes. These results may provide a fair comparison between our health and that of our parents, but it is possible that the trend between our parents and their parents was different entirely. One study that does capture trends during this earlier period is consistent with the health of older people being significantly better than that of their grandparents and great-grandparents (*18*). This found lower age-specific prevalence rates of specific chronic diseases in United States army recruits across the 20th century when compared with those recruited during the Civil War (*18*).

Finally, older populations are characterized by great diversity. Trends within different subclasses in each population may be quite distinct. In the United States, for example, the life expectancy of poorly educated African-American adults may have changed little since the 1950s (*19, 20*).

While the evidence from high-income countries is confusing, data from low- and middle-income countries are largely absent. One exception is China, where a comparison of large representative surveys conducted in 1987 and 2006 found significant increases in both physical and mental limitations during the past two decades, but significant decreases in limitations in vision, hearing, speech and intellect (*21*).

Low- and middle-income countries are currently experiencing the epidemiological transition shown in Fig. 3.4 and Fig. 3.5. Countries such as China are nearing the end of this transition, and the changing age-standardized disability rates described by this study reflect this, with falls in disability related to infectious diseases and marked increases in disability related to cerebrovascular disease and arthritis (which were included in the category of physical disabilities) (*21*). Population diversity is also obvious in these findings, with falls in disability largely observed in urban areas.

Low- and middle-income countries that are earlier in this transition continue to experience a double burden of disease, with high rates of both communicable and noncommunicable diseases, and many people in these countries face far higher exposures to environmental and occupational toxins, and stressors than people in high-income settings. It is possible that this combination of diseases and environmental stressors may impact in unpredictable ways on subsequent morbidity in older adults. Impacts could occur, for example, if these exposures enhanced "inflammageing", which has been suggested as a possible driver of cardiovascular disease (*22, 23*). Therefore, it is not appropriate to simply extrapolate morbidity trends observed in higher-income countries to lower-income settings.

Health characteristics in older age

The remainder of this chapter explores in more detail some of the health-related characteristics of the second half of life and the impact they ultimately have on intrinsic capacity and functional ability. Given the complexity of these changes, the discussion does not attempt to summarize every condition and trend, but highlights key issues that can provide a frame for understanding health trends in older age.

Underlying changes

As described in Chapter 1, at a biological level, ageing is characterized by a gradual, lifelong accumulation of molecular and cellular damage that results in a progressive, generalized impairment in many body functions, an increased vulnerability to environmental challenges and a growing risk of disease and death (24). This is accompanied by a broad range of psychosocial changes.

We summarize below some of the underlying changes that tend to occur to some degree in all humans as they age. Although there is marked diversity in how these changes are experienced at an individual level, general trends are seen when the population as a whole is considered (25). However, these losses in intrinsic capacity can be compensated for by adaptation, and are often accompanied by gains in experience and knowledge. This might explain why workplace productivity does not seem to fall with age (Box 3.1).

Moreover, it is difficult to disentangle the impact on functioning of these underlying trends

Box 3.1. Ageing and productivity

The effects of underlying age-related changes in intrinsic capacity on productivity in the workplace have only just begun to be studied. One reason why is that productivity is difficult to measure objectively, with ratings by peers and supervisors often representing stereotypical conceptions rather than the actual performance of older workers (26). Second, not all occupations lend themselves to the objective measurement of productivity. Because of this, the small amount of research that has been undertaken is often limited to workplaces that enable objective measurements, such as the number of errors or amount of sales.

Overall, productivity does not seem to fall with age, although it may decrease as time spent in a particular job increases, with routinization leading to falls in motivation, or overuse leading to physical harm (27). Thus, one study found that the number of errors committed by each team on the assembly line in a car factory fell slightly with age after controlling for downward selectivity (that is, early retirement, disability) and upward selectivity (that is, promotion). The authors concluded that "older workers are especially able to grasp difficult situations and then concentrate on vital tasks " (28).

This finding highlights the fact that age-related losses, such as a slowing of the speed of information processing or the loss of the ability to multitask, need not have negative impacts on work productivity because up to a certain point, they can be compensated for by the life and work experiences of older people. Furthermore, some declines in physical capacity may be delayed by occupation. For example, falls in grip strength that are observed at the population level may not be seen in subpopulations that have to use their hands for everyday work, although this difference may reverse in later life. Thus, after the age of 80 years, manual labourers have lower levels of physical strength than white-collar workers (29). This may reflect the accrual of physical damage in these occupations.

Age heterogeneity in work teams may also be a determinant of productivity. An intermediate amount of age diversity has been positively related to productivity, possibly reflecting the fact that age diversity has costs (in terms of communication and social integration) as well as benefits (in terms of having a larger knowledge pool to draw from for solutions). This effect was also moderated by the type of work task prevalent in a company. Companies emphasizing creative work profited from age diversity, whereas companies focusing on routine tasks did worse under conditions of age diversity (30).

from the consequences of the diseases individuals may also face across their life course. Thus, where trends across the life course are shown in this chapter for the general population, for example for grip strength and gait speed, these reflect both underlying trends in musculoskeletal functioning and the additional influences of patterns of activity and nutrition, as well as health conditions.

Movement functions

After a peak in early adulthood, muscle mass tends to decline with increasing age, and this can be associated with declines in strength and musculoskeletal function (*31*). One way of measuring muscle function is to measure hand grip strength, which is a strong predictor of mortality, independent of any disease-related influences (*32, 33*).

Age-related declines in average grip strength in countries included in SAGE and the Survey of Health, Ageing and Retirement in Europe (SHARE) are shown in Fig. 3.11. Women tend to have weaker grip strength than men, and for both sexes strength declines with increasing age. The rate of deterioration of grip strength was similar across most of the countries studied. However, the peak level reached varies markedly, with people in India and Mexico generally having lower strength across all ages and sexes. These differences may reflect a mix of genetics and early-life factors, such as nutrition.

Ageing is also associated with significant changes in bones and joints. With age, bone mass, or density, tends to fall, particularly among postmenopausal women. This can progress to a point where the risk of fracture is significantly increased (a condition known as osteoporosis), which has

Fig. 3.11.   Hand grip strength, males and females aged 50 years and over

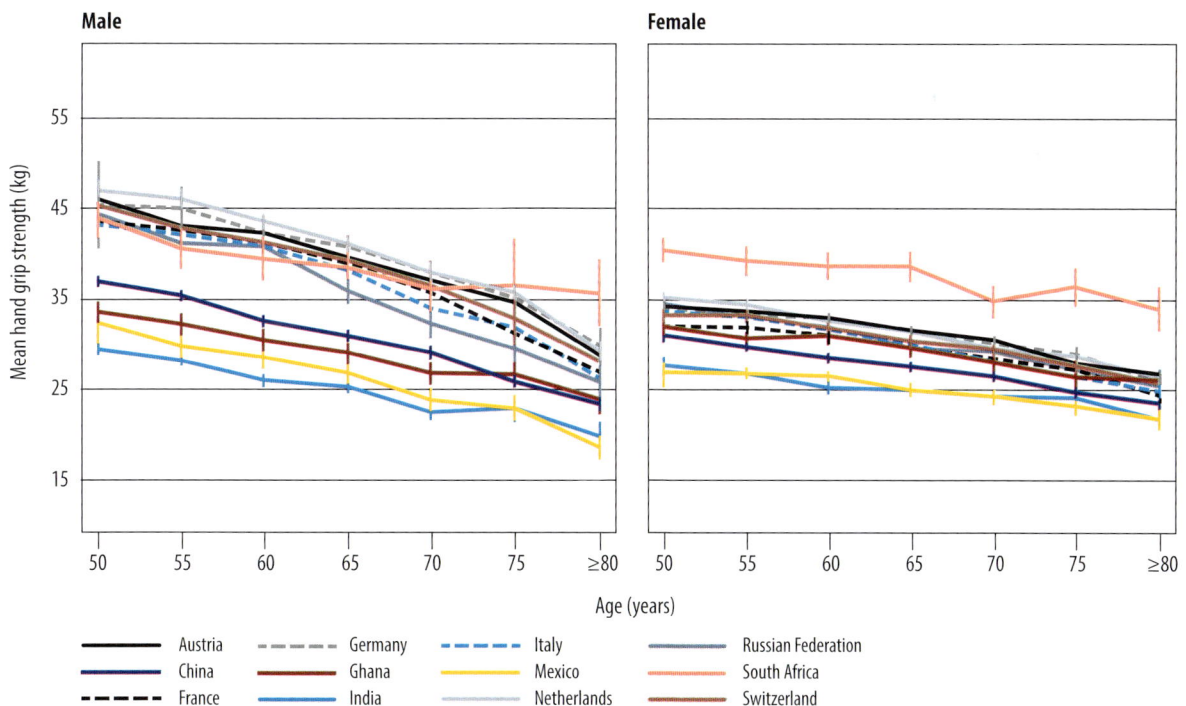

Note: The figure focuses on the fourth wave of SHARE (2010–2011) because the timing of project implementation coincided approximately with the first wave of SAGE (2007–*2010).* Data are not adjusted for height and weight.
Sources: (*16, 34*).

serious implications for disability, reduced quality of life and mortality. Hip fractures are a particularly devastating type of osteoporotic fracture, and as a result of population ageing they will become more common, reaching an estimated annual global incidence of 4.5 million in 2050 (*35*). The median age-standardized rates of fractures related to osteoporosis vary geographically, with the highest observed in North America and Europe, followed by Asia, the Middle East, Oceania, Latin America and Africa (*36*).

Articular cartilage undergoes significant structural, molecular, cellular and mechanical changes with age, increasing the vulnerability of the tissue to degeneration. As cartilage erodes and fluid around the joint decreases, the joint becomes more rigid and fragile (*37*). Although softening of the cartilage commonly occurs with age, this does not universally result in joint pain or the cartilage degeneration responsible for osteoarthritis, although the prevalence of this disorder is strongly associated with age (*38*). Furthermore, regular moderate physical activity has been shown to improve the biomechanical and biological properties of articular cartilage (*37*).

These and other age-related declines ultimately impact on broader musculoskeletal function and movement. This is reflected in a decrease in gait speed – that is, the time someone takes to walk a specified distance. Gait speed is influenced by muscle strength, joint limitations and other factors, such as coordination and proprioception, and has been demonstrated to be one of the most powerful predictors of future outcomes in older age (*39*). Fig. 3.12 demonstrates gait speed at different ages in the six SAGE countries, and shows a general slowing of walking speed with age.

Sensory functions

Ageing is frequently associated with declines in both vision and hearing, although there is marked diversity in how this is experienced at an individual level. Age-related hearing loss (known as presbycusis) is bilateral and most marked

Fig. 3.12. **Gait speed (time needed to walk 4 metres), by age, sex and country**

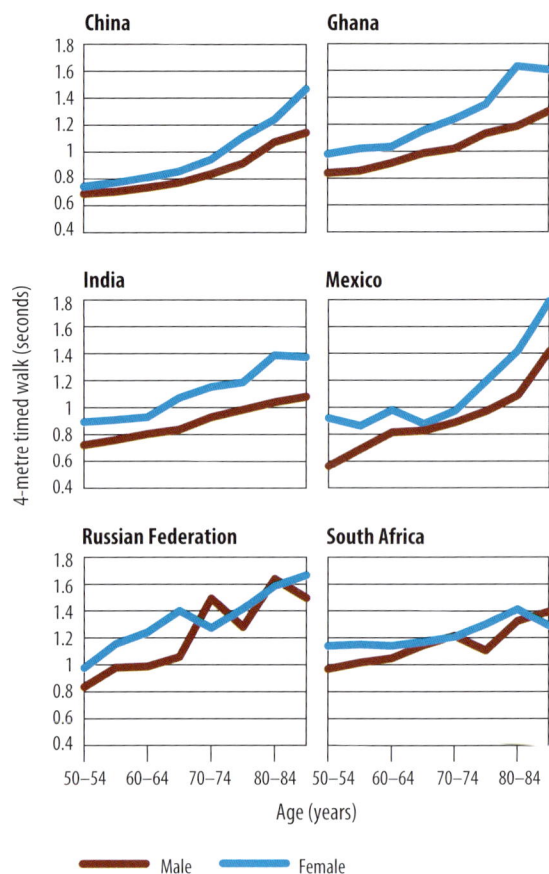

Source: (34).

at higher frequencies. It results from cochlear ageing; environmental exposures, such as noise; genetic predisposition; and increased vulnerability from physiological stressors and modifiable lifestyle behaviours (*40*). Worldwide, more than 180 million people older than 65 years have hearing loss that interferes with understanding normal conversational speech (*41–45*).

Age is also associated with complex functional changes in the eye that result in presbyopia, a decrease in focusing ability that leads to the blurring of near vision, which often becomes apparent in midlife (*46*). Another common change associated with ageing is increasing opacity of the crystalline lens, which can ultimately result in cataract. The age of onset, rate of progression and level of reduced vision vary significantly among individuals, reflecting genetic patterns and environmental exposures (*47*). Ageing is also strongly associated with age-related macular degeneration, which causes retinal damage and leads rapidly to severe visual impairment; it is highly prevalent in people older than 70 years, and a leading cause of blindness in high-income and upper-middle-income countries.

These changes can have important implications for the everyday lives of older adults. Untreated hearing loss affects communication and can contribute to social isolation and loss of autonomy, with associated anxiety, depression and cognitive decline (*48*). The impact of significant hearing loss on an individual's life is often not appreciated by people with normal hearing, and slowness in understanding the spoken word is commonly equated with mental inadequacy, often causing the older individual to withdraw further to avoid being labelled as "slow" or "mentally inadequate" (*49*). Visual impairments can limit mobility, affect interpersonal interactions, trigger depression, become a barrier to accessing information and social media, increase the risk of falls and accidents, and make driving hazardous (*50*). Furthermore, as older people develop strategies to compensate for declining sensory functions, the ways in which they perform other cognitive tasks may also be altered and may be less efficient.

Yet these common limitations in intrinsic capacity can generally be managed effectively. Simple interventions and adaptations for hearing loss include environmental modifications, such as reducing interfering background noise, and behavioural adaptations for the person with hearing loss and for their communication partners (for example, using simple communication techniques, such as speaking clearly). Timely diagnosis and comprehensive eye care and rehabilitation are extremely effective in reducing impairment. Environmental changes such as making improvements in lighting and signage (for example, using high contrast, matte backgrounds placed at eye level) can also help. Assistive technologies, such as listening devices and refractive lenses, are also widely used and effective. These need not be expensive. Even high-quality hearing aids can now be fitted at an affordable cost, and off-the-shelf reading glasses are widely available and generally adequate. Cataracts can best be managed by inexpensive high-quality surgery. Cochlear implants are also effective, but less accessible and affordable.

Cognitive functions

Cognitive functions vary greatly among people and is closely related to years of education. Many cognitive functions begin to decrease at a relatively young age, with different functions decreasing at different rates. As a consequence, functioning becomes increasingly heterogeneous with increasing age (*51*).

Some deterioration in memory and the speed of information processing is common, and complaints about it are frequently reported by older people. However, although ageing is associated with a decrease in the capacity to tackle complex tasks that require dividing or switching attention, it does not appear to reduce the capacity to maintain concentration or to avoid distraction.

Similarly, although ageing is associated with reductions in the capacity to learn and master tasks that involve active manipulation, reorganization, integration or anticipation of various memory items, there is little association with memory for factual information, knowledge of words and concepts, memory related to the personal past, and procedural memory (for example, for the skills needed to ride a bicycle) (*52*). Thus, not all cognitive functions deteriorate with age, and language features, such as comprehension, reading and vocabulary, in particular, remain stable throughout life.

The variation from person to person in the decline in cognitive functions with age is influenced by many factors, including socioeconomic status, lifestyle, the presence of chronic disease and the use of medication, suggesting there are opportunities for public-health interventions across the life course. There is also some evidence that normal age-related cognitive decline can be partially compensated for by practical competence and experience acquired through a lifetime (53), and reduced by mental training and physical activity (54).

Crucially, the subtle and heterogeneous changes in cognitive functioning that are observed in healthy older people are quite distinct from the changes associated with dementia.

Sexuality

Although the data on sexual activity in older age are limited, particularly from lower-income countries, population surveys repeatedly show that people often remain sexually active well into advanced old age. For example, in one longitudinal study, 73% of participants aged 57–64 years, 53% aged 65–74, and 26% aged 75–85 were sexually active. In the oldest age group, 23% of sexually active participants reported having sex once a week or more (55).

Sexuality in older age is influenced by numerous physiological changes that occur as part of the ageing process in both men and women, as well as by multiple psychosocial and socioenvironmental factors (56). Because older age is also a period of increased risk of disease, these underlying changes will often be complicated by the need to deal with diseases that may have physical effects on sexual function. These impacts may be either direct (for example, vascular disease resulting in erectile dysfunction) or indirect (for example, the medication required for an unrelated disease may cause decreased libido), or result from the psychosocial consequences of a disease or its treatment (for example, the changes in self-image in women that may occur after a mastectomy). Indeed, the challenges caused by diseases may be more strongly associated with sexual problems than age itself (55).

In line with predominant sociocultural attitudes, the research on sexuality in older age frequently focuses on these vulnerabilities and sexual dysfunctions rather than on positive aspects of sexuality (57). Thus, a recent survey of middle-aged and older people in 29 countries identified the most common dysfunctions among women as a lack of sexual interest (21%), inability to reach orgasm (16%) and lubrication difficulties (16%) (58). Among men, the most common dysfunctions appeared to be difficulty in achieving or maintaining an erection (37%), lack of interest in sex (28%), climaxing too quickly (28%), anxiety about performance (27%) and an inability to climax (20%).

Despite these challenges, or with the assistance of widely available medical treatments, sexuality remains important in older age and takes many forms. Counter to cisgender stereotypes, the limited research that has been undertaken in this area suggests that higher levels of sexual functioning are important for relationship satisfaction both in older women and older men (although this association may operate in both directions), and physical intimacy involving kissing and cuddling may be even more important for older men than for older women (58).

One often overlooked subject is sexual functioning in older people living in a care home or institution (Chapter 4). This is a complex issue touching on both the rights of these older people to express their sexuality and the need to protect vulnerable individuals from predatory behaviour. Particular ethical dilemmas may arise in relation to sexuality and dementia (59). More research and better guidance on how to manage these delicate and complex situations are urgently needed.

Immune function

Immune function, particularly T-cell activity, declines with age (23, 60, 61). These changes mean that the capacity to respond to new infections (and vaccination) falls in later life, a trend known as immunosenescence (62). There is also some evidence that chronic stress (for example, the need to provide care) can reduce the immune response and the effectiveness of vaccines in older people, and an age-related increase in serum levels of inflammatory cytokines, known as inflammageing, has been linked to a broad range of outcomes, including frailty, atherosclerosis and sarcopenia (22, 23, 63–65). Although the precise association of these trends with the broader physiological changes associated with ageing is still open for debate, immune function clearly has an important role and may present opportunities for future interventions. This possibility has been reinforced by research in mice suggesting that the effective clearance of senescent cells, another role of the immune system, may delay many disorders related to ageing (66).

Functions of the skin

Skin suffers progressive decrements with age that result from damage caused by physiological mechanisms, genetic predisposition and external insults, particularly sun exposure (67, 68). Age-related changes at a cellular level can have numerous affects, including a fall in the skin's ability to act as a barrier (69). Furthermore, the loss of collagen and elastin fibres in the dermis can reduce the tensile strength of the skin, and progressive vascular atrophies can leave patients more susceptible to dermatitis, pressure ulcers and skin tears. Combined, these changes may result in older people having an increased susceptibility to many dermatological disorders (70). Moreover, the cumulative effects of environmental insults, particularly exposure to the sun, contribute to a marked increase in the risk of neoplastic disease.

The potential impacts of these changes are not just physical. Many skin conditions can affect individuals' emotional health or lead to changes in the way they are perceived by others; they may also cause withdrawal from social activity, thus preventing full participation in communities and workplaces.

Health conditions in older age

Age increases the risk of many health disorders, and these can have significant impacts on intrinsic capacity beyond the trends described in the section on Underlying changes. However, it would be wrong to think that the presence of a disease in older age means that someone is no longer healthy (71). Many older adults maintain good functional ability and experience high levels of well-being despite the presence of one or more diseases.

Fig. 3.13 draws on data from the Global Burden of Disease project (2) to identify the common causes of years of healthy life lost due to disability in people older than 60 years; the data are presented for countries grouped according to their level of economic development. These data give an indication of both the incidence and severity of different conditions and the length of time an individual will, on average, be affected by them.

Using these data, the greatest burden of disability is estimated to come from sensory impairments (particularly in low- and lower-middle-income countries), back and neck pain, chronic obstructive pulmonary disease (particularly in low- and lower-middle-income countries), depressive disorders (Box 3.2), falls, diabetes, dementia (particularly in high-income countries) (Box 3.3) and osteoarthritis. The higher burden from dementia in high-income settings is likely to at least partly reflect the older average age in these countries and greater awareness and diagnosis of these conditions. The greater burden from sensory impairments in low- and lower-middle-income countries is likely to reflect many things, including greater exposure to noise and sun across the life course. Higher rates of chronic obstructive pulmonary disease in low- and lower-middle-income countries are likely a consequence of greater exposure to indoor and outdoor air pollutants across the life course.

Box 3.2. Depression and anxiety

Affective disorders, such as depression and anxiety, tend to recur throughout life in a vulnerable proportion of the population.

Episodes of affective disorders might be expected to be more prevalent in older age due to the increased risk of adverse life events. Instead depressive disorders appear to be a little less prevalent among older adults than among younger adults but still affect about 2–3% of older people living in the community (72); however, the prevalence among the most frail and vulnerable older adults living in long-term care facilities is considerably higher, at about 10% (73). Furthermore, compared with younger adults, older people more often suffer from substantial depressive symptomatology without meeting the diagnostic criteria for a depressive disorder. This condition is often referred to as subthreshold depression, and affects nearly 1 in 10 older adults (74). Subthreshold depression also has a major impact on the quality of life of older people, and is a major risk factor for a depressive disorder.

The estimated prevalence of anxiety disorders in the older population ranges from 6% to 10%, which is slightly lower than the estimated prevalence of anxiety disorders in younger adults but still represents a significant cause of disability (75). The prevalence of anxiety disorders in long-term care facilities has been shown to be somewhat lower, and is estimated to be around 5.7% (73). Anxiety disorders and depression often occur together. About 13% of older people with an anxiety disorder also have a depressive disorder, and 36% of older people with depression have a coexisting anxiety disorder (76). Although affective disorders are prevalent in older people, treatment is often effective, including cognitive behavioural therapy (77, 78) and the use of selective serotonin reuptake inhibitors (79).

Mortality patterns also provide an insight into the diseases that are important in older age. Fig 3.14 uses data from the Global Burden of Disease project to show the years of life lost among people older than 60 years with the data presented for countries grouped according to their level of economic development. This is a measure of the disorders that kill older people and the average

potential years of life that they will, on average, be deprived of by these disorders. The greatest burden of mortality in older people all over the world comes from ischaemic heart disease, stroke and chronic obstructive pulmonary disease. The burden from all these conditions is far greater in low- and middle-income countries than in high-income OECD countries. The exceptionally high burden of cardiovascular disease in high-income non-OECD countries is heavily influenced by high rates in the Russian Federation.

Combined, Fig. 3.13 and Fig. 3.14 show that regardless of where people live, the overwhelming disease burden in older age comes from noncommunicable diseases. These are often thought of as diseases of affluence and something that poorer countries will need to give attention to as they develop. What these data show are that for older people, noncommunicable diseases are already causing grossly inequitable burdens in low- and middle-income countries.

Multimorbidity

As people age, they are more likely to experience multimorbidity – that is, the presence of multiple chronic conditions at the same time. This can lead to interactions among conditions; between one condition and the treatment recommendations for another condition; and among the medications prescribed for different conditions. As a result, the impact of multimorbidity on functioning, quality of life and risk of mortality may be significantly greater than the sum of the individual effects that might be expected from these conditions (81). Predictably, multimorbidity is also associated with higher rates of health-care utilization and higher costs (81). Although multimorbidity refers to the presence of two or more chronic conditions, there is no standard definition or consensus on which conditions should be considered. This makes international comparisons of prevalence, or comparisons between or among studies, difficult. Prevalence estimates also vary depending on the identification methods used (for example, self-report versus clinical

Box 3.3. Dementia

In 2015, dementia affected more than 47 million people worldwide. By 2030, it is estimated that more than 75 million people will be living with dementia, and the number is expected to triple by 2050. This is one of the major health challenges for our time. In one Australian study, it was estimated that around 10% of the expected increase in health-care costs during the next 20 years would come from demand for care for this condition alone (*80*).

Contrary to popular belief, dementia is not a natural or inevitable consequence of ageing. It is a condition that impairs the cognitive brain functions of memory, language, perception and thought, and that interferes significantly with the ability to maintain the activities of daily living. The most common types of dementia are Alzheimer's disease and vascular dementia. Evidence suggests that the risks of certain types of dementia may be lowered by reducing risk factors for cardiovascular disease.

The personal, social and economic consequences of dementia are enormous. Dementia leads to increased long-term care costs for governments, communities, families and individuals, and to losses in productivity for economies. The global cost of dementia care in 2010 was estimated to be US$ 604 billion: 1.0% of global gross domestic product. By 2030, the cost of caring for people with dementia worldwide could be US$ 1.2 trillion or more, which could undermine social and economic development throughout the world.

Nearly 60% of people with dementia live in low- and middle-income countries, and this proportion is expected to increase rapidly during the next decade, which may contribute to increasing inequalities among countries and populations. A sustained global effort is thus required to promote action on dementia and address the challenges it poses. No single country, sector or organization can tackle these alone.

The Call for Action by participants in the First WHO Ministerial Conference on Global Action Against Dementia, held in Geneva in March 2015, identified several overarching principles and approaches to guide global efforts. These include making efforts to balance prevention, risk reduction, care and cure so that while efforts are directed towards finding effective treatments, practices and risk-reduction interventions, continual improvements are made in caring for people living with dementia and providing support for their caregivers. The conference noted the incorporation of aspects of dementia prevention, care and rehabilitation in policies related to ageing. The conference emphasized the need to promote a better understanding of dementia and raise public awareness to foster the social inclusion and integration of people living with dementia and their families. In addition, it called for strengthening multisectoral action and partnerships, and increasing collective efforts in research, to accelerate responses to address dementia. As a next step, WHO plans to establish a global dementia observatory to better understand and monitor dementia epidemiology, policy responses, resources across countries, and research efforts to disseminate, advocate for and promote global and national efforts to decrease the burdens associated with dementia. Although this crucial topic will thus be central to any public-health response to population ageing, and care aspects are highlighted in Chapter 5, it is impossible to fully address the needs for improvements in the field of dementia in this report. Further information on dementia can be found in other WHO documents that focus specifically on this topic at http://www.who.int/topics/dementia/en/.

records) and study setting (for example, in the general population or a primary-care setting).

One large systematic review of studies in seven high-income countries concluded that more than half of all older people are affected by multimorbidity, with the prevalence increasing sharply in very old age (*81*). Additional studies in China and Spain yielded similar results, with more than one half of Chinese people aged 70 years or older, and one half to two thirds of Spanish adults older than 65, having two or more chronic conditions (*82, 83*).

In high-income countries, the greatest increases in the prevalence of multimorbidity commonly occur in two periods: between the ages of 50 years and 60 years, and in advanced old age. This can be seen in Fig. 3.15 which shows the prevalence of multimorbidity in different European countries included in SHARE (note that the prevalences are lower than those dis-

Fig. 3.13. **Number of years of healthy life lost due to disability (YLD) per 100 000 population, and top 10 health conditions associated with disability, in populations aged 60 years and older, 2012**

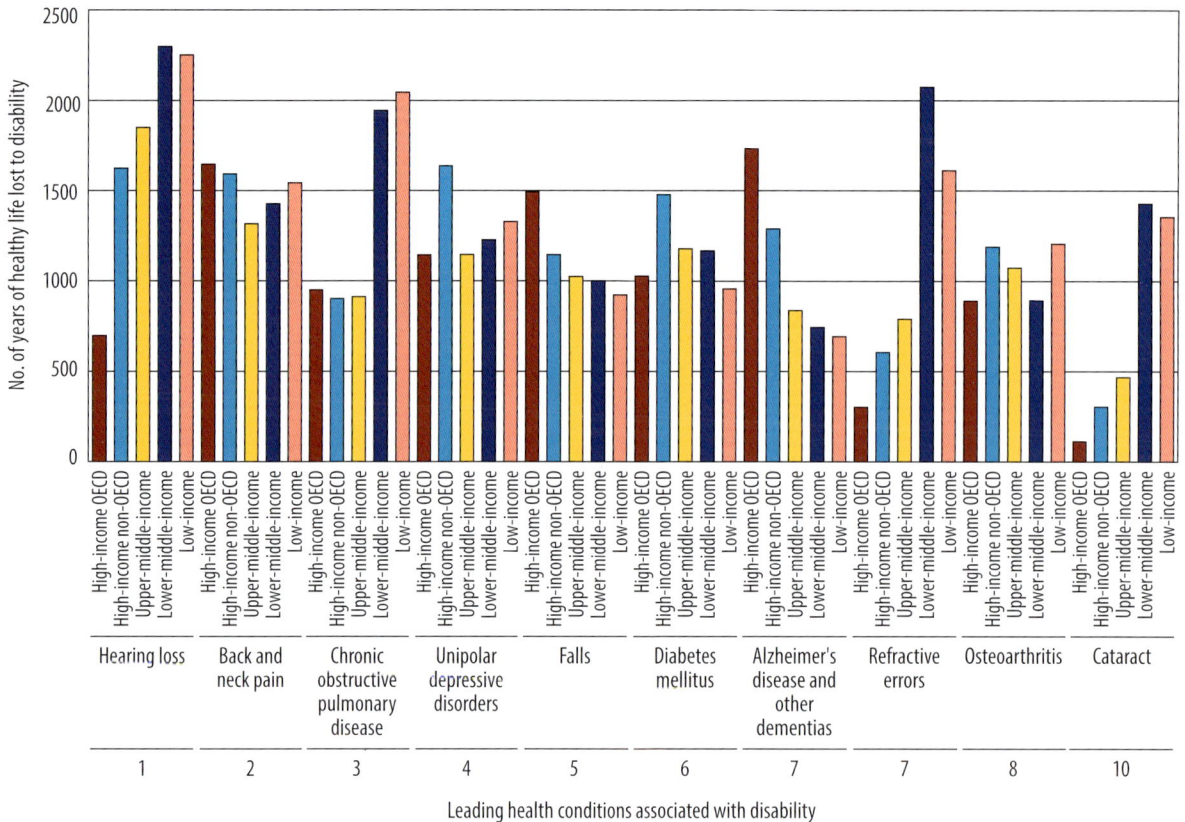

OECD: Organisation for Economic Co-operation and Development.
Source: (*2*).

cussed above due to the exclusion of many conditions, including affective disorders).

However, one large study from Scotland found that the onset of multimorbidity occurred 10–15 years earlier in people living in the most deprived areas compared with the most affluent (*84*). Multimorbidity is also more prevalent in people with low socioeconomic status (*81, 82, 85*). This reinforces the theme repeated throughout this report that good health in older age is closely related to high socioeconomic position. Therefore, ensuring that systems are designed in ways that can equitably meet the needs of older people with comorbidities will be impor-

tant. Although the prevalence of multimorbidity is higher among older women than older men, studies of incidence have found similar rates in both sexes, suggesting that this difference in prevalence reflects a difference in survival rather than risk (*86*). Risk factors that have been identified in the few incidence studies include low socioeconomic status, a higher number of previous diseases, race or ethnicity, and age, although a large-scale historical cohort study in the United States found that a substantial proportion of multimorbidity begins before age 65 years (*81, 86*).

Evidence from low- and middle-income countries is limited. However, given the double

Fig. 3.14.   **Number of years of life lost to mortality (YLL) per 100 000 population for the top 10 causes of lost years, in populations aged 60 years and older, 2012**

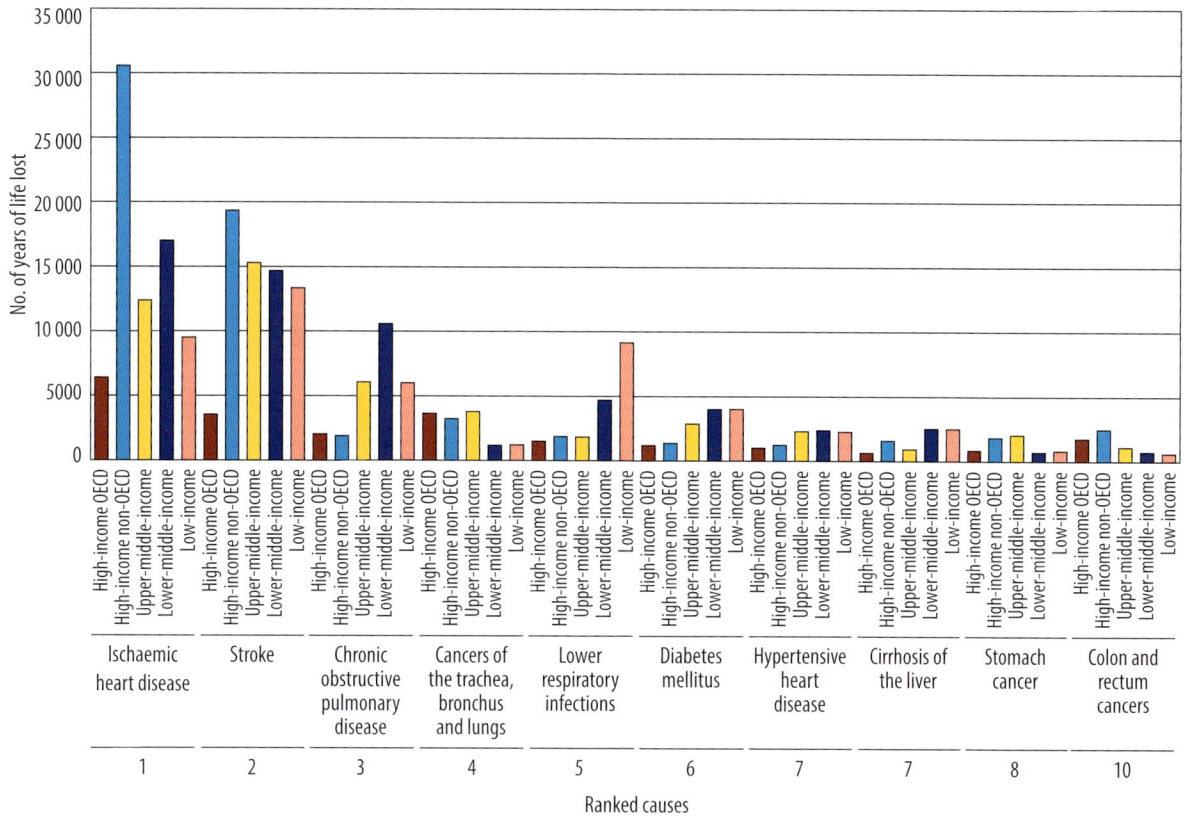

OECD: Organisation for Economic Co-operation and Development.
Source: (2).

burden of communicable and noncommunicable diseases, and the heavier and earlier burden of common disorders described above (Fig. 3.4 and Fig. 3.5), multimorbidity is likely to be even more prevalent. This presents an even greater challenge in these settings, where there may already be difficulties dealing with individual conditions (87).

Furthermore, HIV infection also appears to increase the risk of multimorbidity. As survival improves and HIV infection becomes more of a chronic condition, populations living with HIV are ageing. Research in high-income countries suggests that people with HIV infection may have up to five times the risk of chronic dis-

eases, geriatric syndromes and multimorbidity, even people whose infection is well treated and managed (88, 89). This may be due to immune dysfunction, inflammation, or the cumulative toxicity of treatment, or some combination of these. Countries with a high prevalence of HIV infection may therefore face particularly complex health challenges as their populations age.

Multimorbidity has significant impacts in older age. As the number of chronic conditions increases, so does the risk of declines in capacity (81, 90). However, the impact of multimorbidity on functioning in older age is determined not only by the number of concurrent health conditions but also by the particular diseases involved

Fig. 3.15. **Prevalence of multimorbidity among people aged 50 years and older, 2010–2011**

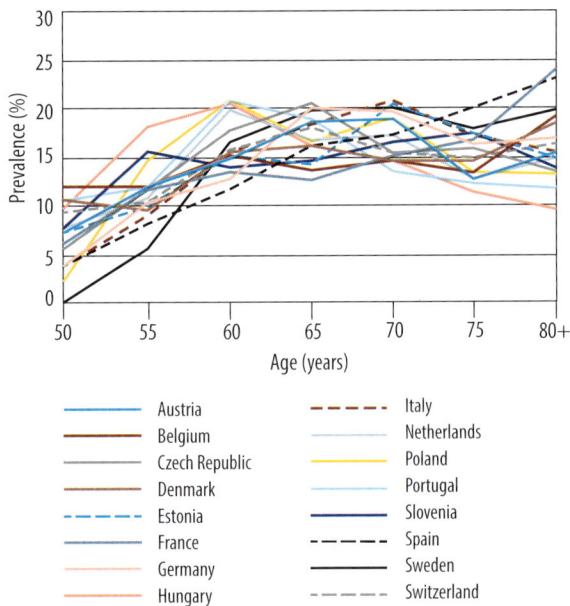

Note: Multimorbidity is generally defined as having two or more chronic morbidities (72). The following health conditions were included in the study: ischaemic heart disease, high blood pressure, stroke, diabetes, chronic obstructive pulmonary disease, asthma, arthritis, osteoporosis, cancer, Parkinson's disease, and Alzheimer's disease and other dementias. *Source*: (16).

health states. Clinical care guidelines typically focus on a single condition, rarely incorporating information on potential comorbidities, and frequently contradicting recommended treatment or lifestyle changes for other conditions (91, 94, 95). One common consequence is polypharmacy, which may be appropriate in terms of the individual conditions being treated, but places the patient at risk of adverse drug interactions and side-effects (94). However, the risk of drug interactions in comorbid and frail older people can limit the use of potentially beneficial pharmacological therapies (96).

Finally, most clinical trials fail to consider the impact of comorbidity, and generally exclude older people entirely, despite their altered physiology (97). This severely limits their usefulness in guiding care and optimizing treatment outcomes in patients at older ages (98). Innovative approaches are therefore needed to identify the best treatments for older people with comorbidities. Until these approaches are in place, improvements in postmarketing research may provide some guidance.

Other complex health issues in older age

Older age is also characterized by the emergence of several complex health states that tend to occur only later in life and that do not fall into discrete disease categories. These are commonly known as geriatric syndromes (99). They are often a consequence of multiple underlying factors and multiple organ systems, and the presenting complaint may not represent the pathological condition underlying it (100). For example, an older person may present with acute cognitive decline or delirium, but this may be a consequence of underlying causes as diverse as an infection or electrolyte disturbance. Similarly, a fall may be a consequence of many underlying characteristics, including drug interactions, environmental factors and muscle weakness.

and how they interact. Furthermore, although the evidence is limited, it appears that comorbidity is not random, and certain conditions tend to occur together (91). This may be at least partly related to the immune changes associated with ageing (92). Some disease combinations have particularly adverse impacts on functioning, with, for example, depression showing a synergistic worsening impact in combination with heart failure, osteoarthritis and cognitive impairment (93).

Despite the large numbers of older people experiencing multimorbidities, most health systems are not equipped to provide the comprehensive care needed to manage these complex

There is still some debate as to which conditions may be considered geriatric syndromes, but they are likely to include frailty, urinary incontinence, falls, delirium and pressure ulcers (99, 101). These appear to be better predictors of survival than the presence or number of specific diseases (102, 103). Yet because of their multisystem nature that crosses many disciplines, they present challenges for traditionally structured health services and are often overlooked in epidemiological research. Innovative approaches to managing these comorbidities and syndromes of older age will need to be central to any societal response to population ageing.

Frailty

The definition of frailty remains contested, but it can be considered as a progressive age-related decline in physiological systems that results in decreased reserves of intrinsic capacity, which confers extreme vulnerability to stressors and increases the risk of a range of adverse health outcomes (104). Frailty, care dependence and comorbidity are distinct but closely related. Thus, one study found comorbidity in 57.7% of cases of frailty and care dependence in 27.2% of cases, with neither being present in 21.5% of frail cases (105).

A large European study estimated the prevalence of frailty at age 50 years to 64 years to be 4.1%, increasing to 17% in those aged 65 and over (106). This same study found the prevalence of being prefrail at these ages was 37.4% and 42.3%, respectively. However, both frailty and prefrailty varied markedly among countries, being more prevalent in southern Europe. These findings are consistent with estimates from Japan and the Republic of Korea, where the prevalence of frailty in both countries has been estimated at around 10% (107, 108). Frailty may be even more prevalent in low-and middle-income countries (109–112). Frailty is more common in women and in people with lower socioeconomic status (113–115).

The course of frailty varies markedly from individual to individual and appears to be reversible, although only a small proportion of frail individuals will return spontaneously to full robustness (116, 117). Because frailty comprises complex decrements occurring in several systems, one key clinical approach is the use of comprehensive geriatric assessments. These assessments, and the person-tailored interventions that derive from them, have been shown to prevent many major negative health-related outcomes, including shortened survival times and care dependence (118, 119). Interventions aimed at increasing physical activity have also been shown to be effective, and may be most effective in more severe cases of frailty (120, 121). Interventions aimed at improving nutrition may also be beneficial, but evidence is limited (122, 123).

Urinary incontinence

Urinary incontinence (that is, the involuntary loss of urine associated with urgency or with effort, physical exertion, sneezing or coughing) is a neglected problem in older people, and a strong predictor of a need for care (124, 125). Urinary incontinence is one of the most common impairments in older age, with the prevalence increasing with age and being much higher in women than men in all age groups (126). In one study conducted in rural China, the prevalence of urinary incontinence was 33.4% among people aged older than 60 years (127). Another population study reported a prevalence among older people with dementia of 19.1% in Latin America, 15.3% in India, and 36.1% in China, and found urinary incontinence to be independently associated with disability (128).

The impact of urinary incontinence can be profound on the quality of life of both older people and caregivers. Urinary incontinence has been associated with depression, care dependence and the self-rated health of older people (129), and it increases the strain and burden on caregivers (130).

Falls

Falls are a major health problem for older adults (*131*). Various reviews and meta-analyses have estimated that 30% of people older than age 65 (*132–141*), and 50% of people older than age 85, who live in the community will fall at least once each year. Falls are even more common in long-term care facilities, occurring annually in more than 50% of people older than age 65 (*136, 141, 142*). Overall, significant injuries occur in 4–15% of falls, and 23–40% of injury-related deaths in older adults are due to falls (*133, 136, 137*). Related injuries can range from minor bruises or lacerations to wrist or hip fractures (*140–142*). Falls are, in fact, the main risk factor for fractures and are even more important than decreased bone mineral density or osteoporosis (80% of low-trauma fractures occur in people who do not have osteoporosis and 95% of hip fractures result from falls) (*136, 143*).

There is an extensive evidence base demonstrating that many falls can be prevented by addressing a wide range of risk factors. These factors include (*132, 134–141, 144–148*):

- individual factors – such as age, gender, ethnicity, poor education and low income;
- health characteristics – such as postural hypotension, chronic conditions, medication use, excessive alcohol use, low levels of physical activity, insufficient sleep, increased body mass index;
- intrinsic capacity – such as declines in physical, emotional and cognitive capacity, and difficulties with vision, balance and mobility;
- environmental – such as inadequate housing (slippery flooring, dim lighting, obstacles and tripping hazards), poor stairway design, uneven streets and footpaths, lack of access to health and social services, improper use of assistive devices, lack of social interaction and community support, inappropriate footwear.

Intrinsic capacity and functional ability

Until this point, this chapter has generally reflected the common epidemiological approaches used to consider health in older age. These focus on causes of mortality and disease, and sometimes the multimorbidities that occur among them. It has also considered underlying physiological trends, as well as geriatric syndromes that are often not classified as disease or disability and so fail to feature in lists of the most significant disorders.

Viewed from the perspective of this increased risk of disease, and considering the major social changes and personal losses often experienced during the second half of life, it might be expected that this is a period of inexorable decline and misery. Yet this is not the case. Multiple studies into trends in subjective well-being across the life course suggest that in many countries overall satisfaction with life actually increases in older age (*149, 150*). There may be a range of explanations for this finding, but it is likely to partly reflect the potential for recovery, adaptation and psychosocial growth in older age.

However, these patterns are not universal, and in some countries older people report worse life satisfaction than younger adults. This highlights the role that environmental characteristics have in enabling people to experience older age in a positive way.

Furthermore, as described in Chapter 2, broad assessments of functioning are far better predictors of positive outcomes in older age than a single disease or even the extent of multimorbidities. This report argues that it is this holistic perspective that provides the appropriate entry point for a public-health response to population ageing.

Healthy Ageing frames this through the concepts of intrinsic capacity and functional ability. The next part of this chapter explores how these might be measured and what the data tell us about how these attributes change across the life course or vary among countries. Unfortunately, data and the methods used to collect this are limited. Disease-based surveillance and research frequently do not collect useful information on functioning, and there are no widely accepted instruments for this purpose, although instruments do exist for measuring specific components of capacity, such as cognitive function or severe limitations in capacity, such as the loss of the ability to perform activities of daily living. The following discussion, therefore, should be viewed as an exploratory exercise in how this significant gap might be filled.

Intrinsic capacity across the life course

The health characteristics and trends described above combine and interact to determine an older person's intrinsic capacity. At present, most information on intrinsic capacity comes from research into the period of life when significant losses in functioning are being experienced, often through the measurement of activities of daily living (ADLs) or instrumental activities of daily living (IADLs). These measures can be useful in identifying the need for social care, and in some longitudinal studies for identifying the predictive value of individual conditions or groups of conditions on functioning more broadly or on future care dependence. The use of ADLs and IADLs fits well with how systems are currently designed. However, these measures are limited to identifying people with serious losses of functioning. Furthermore, they generally assess performance in the real world, which implies some consideration of an older person's environment.

What is missing from this large body of evidence is guidance on the trajectory that may have preceded these significant losses of function or the factors that may have influenced it. As an example of how this trajectory might be constructed, by drawing on data from SAGE we have combined a range of measures, including physical and cognitive assessments and biometric measures, to develop a single vector that summarizes

Fig. 3.16.   Changes in intrinsic capacity across the life course

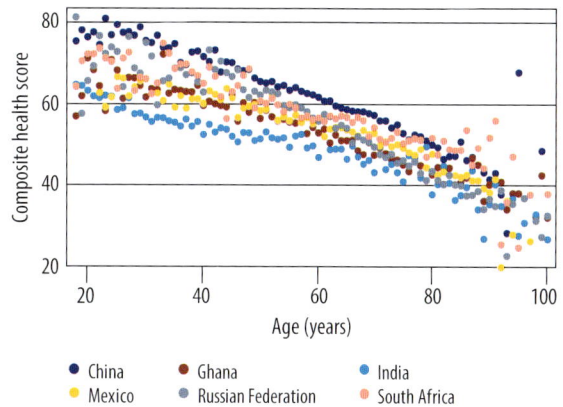

Note: Data on physical and mental capacities were derived from the WHO Study on global AGEing and adult health (SAGE) 2007–2010 (wave 1) (*34*) and then a vector of capacity was developed. Higher scores indicate higher intrinsic capacity.

the key domains of intrinsic capacity (Fig. 3.16) (*34*). What this analysis showed is that for the six countries studied, there was a gradual decline in average capacity that extended across adult life. Of course, for most individuals this decline will not be smooth, but will comprise a range of intermittent setbacks and recoveries. But for the population as a whole, the average decline is gradual: there is no age when most people suddenly have less capacity and become old. Just as importantly, the observed patterns of capacity are different for each country. Measuring these more complex assessments of capacity allows us to ask: why?

Fig. 3.17 shows the mean intrinsic capacity of men and women at different ages in all countries in SAGE. The shading around the means shows the range of capacity across all individuals at these ages. Although there is a distinct trend for intrinsic capacity to decline with age, there are some exceptional individuals aged 80 years or older who maintain intrinsic capacity at significantly higher than the mean level observed in young adults. The figure also highlights the fact that although capacity in early adulthood is, on average, higher, there are some individuals with very low levels. In high-income countries it is likely that there would be significantly fewer of these younger adults with marked limitations in capacity (which thus explains the differences between Fig. 3.17 and Fig. 1.1).

As suggested in Chapter 1, this wide distribution of intrinsic capacity across the life course is not random. Fig. 3.18 uses aggregated SAGE data to explore the relationship between the vector of intrinsic capacity and socioeconomic status. This demonstrates that intrinsic capacity in someone with a low socioeconomic position peaks at a far lower level than it does in someone with a higher socioeconomic position, and this differential is maintained across the life course. This is consistent with the longitudinal data from the Australian Longitudinal Study on Women's Health shown in Fig. 1.19 (*151*).

What explains these patterns? Around 25% of the diversity of intrinsic capacity in older age is explained by genetic factors (*152*). The other 75% of this diversity is largely the result of the cumulative impact of behaviours and exposures

Fig. 3.18. Intrinsic capacity, by wealth quintile and age

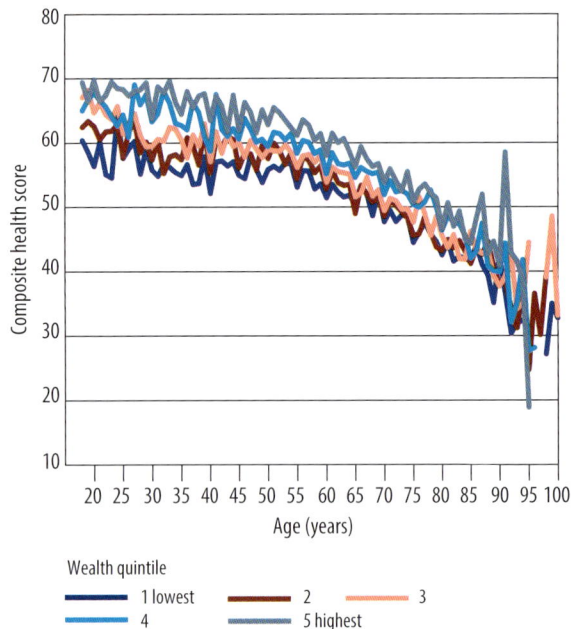

Note: Higher scores indicate better health.
Source: (*34*).

during a person's life course. Many of these experiences are strongly influenced by personal factors, such as the social position into which someone was born (*153*). Fig. 1.1, Fig. 3.17 and Fig. 3.18 thus reflect the powerful impact of these social determinants on functioning in older age.

Patterns of functioning in countries at different levels of socioeconomic development

These analyses are possible because of the broad array of measures included in SAGE. Unfortunately, this comprehensive information is generally not available from population surveillance or even most research studies of older people. For these purposes, simple instruments are required that can be used in large samples and that can distinguish between the intrinsic

Fig. 3.17. Range and mean intrinsic capacity of men and women in all countries in SAGE

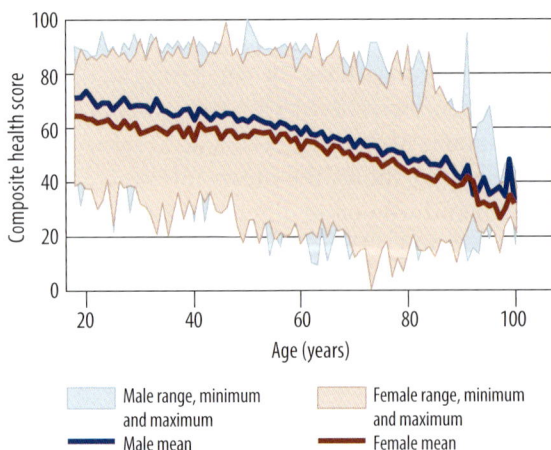

Note: Data on physical and mental capacities were derived from SAGE and a composite health score was calculated. Higher scores indicate better health.
Source: (*34*).

capacity of the individual and the influence of the environment they live in (that is, their functional ability).

Although there are no generally accepted instruments to measure these characteristics, several instruments that have been developed to estimate broad aspects of disability provide a useful starting point for further analyses. In the WHO World Health Survey conducted during 2002–2004, a set of questions across eight domains was used in each country to estimate the health state (Fig. 3.19) (*154*). These measured difficulties engaging in work or household activities, moving around, engaging in vigorous activities, washing or dressing, maintaining general appearance, concentrating or remembering things, learning a new task, maintaining personal relationships or participating in the community and dealing with conflicts. Thus, the health state score can be considered to reflect some aspects of both intrinsic capacity and functional ability. However, unlike the measure used as the basis for the analysis in Fig. 3.16, this instrument relies on self-reported health status and includes no biometric measures.

Fig. 3.19 shows the average scores for these items across the life course and how these vary among high-, middle- and low-income countries. The figure shows that in all but the low-income countries, average functioning remains relatively high until the age of 60 years, when an underlying slow rate of decline accelerates. The higher the level of socioeconomic development, the later this acceleration tends to occur. Individuals in high-income OECD countries tend to reach a slightly higher peak of functioning than those in low- and middle-income countries, and generally maintain this differential. This may reflect better nutrition and more supportive environments in high-income settings during childhood that allow a higher peak of intrinsic capacity to be achieved, while greater exposure to stressors and higher burdens of disease in low- and middle-income countries may result in a more rapid decline with age.

Fig. 3.19.   Health state by age, 2002–2004

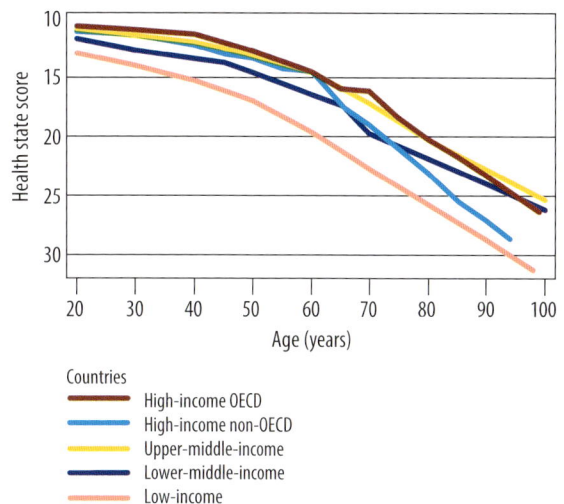

OECD: Organisation for Economic Co-operation and Development.
Note: The variables used in the analysis were difficulties engaging in work or household activities, moving around, engaging in vigorous activities, washing or dressing, maintaining general appearance, concentrating or remembering things, learning a new task, maintaining personal relationships or participating in the community and dealing with conflicts. A higher score implies higher disability.
Source: (*154*).

Fig. 3.19 shows an unexpected late drop for high-income OECD countries compared with upper-middle-income countries. This may reflect the absence of the most developed countries, such as Germany, the United Kingdom and the United States, from this analysis because not all questions were asked in all settings. The more rapid decline in scores for high-income non-OECD countries may reflect particular epidemiological patterns in the Russian Federation.

Significant loss of functional ability, and care dependence

The word dependence is widely used in relation to ageing, although there is neither agreement on what this term actually means nor whether it is a positive or negative state (*155*). Thus, although in economic discussions old-age dependence is generally portrayed as a negative state resulting in the transfer of benefits from younger presumably more productive generations to older ones, others have suggested that the relationship between younger and older generations is better conceptualized as a two-way interdependency (156–158). In many Asian and other cultures this interdependency is viewed as a fundamental social good (159).

This report therefore limits the use of the term dependence to the concept of "care dependence", which arises when functional ability has fallen to a point where an individual is no longer able to undertake the basic tasks that are necessary for daily life without the assistance of others. It is a reflection of decrements in capacity that cannot be compensated for by other aspects of the older person's environments or the use of available assistive devices. The provision of this care increases functional ability to the point where these basic tasks can be achieved. Crucially, autonomy can be maintained despite dependence on care if individuals retain the ability to make decisions on matters that affect them and can direct the execution of these choices.

Care dependence has often been assessed using instruments that determine when an individual requires assistance with ADLs. These measure a range of basic domains of functioning, including urinary and faecal continence, and the ability to independently perform personal care activities (such as tooth brushing), using the toilet, feeding yourself, transferring (for example, moving to a chair), getting around the home, dressing, walking upstairs and bathing. Unfortunately, several variations of these instruments exist (for example, some require simple yes/no responses, others use scaled responses). This needs to be considered when making comparisons among studies or settings.

Fig. 3.20 summarizes information from SHARE and SAGE on the prevalence among older people of needing assistance with at least one of five ADLs (eating, bathing, dressing, getting in and out of bed, using the toilet). The figure

Fig. 3.20. **Percentage of the population aged 65–74 years and aged 75 years or older with a limitation in one or more of five basic activities of daily living (ADL), by country**

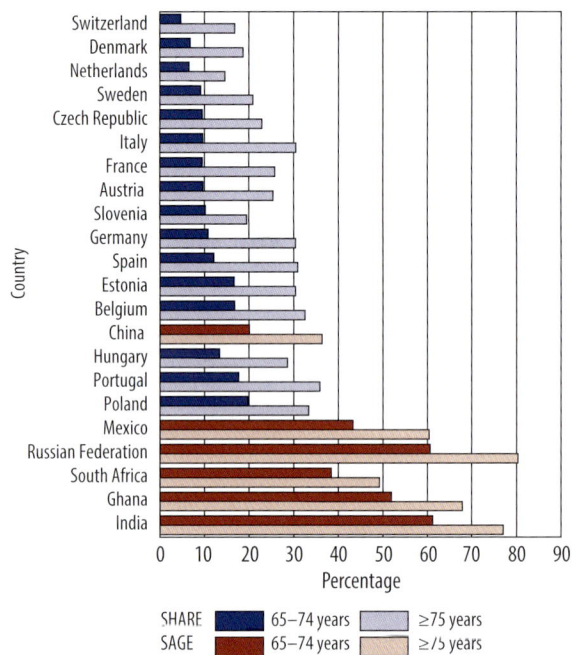

Note: The five basic ADL items included in the analysis were eating, bathing, dressing, getting in and out of bed, and using the toilet.
Sources: (16, 34).

shows there are marked differences among countries in the percentage of people requiring assistance with at least one basic ADL. It also clearly demonstrates the impact of age, with those aged 65 years to 74 years having far less need for assistance than those aged 75 years or older.

The marked difference among countries at the bottom of the list (where a higher percentage of the population has a limitation) and those higher on the list is likely to reflect both the economic situation in different settings as well as differences in the instruments used (the five countries at the bottom of the list are all from SAGE where the threshold for a positive response may have been lower). Furthermore, some of these variations may be due to differing social expectations (and hence reporting) in different cultures and income settings. But it is likely that a significant proportion of these trends reflects genuine underlying differences in intrinsic capacity. This is important for two reasons. First, ADLs are used in many settings as indicators of eligibility for care services and they are likely to reflect a significant need for care. This need for assistance ranges from around 17% of people 75 years and older in Switzerland to well over 40% of people of the same age in Ghana, India, Mexico and the Russian Federation. Many of the countries with the highest need also have the least infrastructure and services in place to address this care dependence and default to relying on families to provide care. How this gap might start to be filled is expanded on in Chapter 4.

But these dramatic variations also raise the question: why? What are the factors that lead to a 65–74-year-old in China being three times less likely to require care than one in India? Why is a 65–74-year-old in Belgium almost twice as likely to require care as someone of a similar age in the neighbouring country of the Netherlands? Assuming some of this variation reflects real differences, identifying the answers can inform how we might develop a better public-health response to delay or avert this need.

Fig. 3.21 summarizes information about IADLs from SHARE (these domains were not considered in SAGE). The same increasing prevalence with age is seen, and the overall prevalence is somewhat higher. These individuals might not be care-dependent, but are at high risk of becoming so. In the approach this report proposes for long-term care, these older people would be potential recipients of interventions to improve their capacity and avoid care dependence.

Because care dependency increases with age, population ageing will dramatically increase the proportion and number of people needing social care in countries at all levels of development. This will occur at the same time as the proportion of people at younger ages who might be available to

Fig. 3.21. **Percentage of the population aged 65–74 years and aged 75 years or older with a limitation in one or more instrumental activities of daily living, by country**

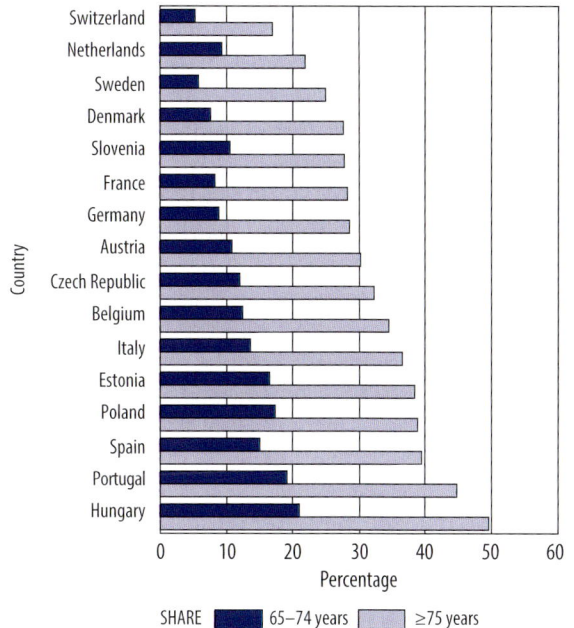

Note: These activities include difficulties using the telephone, taking medications, managing money, shopping for groceries, preparing meals and using a map.
Source: (16).

provide this care will be falling, and the role of women, who have until now been the main care providers, is changing.

Key behaviours that influence *Healthy Ageing*

Because most of the disease burden in older age is due to noncommunicable diseases, risk factors for these conditions are important targets for health promotion. Strategies to reduce the burden of disability and mortality in older age by enabling healthy behaviours and controlling metabolic risk factors can therefore start early in life and should continue across the life course

(*160*). The risks associated with these behaviours and metabolic risk factors continue into older ages, although this relationship may attenuate (*161–163*). Strategies to reduce their impact continue to be effective in older age, particularly for reducing hypertension (*164*), improving nutrition (*160, 165*) and stopping smoking (*166*), although evidence in advanced old age is limited. Furthermore, there is some evidence that reducing exposure to cardiovascular risk factors can also reduce the risk of at least some types of dementia (*167*).

Yet despite this clear evidence of the importance of the need to continue to modify risk factors into older age, surveys of older populations suggest that behaviours that put older people at risk of cardiovascular diseases are widespread (Fig. 3.22) (*168*). The great variation among countries in the prevalence of these unhealthy behaviours suggests that many opportunities exist for intervention.

Moreover, there is growing evidence that key health-related behaviours, such as engaging in physical activity and maintaining adequate nutrition, may exert powerful influences on intrinsic capacity in older age that are quite separate from their action in reducing the risk of noncommunicable diseases. These broader impacts on intrinsic capacity have been less well researched, but may be central to strategies to reverse or delay declines in capacity and even conditions such as frailty. This section explores in more detail the relationship between two of these behaviours and functional ability.

Physical activity

Engaging in physical activity across the life course has many benefits, including increasing longevity. For example, a recent pooled analysis of large longitudinal studies found that people who engaged in 150 minutes per week of physical activity at moderate intensity had a 31% reduction in mortality compared with those who were less active. The benefit was greatest in those older than 60 years (*169*).

Physical activity has multiple other benefits in older age. These include improving physical and mental capacities (for example, by maintaining muscle strength and cognitive function, reducing anxiety and depression, and improving self-esteem); preventing disease and reducing risk (for example, of coronary heart disease, diabetes and stroke); and improving social outcomes (for example, by increasing community involvement, and maintaining social networks and intergenerational links).

Fig. 3.22. **Age-adjusted prevalence of physical inactivity in people aged 60 years and older, by country**

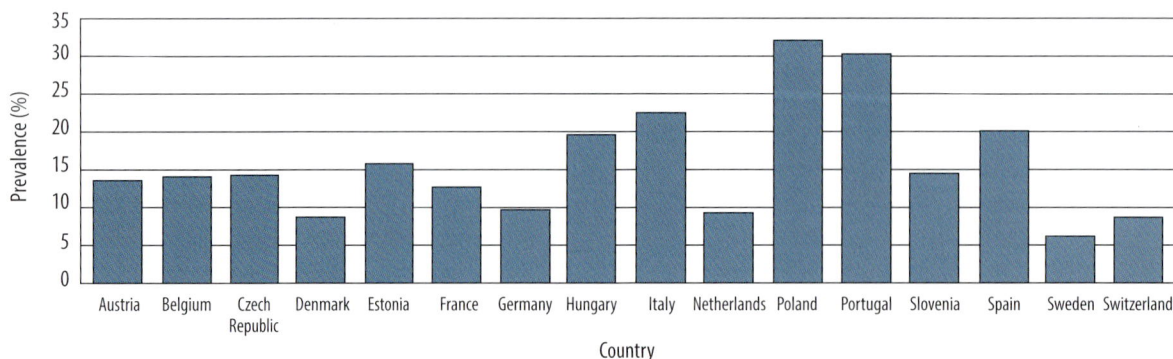

Source: (*16*).

These benefits can be substantial. For example, both cross-sectional and longitudinal studies have suggested there is a 50% reduction in the relative risk of developing functional limitations among those reporting regular and at least moderate-intensity physical activity (170, 171). Randomized controlled trials have shown similar benefits (121, 170), and progressive resistance training may give independent benefits (172). Physical activity also appears to preserve, and may even improve, cognitive function in people without dementia (170, 173), reducing cognitive decline by around one third (174).

In addition, physical activity protects against some of the most important health conditions in older age. Physical inactivity may account for up to 20% of the population-attributable risk of dementia, and it has been estimated that 10 million new cases globally might be avoided each year if older adults met recommendations for physical activity (175). Similarly, stroke causes some of the greatest burden of disease in older age, and moderate physical activity may reduce the risk by 11–15%, and vigorous physical activity has even greater benefits, reducing the risk by 19–22% (176).

Yet despite the clear benefits of physical activity, the proportion of the population meeting recommended levels falls with age, and analyses of data from SAGE and the WHO World Health Survey suggest that around one third of 70–79-year-olds and one half of people aged 80 years or older fail to meet basic WHO guidelines for physical activity in older age (177).

However, since the prevalence of inactivity varies significantly among countries, this suggests that cultural and environmental factors that may be amenable to change are likely to be among the underlying drivers of these patterns. Furthermore, interventions at both a programmatic level and at a broad population level appear to be effective in improving levels of physical activity (178). Interventions to promote muscle strength and endurance have also been shown to be effective (172).

Essentially all domains of fitness – aerobic, strength and neuromotor (balance) – are important for older populations. Yet it is prudent to consider that strength and balance training should precede aerobic exercise, with new evidence showing that progressive resistance training has favourable effects not only on muscular strength, physical capacity and the risk of falls (172) but also that its benefits extend to cardiovascular function, metabolism and coronary risk factors (179) for those without or with cardiovascular disease. However, the benefits of aerobic physical activities, such as walking, which is the main mode of aerobic exercise among older adults, cannot be transferred to improving balance (180), have no effect on preventing falls (181, 182), and no clear benefit in relation to strength. Therefore, it is logical and possibly safer to suggest that older adults whose mobility is compromised start by increasing their strength and improving their balance before embarking on aerobic training.

Nutrition

Ageing is accompanied by physiological changes that can negatively impact nutritional status. Sensory impairments, such as a decreased sense of taste or smell, or both, may result in reduced appetite. Poor oral health and dental problems can lead to difficulty chewing, inflammation of the gums and a monotonous diet that is poor in quality, all of which increase the risk of malnutrition (183) (Box 3.4). Gastric acid secretion may be impaired, leading to reduced absorption of iron and vitamin B12. The progressive loss of vision and hearing, as well as osteoarthritis, may limit mobility and affect elderly people's ability to shop for food and prepare meals. Along with these physiological changes, ageing may also be associated with profound psychosocial and environmental changes, such as isolation, loneliness, depression and inadequate finances, which may also have significant impacts on diet.

Box 3.4. Oral health in older people

One crucial and often neglected area of *Healthy Ageing* is oral health. This is particularly important in relation to disadvantaged older people, regardless of whether they live in developing or developed countries. Poor oral health can have a profound bearing on general health and well-being, for example, through its influence on nutrition. Moreover, the experience of pain, and problems with eating, chewing, smiling and communicating due to missing, discoloured or damaged teeth have a major impact on functional ability and older people's daily lives.

Poor oral health among older people is reflected in high levels of dental caries (or tooth decay), a high prevalence of periodontal disease (or gum disease), tooth loss, dry mouth and oral precancer or cancer. Avoiding tooth loss is crucial for *Healthy Ageing*. Yet the complete loss of natural teeth is highly prevalent among older people all over the world, with severe dental caries and advanced periodontal disease being the major causes. Furthermore, although tooth loss is declining in many high-income countries, and older people are increasingly preserving their teeth in a functional condition, tooth loss may be increasing in low- and middle-income countries. This is reflected in the prevalence of reported problems with the mouth and teeth among older people ranging from 42% in low-income countries to 29% in high-income countries (*184*).

The major chronic diseases and oral diseases have risk factors in common. Unhealthy diets rich in sugars are a cause of dental caries and in addition to poor oral hygiene, periodontal disease is related to tobacco use, excessive consumption of alcohol, obesity and diabetes. The use of tobacco or alcohol, or both, are the key risk factors for oral cancer. Therefore, the prevention of chronic and oral diseases can be strengthened by integrating oral health into general health-promotion activities. As for other determinants of intrinsic capacity, disadvantaged older people have an increased risk of oral diseases, and they are largely underserved in terms of dental care.

Combined, these trends increase the risk of malnutrition in older age because although energy needs decrease with age, the need for most nutrients remains relatively unchanged. Malnutrition in older age interacts with the underlying age-related changes described above, often taking the form of reduced muscle and bone mass, and increases the risk of frailty. Malnutrition has also been associated with diminished cognitive function, a diminished ability to care for oneself, and a higher risk of becoming care-dependent.

However, malnutrition in older age often goes undiagnosed, and thorough assessments of the global prevalence of the different forms of malnutrition are limited. The evidence suggests that worldwide a sizeable proportion of older people may be affected by malnutrition.

A thorough nutritional assessment of older people requires performing anthropometric measurements, clinical biochemistry and dietary assessment. One study from the United Kingdom using these comprehensive approaches showed that the risk of protein–energy malnutrition was between 11% and 19%, and found that it was accompanied by deficiencies of vitamins C and D, and low levels of carotenoids (*185*). In a study from the Philippines conducted among older people living in the community, energy intake was approximately 65% of the amount required based on total energy expenditure (*186*). A study from rural Malaysia identified problems related to both undernutrition and overnutrition, as well as low levels of thiamin, riboflavin and calcium (*187*). Furthermore, higher levels of malnutrition (15–60%) have been documented in many countries in older patients who are hospitalized, live in nursing homes or are in home-care programmes (*188–191*).

A questionnaire-based approach has been used in several studies to provide a simple assessment of older patients in outpatient clinics, hospitals and nursing homes (*192*). A study among older people living in rural areas of South India used this approach and found that more than 60% of the participants had low protein–energy intakes (*192*). A study from the Islamic Republic of Iran revealed a 12% prevalence of malnutrition among older people, with higher prevalence in lower socioeconomic groups (*193*).

As with other aspects of geriatric care, the management of malnutrition in older age needs to be multidimensional. Various types of interventions are effective in reversing these patterns of malnutrition, and have been shown to delay care dependency, improve intrinsic capacity and revert frail states (123). The nutrient density of food should be improved, particularly that of vitamins and minerals, but energy and protein intake are important targets. Individualized nutritional counselling has been shown to improve the nutritional status of older people within 12 weeks (194).

Key environmental risks

Emergency situations

Functional ability is determined by the intrinsic capacity of the individual, the relevant characteristics of their environment and the interaction between them. The influence of the environment may be particularly strong in the event of natural or technological disasters and human-induced conflict. Yet although responses to these events typically prioritize assistance to vulnerable or marginalized groups, the needs of older adults are frequently overlooked. This occurs despite a significantly elevated risk of death, injury, illness and loss of function among older people that may extend long after the event itself (195, 196).

This increased risk is reflected in data from five major natural disasters that show more than half of the deaths associated with these events occurred among people aged 60 years and older. For example, despite comprising only 23% of the general population, 56% of those who lost their lives during the 2011 Great East Japan earthquake were aged 65 and older (197). Furthermore, many of these deaths may have occurred after the event itself, reflecting failings in the emergency response.

The vulnerability of older people in emergency situations derives partly from the diminished intrinsic capacity generally associated with ageing and partly from a greater reliance on environmental characteristics to maintain functional ability. As a consequence, mild deficits in intrinsic capacity that had been compensated for in various ways in an older person's normal environment quickly become a major burden.

At a physiological level, older adults may be more susceptible to dehydration, hypothermia and hyperthermia. Limitations in intrinsic capacity may be exacerbated by malnutrition or interrupted health care. Given the high prevalence of chronic disease and multimorbidity in older adults, interruptions in health care and access to essential medicines can have severe and life-threatening consequences. Yet chronic disease management is not typically part of the health response to humanitarian emergencies.

Furthermore, older people may be more susceptible to injuries and to communicable diseases, both of which are common risks in emergency situations. Mobility impairments may restrict the ability of older people to evacuate or to gain access to water, food, essential medicines and health services after a disaster. Sensory impairments may limit their ability to gain access to services or be aware of services that may be available, and many may have lost essential assistive devices, such as glasses or hearing aids, during the event.

One reason for the failure to prioritize the needs of older people during emergency situations may be that older people are often not visible due to mobility limitations and social isolation. For their needs to be identified and addressed, those responsible for emergency response must actively search for older people, and not assume that they will be cared for by family. More fundamentally, all data collected in emergency situations should be disaggregated by age and sex. However, it is wrong to assume that all older people are vulnerable or helpless. During times of disaster, many provide invaluable support to their families and communities. Indeed, many of those who volunteered during the response to the 2011 earthquake in Japan were older people.

Chapter 6 explores how the vulnerability of older people can be reduced and how responses in emergency situations can be better designed to meet the needs of older people.

Elder abuse

Older adults frequently find themselves mistreated in various ways by people they trust, with significant, lasting consequences. This is elder abuse: "a single or repeated act, or lack of appropriate action, occurring within any relationship where there is an expectation of trust, which causes harm or distress to an older person" (198).

Elder abuse takes many forms including physical, sexual, psychological, emotional, financial and material abuse, abandonment, neglect and serious losses of dignity and respect. It occurs both within and outside a caregiving context – for example, between two spouses with high functional ability, or at the hands of an adult child who depends on the older person for housing or financial security (199). But it is distinct from interpersonal violence that is unrelated to close relationships, such as violent crime occurring in the community.

Elder abuse has severe physical consequences, including pain, injury and even death; psychological effects, such as stress and depression; and it increases the risk of nursing home placement and hospitalization (200–204). These impacts may be particularly significant in older people who have reduced intrinsic capacity and less resilience to cope with the physical and psychological injuries that may result from abuse. Although rigorous data are limited, particularly from institutional contexts, a background review commissioned for this report found that the prevalence of elder abuse in high- or middle-income countries ranged from 2.2% to 14% (205). According to the analysis, the most common types included:

- physical abuse (prevalence, 0.2–4.9%);
- sexual abuse (prevalence, 0.04–0.82%);
- psychological abuse, above a threshold for frequency or severity (prevalence, 0.7–6.3%);
- financial abuse (prevalence, 1.0–9.2%);
- neglect (prevalence, 0.2–5.5%).

Table 3.1. **Risk factors for elder abuse and strength of evidence for the risk factor**

Level	Risk factors	Strength of evidence
Individual (victim)	Gender: female	Low–moderate
	Age: older than 74 years	Low–moderate
	Dependence: significant disability	Strong
	Poor physical health	Strong
	Mental disorders: depression	Strong
	Low income or socioeconomic status	Strong
	Financial dependence	Low–moderate
	Race	Low–moderate
	Cognitive impairment	Strong
	Social isolation	Strong
Individual (perpetrator)	Mental disorders: depression	Strong
	Substance abuse: alcohol and drug misuse	Strong
	Dependence on the abused: financial, emotional, relational	Strong
Relationship	Victim–perpetrator relationship	Low–moderate
	Living arrangement: victim lives alone with perpetrator	Strong
	Marital status	Low–moderate
Community	Geographical location: socially isolated	Low–moderate
Societal	Negative stereotypes about ageing	Insufficient data
	Cultural norms	Insufficient data

Crucially, these rates exclude both older adults with cognitive impairments and those living in nursing homes or long-term care facilities. Yet these groups may be at particular risk of abuse. For example, one review found that psychological abuse of older adults with dementia ranged from 28% to 62%, and physical abuse affected 3.5% to 23% of older adults with dementia (*203*).

Victims of elder abuse are more likely to be female and to have a physical disability; be care-dependent; have poor physical or mental health, or both; have a low income; and lack social support (*205*, *206*). The quality of close relationships and shared living arrangements also appear to affect risk. Family members who abuse older people are more likely to have mental health issues, (for example, personality disorders) and substance abuse disorders, than family members or caregivers who do not abuse. Abusers are themselves often dependent on the abused person (*199*, *206*). Table 3.1 summarizes the strength of the evidence for risk factors for elder abuse at the level of the older person, the perpetrator, the type of relationship between them, and community or societal factors. Although a public-health response to elder abuse is hampered by the almost complete absence of reliable evidence on the effectiveness of prevention programmes, Chapter 5 explores some of the options being considered across sectors.

References

1. Aboderin IA, Beard JR. Older people's health in sub-Saharan Africa. Lancet. 2015 Feb 14;385(9968):e9–11. doi: http://dx.doi.org/10.1016/S0140-6736(14)61602-0 PMID: 25468150

2. Global health estimates 2013: deaths by cause, age, sex and regional grouping, 2000–2012. In: World Health Organization, Global health estimates [website]. Geneva: World Health Organization; 2015 (http://www.who.int/healthinfo/global_burden_disease/en, accessed 24 July 2015).

3. Christensen K, Doblhammer G, Rau R, Vaupel JW. Ageing populations: the challenges ahead. Lancet. 2009 Oct 3;374(9696):1196–208. doi: http://dx.doi.org/10.1016/S0140-6736(09)61460-4 PMID: 19801098

4. Global health estimates: life expectancy trends by country. In: World Health Organization, Global health estimates [website]. Geneva: World Health Organization; 2015 (http://www.who.int/healthinfo/global_burden_disease/en, accessed 24 July 2015).

5. Fertility rates, total (births per woman). In: The World Bank [website]. Washington (DC): World Bank; 2015 (http://data.worldbank.org/indicator/SP.DYN.TFRT.IN, accessed 12 March 2015).

6. Crimmins EM, Beltrán-Sánchez H. Mortality and morbidity trends: is there compression of morbidity? J Gerontol B Psychol Sci Soc Sci. 2011 Jan;66(1):75–86. doi: http://dx.doi.org/10.1093/geronb/gbq088 PMID: 21135070

7. Manton KG, Gu X, Lamb VL. Change in chronic disability from 1982 to 2004/2005 as measured by long-term changes in function and health in the U.S. elderly population. Proc Natl Acad Sci U S A. 2006 Nov 28;103(48):18374–9. doi: http://dx.doi.org/10.1073/pnas.0608483103 PMID: 17101963

8. Seeman TE, Merkin SS, Crimmins EM, Karlamangla AS. Disability trends among older Americans: National Health And Nutrition Examination Surveys, 1988–1994 and 1999–2004. Am J Public Health. 2010 Jan;100(1):100–7. doi: http://dx.doi.org/10.2105/AJPH.2008.157388 PMID: 19910350

9. Liao Y, McGee DL, Cao G, Cooper RS. Recent changes in the health status of the older U.S. population: findings from the 1984 and 1994 supplement on aging. J Am Geriatr Soc. 2001 Apr;49(4):443–9. doi: http://dx.doi.org/10.1046/j.1532-5415.2001.49089.x PMID: 11347789

10. Hung WW, Ross JS, Boockvar KS, Siu AL. Recent trends in chronic disease, impairment and disability among older adults in the United States. BMC Geriatr. 2011;11(1):47. doi: http://dx.doi.org/10.1186/1471-2318-11-47 PMID: 21851629

11. Lin S-F, Beck AN, Finch BK, Hummer RA, Masters RK. Trends in US older adult disability: exploring age, period, and cohort effects. Am J Public Health. 2012 Nov;102(11):2157–63. doi: http://dx.doi.org/10.2105/AJPH.2011.300602 PMID: 22994192

12. Stewart ST, Cutler DM, Rosen AB. US trends in quality-adjusted life expectancy from 1987 to 2008: combining national surveys to more broadly track the health of the nation. Am J Public Health. 2013 Nov;103(11):e78–87. doi: http://dx.doi.org/10.2105/AJPH.2013.301250 PMID: 24028235

13. Jagger C, Gillies C, Moscone F, Cambois E, Van Oyen H, Nusselder W, et al.; EHLEIS team. Inequalities in healthy life years in the 25 countries of the European Union in 2005: a cross-national meta-regression analysis. Lancet. 2008 Dec 20;372(9656):2124–31. doi: http://dx.doi.org/10.1016/S0140-6736(08)61594-9 PMID: 19010526

14. Balestat G, Lafortune G. Trends in severe disability among elderly people: assessing the evidence in 12 OECD countries and the future implications. Paris: OECD Publishing; 2007 (OECD Health Working Papers No. 26). doi: http://dx.doi.org/http://dx.doi.org/10.1787/217072070078 doi: http://dx.doi.org/10.1787/217072070078

15. Chatterji S, Byles J, Cutler D, Seeman T, Verdes E. Health, functioning, and disability in older adults–present status and future implications. Lancet. 2015 Feb 7;385(9967):563–75. doi: http://dx.doi.org/10.1016/S0140-6736(14)61462-8 PMID: 25468158

16. Wave 4, release 1.1.1 (28 March 2013). In: Survey of Health, Ageing and Retirement in Europe (SHARE) [website]. Munich: Munich Center for the Economics of Aging; 2013 (http://www.share-project.org/home0/wave-4.html, accessed 27 July 2015).

17. International classification of functioning, disability and health. Geneva: World Health Organization; 2001.

18. Fogel RW. Changes in the process of aging during the twentieth century: findings and procedures of the early indicators project. Cambridge (MA): National Bureau of Economic Research; 2003.

19. Cheng ER, Kindig DA. Disparities in premature mortality between high- and low-income US counties. Prev Chronic Dis. 2012;9:E75. PMID: 22440549

20. Olshansky SJ, Antonucci T, Berkman L, Binstock RH, Boersch-Supan A, Cacioppo JT, et al. Differences in life expectancy due to race and educational differences are widening, and many may not catch up. Health Aff (Millwood). 2012 Aug;31(8):1803–13. doi: http://dx.doi.org/10.1377/hlthaff.2011.0746 PMID: 22869659

21. Zheng X, Chen G, Song X, Liu J, Yan L, Du W, et al. Twenty-year trends in the prevalence of disability in China. Bull World Health Organ. 2011 Nov 1;89(11):788–97. doi: http://dx.doi.org/10.2471/BLT.11.089730 PMID: 22084524

22. Macaulay R, Akbar AN, Henson SM. The role of the T cell in age-related inflammation. Age (Dordr). 2013 Jun;35(3):563–72. doi: http://dx.doi.org/10.1007/s11357-012-9381-2 PMID: 22252437

23. McElhaney JE, Zhou X, Talbot HK, Soethout E, Bleackley RC, Granville DJ, et al. The unmet need in the elderly: how immu-nosenescence, CMV infection, co-morbidities and frailty are a challenge for the development of more effective influenza vaccines. Vaccine. 2012 Mar 9;30(12):2060–7. doi: http://dx.doi.org/10.1016/j.vaccine.2012.01.015 PMID: 22289511

24. Kirkwood TB. A systematic look at an old problem. Nature. 2008 Feb 7;451(7179):644–7. doi: http://dx.doi.org/10.1038/451644a PMID: 18256658

25. Sehl ME, Yates FE. Kinetics of human aging: I. Rates of senescence between ages 30 and 70 years in healthy people. J Gerontol A Biol Sci Med Sci. 2001 May;56(5):B198–208. doi: http://dx.doi.org/10.1093/gerona/56.5.B198 PMID: 11320100

26. Heidemeier H, Moser K. Self-other agreement in job performance ratings: a meta-analytic test of a process model. J Appl Psychol. 2009 Mar;94(2):353–70. doi: http://dx.doi.org/10.1037/0021-9010.94.2.353 PMID: 19271795

27. Staudinger U, Bowen C. A systemic approach to aging in the work context. Zeitschrift für Arbeitsmarktforschung. 2011;44(4):295–306. doi: http://dx.doi.org/10.1007/s12651-011-0086-2

28. Börsch-Supan A, Weiss M. Productivity and age: evidence from work teams at the assembly line. Munich: Munich Center for the Economics of Aging; 2013 (MEA discussion papers).

29. Russo A, Onder G, Cesari M, Zamboni V, Barillaro C, Capoluongo E, et al. Lifetime occupation and physical function: a prospective cohort study on persons aged 80 years and older living in a community. Occup Environ Med. 2006 Jul;63(7):438–42. PMID: 16782827

30. Backes-Gellner U, Veen S. Positive effects of ageing and age diversity in innovative companies – large-scale empirical evidence on company productivity. Hum Resour Manage J. 2013;23(3):279–95. doi: http://dx.doi.org/10.1111/1748-8583.12011

31. Cruz-Jentoft AJ, Baeyens JP, Bauer JM, Boirie Y, Cederholm T, Landi F, et al.; European Working Group on Sarcopenia in Older People. Sarcopenia: European consensus on definition and diagnosis: Report of the European Working Group on Sarcopenia in Older People. Age Ageing. 2010 Jul;39(4):412–23. doi: http://dx.doi.org/10.1093/ageing/afq034 PMID: 20392703

32. Rantanen T, Volpato S, Ferrucci L, Heikkinen E, Fried LP, Guralnik JM. Handgrip strength and cause-specific and total mortality in older disabled women: exploring the mechanism. J Am Geriatr Soc. 2003 May;51(5):636–41. doi: http://dx.doi.org/10.1034/j.1600-0579.2003.00207.x PMID: 12752838

33. Leong DP, Teo KK, Rangarajan S, Lopez-Jaramillo P, Avezum A Jr, Orlandini A, et al.; Prospective Urban Rural Epidemiology (PURE) Study investigators. Prognostic value of grip strength: findings from the Prospective Urban Rural Epidemiology (PURE) study. Lancet. 2015 Jul 18;386(9990):266–73. doi: http://dx.doi.org/10.1016/S0140-6736(14)62000-6 PMID: 25982160

34. WHO Study on global AGEing and adult health (SAGE). In: World Health Organization, Health statistics and information systems [website]. Geneva: World Health Organization; 2015 (http://www.who.int/healthinfo/sage/en/, accessed 23 June 2015).

35. Gullberg B, Johnell O, Kanis JA. World-wide projections for hip fracture. Osteoporos Int. 1997;7(5):407–13. doi: http://dx.doi.org/10.1007/PL00004148 PMID: 9425497

36. Cauley JA, Chalhoub D, Kassem AM, Fuleihan Gel-H. Geographic and ethnic disparities in osteoporotic fractures. Nat Rev Endocrinol. 2014 Jun;10(6):338–51. doi: http://dx.doi.org/10.1038/nrendo.2014.51 PMID: 24751883

37. Novelli C. Effects of aging and physical activity on articular cartilage: a literature review. J Morphol Sci. 2012;29(1):1–7. (http://jms.org.br/PDF/v29n1a01.pdf, accessed August 17 2015).

38. Martin JA, Buckwalter JA. Aging, articular cartilage chondrocyte senescence and osteoarthritis. Biogerontology. 2002;3(5):257–64. doi: http://dx.doi.org/10.1023/A:1020185404126 PMID: 12237562

39. Studenski S, Perera S, Patel K, Rosano C, Faulkner K, Inzitari M, et al. Gait speed and survival in older adults. JAMA. 2011 Jan 5;305(1):50–8. doi: http://dx.doi.org/10.1001/jama.2010.1923 PMID: 21205966

40. Yamasoba T, Lin FR, Someya S, Kashio A, Sakamoto T, Kondo K. Current concepts in age-related hearing loss: epidemiology and mechanistic pathways. Hear Res. 2013 Sep;303:30–8. doi: http://dx.doi.org/10.1016/j.heares.2013.01.021 PMID: 23422312

41. Olusanya BO, Neumann KJ, Saunders JE. The global burden of disabling hearing impairment: a call to action. Bull World Health Organ. 2014 May 1;92(5):367–73. PMID: 24839326

42. Prevention of blindness and deafness: estimates. In: World Health Organization, Prevention of blindness and deafness [website]. Geneva: World Health Organization; 2015 (http://www.who.int/pbd/deafness/estimates/en/, accessed 5 June 2015).

43. Davis A, Davis KA. Epidemiology of aging and hearing loss related to other chronic illnesses. Hearing care for adults – the challenge of aging. Chicago: Phonak; 2010. 23–32. (http://www.phonak.com/content/dam/phonak/b2b/Events/conference_proceedings/chicago_2009/proceedings/09_P69344_Pho_Kapitel_2_S23_32.pdf, accessed 5 June 2015).

44. Gates GA, Mills JH. Presbycusis. Lancet. 2005 Sep 24-30;366(9491):1111–20. doi: http://dx.doi.org/10.1016/S0140-6736(05)67423-5 PMID: 16182900

45. Baltes PB, Lindenberger U. Emergence of a powerful connection between sensory and cognitive functions across the adult life span: a new window to the study of cognitive aging? Psychol Aging. 1997 Mar;12(1):12–21. doi: http://dx.doi.org/10.1037/0882-7974.12.1.12 PMID: 9100264

46. Hickenbotham A, Roorda A, Steinmaus C, Glasser A. Meta-analysis of sex differences in presbyopia. Invest Ophthalmol Vis Sci. 2012 May;53(6):3215–20. doi: http://dx.doi.org/10.1167/iovs.12-9791 PMID: 22531698

47. Stuck AE, Walthert JM, Nikolaus T, Büla CJ, Hohmann C, Beck JC. Risk factors for functional status decline in community-living elderly people: a systematic literature review. Soc Sci Med. 1999 Feb;48(4):445–69. doi: http://dx.doi.org/10.1016/S0277-9536(98)00370-0 PMID: 10075171

48. Parham K, McKinnon BJ, Eibling D, Gates GA. Challenges and opportunities in presbycusis. Otolaryngol Head Neck Surg. 2011 Apr;144(4):491–5. doi: http://dx.doi.org/10.1177/0194599810395079 PMID: 21493222

49. Ryan EB, Giles H, Bartolucci G, Henwood K. Psycholinguistic and social psychological components of communication by and with the elderly. Lang Commun. 1986;6(1):1–24. doi: http://dx.doi.org/10.1016/0271-5309(86)90002-9

50. Turano K, Rubin GS, Herdman SJ, Chee E, Fried LP. Visual stabilization of posture in the elderly: fallers vs. nonfallers. Optom Vis Sci. 1994 Dec;71(12):761–9. doi: http://dx.doi.org/10.1097/00006324-199412000-00006 PMID: 7898883

51. Park DC. The basic mechanism accounting for age-related decline in cognitive function. In: Park DC, Schwarz N, editors. Cognitive aging: a primer. New York: Psychology Press; 2000:3–21.

52. Henry JD, MacLeod MS, Phillips LH, Crawford JR. A meta-analytic review of prospective memory and aging. Psychol Aging. 2004 Mar;19(1):27–39. doi: http://dx.doi.org/10.1037/0882-7974.19.1.27 PMID: 15065929

53. Baltes P, Freund A, Li S-C. The psychological science of human ageing. In: Johnson ML, Bengtson VL, Coleman PG, Kirkwood TBL, editors. The Cambridge handbook of age and ageing. Cambridge: Cambridge University Press; 2005:47–71.

54. Muscari A, Giannoni C, Pierpaoli L, Berzigotti A, Maietta P, Foschi E, et al. Chronic endurance exercise training prevents aging-related cognitive decline in healthy older adults: a randomized controlled trial. Int J Geriatr Psychiatry. 2010 Oct;25(10):1055–64. doi: http://dx.doi.org/10.1002/gps.2462 PMID: 20033904

55. Lindau ST, Schumm LP, Laumann EO, Levinson W, O'Muircheartaigh CA, Waite LJ. A study of sexuality and health among older adults in the United States. N Engl J Med. 2007 Aug 23;357(8):762–74. doi: http://dx.doi.org/10.1056/NEJMoa067423 PMID: 17715410

56. Lochlainn MN, Kenny RA. Sexual activity and aging. J Am Med Dir Assoc. 2013 Aug;14(8):565–72. doi: http://dx.doi.org/10.1016/j.jamda.2013.01.022 PMID: 23540950

57. Lusti-Narasimhan M, Beard JR. Sexual health in older women. Bull World Health Organ. 2013 Sep 1;91(9):707–9. PMID: 24101788

58. Nicolosi A, Laumann EO, Glasser DB, Moreira ED Jr, Paik A, Gingell C; Global Study of Sexual Attitudes and Behaviors Investigators' Group. Sexual behavior and sexual dysfunctions after age 40: the global study of sexual attitudes and behaviors. Urology. 2004 Nov;64(5):991–7. doi: http://dx.doi.org/10.1016/j.urology.2004.06.055 PMID: 15533492

59. Brenoff A. Dementia and sex: what was really on trial with Henry Rayhons. Huffington Post. 23 April 2015 (http://www.huffingtonpost.com/ann-brenoff/dementia-and-sex-henry-rayhons_b_7122460.html, accessed 5 June 2015).

60. Castelo-Branco C, Soveral I. The immune system and aging: a review. Gynecol Endocrinol. 2014 Jan;30(1):16–22. doi: http://dx.doi.org/10.3109/09513590.2013.852531 PMID: 24219599

61. Lang PO, Govind S, Aspinall R. Reversing T cell immunosenescence: why, who, and how. Age (Dordr). 2013 Jun;35(3):609–20. doi: http://dx.doi.org/10.1007/s11357-012-9393-y PMID: 22367580

62. Lang PO, Mendes A, Socquet J, Assir N, Govind S, Aspinall R. Effectiveness of influenza vaccine in aging and older adults: comprehensive analysis of the evidence. Clin Interv Aging. 2012;7:55–64. PMID: 22393283

63. Wong SY, Wong CK, Chan FW, Chan PK, Ngai K, Mercer S, et al. Chronic psychosocial stress: does it modulate immunity to the influenza vaccine in Hong Kong Chinese elderly caregivers? Age (Dordr). 2013 Aug;35(4):1479–93. doi: http://dx.doi.org/10.1007/s11357-012-9449-z PMID: 22772580

64. Macaulay R, Akbar AN, Henson SM. The role of the T cell in age-related inflammation. Age (Dordr). 2013 Jun;35(3):563–72. doi: http://dx.doi.org/10.1007/s11357-012-9449-z PMID: 22252437

65. Salvioli S, Monti D, Lanzarini C, Conte M, Pirazzini C, Bacalini MG, et al. Immune system, cell senescence, aging and longevity–inflamm-aging reappraised. Curr Pharm Des. 2013;19(9):1675–9. PMID: 23589904

66. Baker DJ, Wijshake T, Tchkonia T, LeBrasseur NK, Childs BG, van de Sluis B, et al. Clearance of p16Ink4a-positive senescent cells delays ageing-associated disorders. Nature. 2011 Nov 10;479(7372):232–6. doi: http://dx.doi.org/10.1038/nature10600 PMID: 22048312

67. White-Chu EF, Reddy M. Dry skin in the elderly: complexities of a common problem. Clin Dermatol. 2011 Jan-Feb;29(1):37–42. doi: http://dx.doi.org/10.1016/j.clindermatol.2010.07.005 PMID: 21146730

68. Lorencini M, Brohem CA, Dieamant GC, Zanchin NI, Maibach HI. Active ingredients against human epidermal aging. Ageing Res Rev. 2014 May;15:100–15. PMID: 24675046

69. Farage MA, Miller KW, Berardesca E, Maibach HI. Clinical implications of aging skin: cutaneous disorders in the elderly. Am J Clin Dermatol. 2009;10(2):73–86. doi: http://dx.doi.org/10.2165/00128071-200910020-00001 PMID: 19222248

70. Patel T, Yosipovitch G. The management of chronic pruritus in the elderly. Skin Therapy Lett. 2010 Sep;15(8):5–9. PMID: 20844849

71. Young Y, Frick KD, Phelan EA. Can successful aging and chronic illness coexist in the same individual? A multidimensional concept of successful aging. J Am Med Dir Assoc. 2009 Feb;10(2):87–92. doi: http://dx.doi.org/10.1016/j.jamda.2008.11.003 PMID: 19187875

72. Beekman AT, Copeland JR, Prince MJ. Review of community prevalence of depression in later life. Br J Psychiatry. 1999 Apr;174(4):307–11. doi: http://dx.doi.org/10.1192/bjp.174.4.307 PMID: 10533549

73. Seitz D, Purandare N, Conn D. Prevalence of psychiatric disorders among older adults in long-term care homes: a systematic review. Int Psychogeriatr. 2010 Nov;22(7):1025–39. PMID: 20522279

74. Meeks TW, Vahia IV, Lavretsky H, Kulkarni G, Jeste DV. A tune in "a minor" can "b major": a review of epidemiology, illness course, and public health implications of subthreshold depression in older adults. J Affect Disord. 2011 Mar;129(1-3):126–42. doi: http://dx.doi.org/10.1016/j.jad.2010.09.015 PMID: 20926139

75. Schuurmans J, van Balkom A. Late-life anxiety disorders: a review. Curr Psychiatry Rep. 2011 Aug;13(4):267–73. doi: http://dx.doi.org/10.1007/s11920-011-0204-4 PMID: 21538031

76. van Balkom AJ, Beekman AT, de Beurs E, Deeg DJ, van Dyck R, van Tilburg W. Comorbidity of the anxiety disorders in a community-based older population in The Netherlands. Acta Psychiatr Scand. 2000 Jan;101(1):37–45. doi: http://dx.doi.org/10.1034/j.1600-0447.2000.101001037.x PMID: 10674949

77. Jayasekara R, Procter N, Harrison J, Skelton K, Hampel S, Draper R, et al. Cognitive behavioural therapy for older adults with depression: a review. J Ment Health. 2015 Jun;24(3):168–71. PMID: 25358075

78. Thorp SR, Ayers CR, Nuevo R, Stoddard JA, Sorrell JT, Wetherell JL. Meta-analysis comparing different behavioral treatments for late-life anxiety. Am J Geriatr Psychiatry. 2009 Feb;17(2):105–15. doi: http://dx.doi.org/10.1097/JGP.0b013e31818b3f7e PMID: 19155744

79. Tedeschini E, Levkovitz Y, Iovieno N, Ameral VE, Nelson JC, Papakostas GI. Efficacy of antidepressants for late-life depression: a meta-analysis and meta-regression of placebo-controlled randomized trials. J Clin Psychiatry. 2011 Dec;72(12):1660–8. doi: http://dx.doi.org/10.4088/JCP.10r06531 PMID: 22244025

80. Vos T, Goss J, Begg S, Mann N. Projection of health care expenditure by disease: a case study from Australia. New York: United Nations; 2007 (Background paper for the United Nations).

81. Marengoni A, Angleman S, Melis R, Mangialasche F, Karp A, Garmen A, et al. Aging with multimorbidity: a systematic review of the literature. Ageing Res Rev. 2011 Sep;10(4):430–9.http://www.goldcopd.it/gruppi_lavoro/2013/ageingmulti-morbidityreviw2011.pdf Available from: accessed August 17 2015). PMID: 21402176

82. Wang HH, Wang JJ, Wong SY, Wong MC, Li FJ, Wang PX, et al. Epidemiology of multimorbidity in China and implications for the healthcare system: cross-sectional survey among 162,464 community household residents in southern China. BMC Med. 2014;12(1):188. doi: http://dx.doi.org/10.1186/s12916-014-0188-0 PMID: 25338506

83. Garin N, Olaya B, Perales J, Moneta MV, Miret M, Ayuso-Mateos JL, et al. Multimorbidity patterns in a national representative sample of the Spanish adult population. PLoS One. 2014;9(1):e84794. doi: http://dx.doi.org/10.1371/journal.pone.0084794 PMID: 24465433

84. Barnett K, Mercer SW, Norbury M, Watt G, Wyke S, Guthrie B. Epidemiology of multimorbidity and implications for health care, research, and medical education: a cross-sectional study. Lancet. 2012 Jul 7;380(9836):37–43. doi: http://dx.doi.org/10.1016/S0140-6736(12)60240-2 PMID: 22579043

85. Uijen AA, van de Lisdonk EH. Multimorbidity in primary care: prevalence and trend over the last 20 years. Eur J Gen Pract. 2008;14 Suppl 1:28–32. doi: http://dx.doi.org/10.1080/13814780802436093 PMID: 18949641

86. St Sauver JL, Boyd CM, Grossardt BR, Bobo WV, Finney Rutten LJ, Roger VL, et al. Risk of developing multimorbidity across all ages in an historical cohort study: differences by sex and ethnicity. BMJ Open. 2015;5(2):e006413. doi: http://dx.doi.org/10.1136/bmjopen-2014-006413 PMID: 25649210

87. Beran D. Difficulties facing the provision of care for multimorbidity in low-income countries. In: Sartorius N, Holt R, Maj M, editors. Comorbidity of mental and physical disorders: key issues in mental health. Basel: Karger; 2015:33–41.

88. Deeks SG, Lewin SR, Havlir DV. The end of AIDS: HIV infection as a chronic disease. Lancet. 2013 Nov 2;382(9903):1525–33. doi: http://dx.doi.org/10.1016/S0140-6736(13)61809-7 PMID: 24152939

89. Guaraldi G, Zona S, Brothers TD, Carli F, Stentarelli C, Dolci G, et al. Aging with HIV vs. HIV seroconversion at older age: a diverse population with distinct comorbidity profiles. PLoS One. 2015;10(4):e0118531. doi: http://dx.doi.org/10.1371/journal.pone.0118531 PMID: 25874806

90. Garin N, Olaya B, Moneta MV, Miret M, Lobo A, Ayuso-Mateos JL, et al. Impact of multimorbidity on disability and quality of life in the Spanish older population. PLoS One. 2014;9(11):e111498. doi: http://dx.doi.org/10.1371/journal.pone.0111498 PMID: 25375890

91. Sinnige J, Braspenning J, Schellevis F, Stirbu-Wagner I, Westert G, Korevaar J. The prevalence of disease clusters in older adults with multiple chronic diseases–a systematic literature review. PLoS One. 2013;8(11):e79641. doi: http://dx.doi.org/10.1371/journal.pone.0079641 PMID: 24244534

92. Fulop T, Larbi A, Witkowski JM, McElhaney J, Loeb M, Mitnitski A, et al. Aging, frailty and age-related diseases. Biogerontology. 2010 Oct;11(5):547–63. doi: http://dx.doi.org/10.1007/s10522-010-9287-2 PMID: 20559726

93. Tinetti ME, McAvay GJ, Chang SS, Newman AB, Fitzpatrick AL, Fried TR, et al. Contribution of multiple chronic conditions to universal health outcomes. J Am Geriatr Soc. 2011 Sep;59(9):1686–91. doi: http://dx.doi.org/10.1111/j.1532-5415.2011.03573.x PMID: 21883118

94. Guthrie B, Payne K, Alderson P, McMurdo ME, Mercer SW. Adapting clinical guidelines to take account of multimorbidity. BMJ. 2012;345 oct04 1:e6341. doi: http://dx.doi.org/10.1136/bmj.e6341 PMID: 23036829

95. Uhlig K, Leff B, Kent D, Dy S, Brunnhuber K, Burgers JS, et al. A framework for crafting clinical practice guidelines that are relevant to the care and management of people with multimorbidity. J Gen Intern Med. 2014 Apr;29(4):670–9. doi: http://dx.doi.org/10.1007/s11606-013-2659-y PMID: 24442332

96. DuBeau CE, Kuchel GA, Johnson T 2nd, Palmer MH, Wagg A; Fourth International Consultation on Incontinence. Incontinence in the frail elderly: report from the 4th International Consultation on Incontinence. Neurourol Urodyn. 2010;29(1):165–78. doi: http://dx.doi.org/10.1002/nau.20842 PMID: 20025027

97. Gurwitz JH, Goldberg RJ. Age-based exclusions from cardiovascular clinical trials: implications for elderly individuals (and for all of us): comment on "the persistent exclusion of older patients from ongoing clinical trials regarding heart failure". Arch Intern Med. 2011 Mar 28;171(6):557–8. PMID: 21444845

98. Boyd CM, Vollenweider D, Puhan MA. Informing evidence-based decision-making for patients with comorbidity: availability of necessary information in clinical trials for chronic diseases. PLoS One. 2012;7(8):e41601. doi: http://dx.doi.org/10.1371/journal.pone.0041601 PMID: 22870234

99. Inouye SK, Studenski S, Tinetti ME, Kuchel GA. Geriatric syndromes: clinical, research, and policy implications of a core geriatric concept. J Am Geriatr Soc. 2007 May;55(5):780–91. doi: http://dx.doi.org/10.1111/j.1532-5415.2007.01156.x PMID: 17493201

100. Fried LP, Storer DJ, King DE, Lodder F. Diagnosis of illness presentation in the elderly. J Am Geriatr Soc. 1991 Feb;39(2):117–23. doi: http://dx.doi.org/10.1111/j.1532-5415.1991.tb01612.x PMID: 1991942

101. Fernández-Garrido J, Ruiz-Ros V, Buigues C, Navarro-Martinez R, Cauli O. Clinical features of prefrail older individuals and emerging peripheral biomarkers: a systematic review. Arch Gerontol Geriatr. 2014 Jul-Aug;59(1):7–17. doi: http://dx.doi.org/10.1016/j.archger.2014.02.008 PMID: 24679669

102. Kane RL, Shamliyan T, Talley K, Pacala J. The association between geriatric syndromes and survival. J Am Geriatr Soc. 2012 May;60(5):896–904. doi: http://dx.doi.org/10.1111/j.1532-5415.2012.03942.x PMID: 22568483

103. Lordos EF, Herrmann FR, Robine JM, Balahoczky M, Giannelli SV, Gold G, et al. Comparative value of medical diagnosis versus physical functioning in predicting the 6-year survival of 1951 hospitalized old patients. Rejuvenation Res. 2008 Aug;11(4):829–36. doi: http://dx.doi.org/10.1089/rej.2008.0721 PMID: 18729815

104. Cesari M, Prince M, Bernabei R, Chan P, Gutierrez-Robledo LM, Michel JP, et al. Frailty – an emerging public health priority. Gerontologist. 2016. (In press.)

105. Fried LP, Ferrucci L, Darer J, Williamson JD, Anderson G. Untangling the concepts of disability, frailty, and comorbidity: implications for improved targeting and care. J Gerontol A Biol Sci Med Sci. 2004 Mar;59(3):255–63. doi: http://dx.doi.org/10.1093/gerona/59.3.M255 PMID: 15031310

106. Santos-Eggimann B, Cuénoud P, Spagnoli J, Junod J. Prevalence of frailty in middle-aged and older community-dwelling Europeans living in 10 countries. J Gerontol A Biol Sci Med Sci. 2009 Jun;64(6):675–81. doi: http://dx.doi.org/10.1093/gerona/glp012 PMID: 19276189

107. Han ES, Lee Y, Kim J. Association of cognitive impairment with frailty in community-dwelling older adults. Int Psychogeriatr. 2014 Jan;26(1):155–63. PMID: 24153029

108. Shimada H, Makizako H, Doi T, Yoshida D, Tsutsumimoto K, Anan Y, et al. Combined prevalence of frailty and mild cognitive impairment in a population of elderly Japanese people. J Am Med Dir Assoc. 2013 Jul;14(7):518–24. PMID: 23669054

109. Alvarado BE, Zunzunegui MV, Béland F, Bamvita JM. Life course social and health conditions linked to frailty in Latin American older men and women. J Gerontol A Biol Sci Med Sci. 2008 Dec;63(12):1399–406. doi: http://dx.doi.org/10.1093/gerona/63.12.1399 PMID: 19126855

110. Rosero-Bixby L, Dow WH. Surprising SES Gradients in mortality, health, and biomarkers in a Latin American population of adults. J Gerontol B Psychol Sci Soc Sci. 2009 Jan;64(1):105–17. doi: http://dx.doi.org/10.1093/geronb/gbn004 PMID: 19196695

111. Llibre JdeJ, López AM, Valhuerdi A, Guerra M, Llibre-Guerra JJ, Sánchez YY, et al. Frailty, dependency and mortality predictors in a cohort of Cuban older adults, 2003–2011. MEDICC Rev. 2014 Jan;16(1):24–30. PMID: 24487672

112. Aguilar-Navarro S, Gutierrez-Robledo LM, Garcia-Lara JMA, Payette H, Amieva H. Avila- Funes JA. The phenotype of frailty predicts disability and mortality among Mexican community-dwelling elderly. J Frailty Aging. 2012;1(3):111–7. (http://www.jfrailtyaging.com/all-issues.html?article=60, accessed August 17 2015).

113. Fried LP, Tangen CM, Walston J, Newman AB, Hirsch C, Gottdiener J, et al.; Cardiovascular Health Study Collaborative Research Group. Frailty in older adults: evidence for a phenotype. J Gerontol A Biol Sci Med Sci. 2001 Mar;56(3):M146–56. doi: http://dx.doi.org/10.1093/gerona/56.3.M146 PMID: 11253156

114. Newman AB, Gottdiener JS, Mcburnie MA, Hirsch CH, Kop WJ, Tracy R, et al.; Cardiovascular Health Study Research Group. Associations of subclinical cardiovascular disease with frailty. J Gerontol A Biol Sci Med Sci. 2001 Mar;56(3):M158–66. doi: http://dx.doi.org/10.1093/gerona/56.3.M158 PMID: 11253157

115. Shlipak MG, Stehman-Breen C, Fried LF, Song X, Siscovick D, Fried LP, et al. The presence of frailty in elderly persons with chronic renal insufficiency. Am J Kidney Dis. 2004 May;43(5):861–7. doi: http://dx.doi.org/10.1053/j.ajkd.2003.12.049 PMID: 15112177

116. Borrat-Besson C, Ryser V-A, Wernli B. Transitions between frailty states – a European comparison. In: Börsch-Supan A, Brandt M, Litwin H, Weber GW, editors. Active ageing and solidarity between generations in Europe: first results from SHARE after the economic crisis. Berlin: De Gruyter; 2013:175–86.

117. Gill TM, Gahbauer EA, Allore HG, Han L. Transitions between frailty states among community-living older persons. Arch Intern Med. 2006 Feb 27;166(4):418–23. doi: http://dx.doi.org/10.1001/archinte.166.4.418 PMID: 16505261

118. Daniels R, van Rossum E, de Witte L, Kempen GI, van den Heuvel W. Interventions to prevent disability in frail community-dwelling elderly: a systematic review. BMC Health Serv Res. 2008;8(1):278. doi: http://dx.doi.org/10.1186/1472-6963-8-278 PMID: 19115992

119. Stuck AE, Siu AL, Wieland GD, Adams J, Rubenstein LZ. Comprehensive geriatric assessment: a meta-analysis of controlled trials. Lancet. 1993 Oct 23;342(8878):1032–6. doi: http://dx.doi.org/10.1016/0140-6736(93)92884-V PMID: 8105269

120. Cesari M, Vellas B, Hsu FC, Newman AB, Doss H, King AC, et al.; LIFE Study Group. A physical activity intervention to treat the frailty syndrome in older persons-results from the LIFE-P study. J Gerontol A Biol Sci Med Sci. 2015 Feb;70(2):216–22. doi: http://dx.doi.org/10.1093/gerona/glu099 PMID: 25387728

121. Pahor M, Guralnik JM, Ambrosius WT, Blair S, Bonds DE, Church TS, et al.; LIFE study investigators. Effect of structured physical activity on prevention of major mobility disability in older adults: the LIFE study randomized clinical trial. JAMA. 2014 Jun 18;311(23):2387–96. doi: http://dx.doi.org/10.1001/jama.2014.5616 PMID: 24866862

122. Kelaiditi E, van Kan GA, Cesari M. Frailty: role of nutrition and exercise. Curr Opin Clin Nutr Metab Care. 2014 Jan;17(1):32–9. PMID: 24281373

123. Dorner TE, Lackinger C, Haider S, Luger E, Kapan A, Luger M, et al. Nutritional intervention and physical training in malnourished frail community-dwelling elderly persons carried out by trained lay "buddies": study protocol of a randomized controlled trial. BMC Public Health. 2013;13(1):1232. doi: http://dx.doi.org/10.1186/1471-2458-13-1232 PMID: 24369785

124. Yuan HB, Williams BA, Liu M. Attitudes toward urinary incontinence among community nurses and community-dwelling older people. J Wound Ostomy Continence Nurs. 2011 Mar-Apr;38(2):184–9. PMID: 21326113

125. Abrams P, Cardozo L, Fall M, Griffiths D, Rosier P, Ulmsten U, et al.; Standardisation Sub-committee of the International Continence Society. The standardisation of terminology of lower urinary tract function: report from the Standardisation Sub-committee of the International Continence Society. Neurourol Urodyn. 2002;21(2):167–78. doi: http://dx.doi.org/10.1002/nau.10052 PMID: 11857671

126. Milsom I, Coyne KS, Nicholson S, Kvasz M, Chen CI, Wein AJ. Global prevalence and economic burden of urgency urinary incontinence: a systematic review. Eur Urol. 2014 Jan;65(1):79–95. doi: http://dx.doi.org/10.1016/j.eururo.2013.08.031 PMID: 24007713

127. Yu PL, Shi J, Liu XR, Xia CW, Liu DF, Wu ZL, et al. [Study on the prevalence of urinary incontinence and its related factors among elderly in rural areas, Jixian county, Tianjin]. Zhonghua Liu Xing Bing Xue Za Zhi. 2009 Aug;30(8):766–71. PMID: 20193194

128. Prince M, Acosta D, Ferri CP, Guerra M, Huang Y, Jacob KS, et al. The association between common physical impairments and dementia in low and middle income countries, and, among people with dementia, their association with cognitive function and disability. A 10/66 Dementia Research Group population-based study. Int J Geriatr Psychiatry. 2011 May;26(5):511–9. doi: http://dx.doi.org/10.1002/gps.2558 PMID: 20669334

129. Sims J, Browning C, Lundgren-Lindquist B, Kendig H. Urinary incontinence in a community sample of older adults: prevalence and impact on quality of life. Disabil Rehabil. 2011;33(15-16):1389–98. doi: http://dx.doi.org/10.3109/09638288.2010.532284 PMID: 21692622

130. Tamanini JT, Santos JL, Lebrão ML, Duarte YA, Laurenti R. Association between urinary incontinence in elderly patients and caregiver burden in the city of Sao Paulo/Brazil: Health, Wellbeing, and Ageing Study. Neurourol Urodyn. 2011 Sep;30(7):1281–5. PMID: 21560151

131. Perracini M, Clemson L, Tiedmann A, Kalula S, Scott V, Sherrington C. Falls in older adults: current evidence, gaps and priorities. Gerontologist. 2016. (In press).

132. Chang JT, Morton SC, Rubenstein LZ, Mojica WA, Maglione M, Suttorp MJ, et al. Interventions for the prevention of falls in older adults: systematic review and meta-analysis of randomised clinical trials. BMJ. 2004 Mar 20;328(7441):680. doi: http://dx.doi.org/10.1136/bmj.328.7441.680 PMID: 15031239

133. Gillespie LD, Robertson MC, Gillespie WJ, Lamb SE, Gates S, Cumming RG, et al. Interventions for preventing falls in older people living in the community. Cochrane Database Syst Rev. 2009; (2):CD007146. PMID: 19370674

134. Hoops ML, Rosenblatt NJ, Hurt CP, Crenshaw J, Grabiner MD. Does lower extremity osteoarthritis exacerbate risk factors for falls in older adults? Womens Health (Lond Engl). 2012 Nov;8(6):685–96, quiz 697–8. doi: http://dx.doi.org/10.2217/whe.12.53 PMID: 23181533

135. Dhital A, Pey T, Stanford MR. Visual loss and falls: a review. Eye (Lond). 2010 Sep;24(9):1437–46. doi: http://dx.doi.org/10.1038/eye.2010.60 PMID: 20448666

136. Karlsson MK, Magnusson H, von Schewelov T, Rosengren BE. Prevention of falls in the elderly–a review. Osteoporos Int. 2013 Mar;24(3):747–62. PMID: 23296743

137. Lee WK, Kong KA, Park H. Effect of preexisting musculoskeletal diseases on the 1-year incidence of fall-related injuries. J Prev Med Public Health. 2012 Sep;45(5):283–90. PMID: 23091653

138. Mager DR. Orthostatic hypotension: pathophysiology, problems, and prevention. Home Healthc Nurse. 2012 Oct;30(9):525–30, quiz 530–2. doi: http://dx.doi.org/10.1097/NHH.0b013e31826a6805 PMID: 23026987

139. Shaw BH, Claydon VE. The relationship between orthostatic hypotension and falling in older adults. Clin Auton Res. 2014 Feb;24(1):3–13. PMID: 24253897

140. Tinetti ME, Kumar C. The patient who falls: "It's always a trade-off". JAMA. 2010 Jan 20;303(3):258–66. doi: http://dx.doi.org/10.1001/jama.2009.2024 PMID: 20085954

141. Ungar A, Rafanelli M, Iacomelli I, Brunetti MA, Ceccofiglio A, Tesi F, et al. Fall prevention in the elderly. Clin Cases Miner Bone Metab. 2013 May;10(2):91–5. PMID: 24133524

142. Cameron ID, Gillespie LD, Robertson MC, Murray GR, Hill KD, Cumming RG, et al. Interventions for preventing falls in older people in care facilities and hospitals. Cochrane Database Syst Rev. 2012;12(12):CD005465. PMID: 23235623

143. Järvinen TL, Sievänen H, Khan KM, Heinonen A, Kannus P. Shifting the focus in fracture prevention from osteoporosis to falls. BMJ. 2008 Jan 19;336(7636):124–6. doi: http://dx.doi.org/10.1136/bmj.39428.470752.AD PMID: 18202065

144. Grundstrom AC, Guse CE, Layde PM. Risk factors for falls and fall-related injuries in adults 85 years of age and older. Arch Gerontol Geriatr. 2012 May-Jun;54(3):421–8. doi: http://dx.doi.org/10.1016/j.archger.2011.06.008 PMID: 21862143

145. Low PA. Prevalence of orthostatic hypotension. Clin Auton Res. 2008 Mar;18 Suppl 1:8–13. PMID: 18368301

146. Muraki S, Akune T, Ishimoto Y, Nagata K, Yoshida M, Tanaka S, et al. Risk factors for falls in a longitudinal population-based cohort study of Japanese men and women: the ROAD Study. Bone. 2013 Jan;52(1):516–23. doi: http://dx.doi.org/10.1016/j.bone.2012.10.020 PMID: 23103329

147. Patino CM, McKean-Cowdin R, Azen SP, Allison JC, Choudhury F, Varma R; Los Angeles Latino Eye Study Group. Central and peripheral visual impairment and the risk of falls and falls with injury. Ophthalmology. 2010 Feb;117(2):199–206.e1. PMID: 20031225

148. Reed-Jones RJ, Solis GR, Lawson KA, Loya AM, Cude-Islas D, Berger CS. Vision and falls: a multidisciplinary review of the contributions of visual impairment to falls among older adults. Maturitas. 2013 May;75(1):22–8. doi: http://dx.doi.org/10.1016/j.maturitas.2013.01.019 PMID: 23434262

149. Blanchflower DG, Oswald AJ. Is well-being U-shaped over the life cycle? Soc Sci Med. 2008 Apr;66(8):1733–49. doi: http://dx.doi.org/10.1016/j.socscimed.2008.01.030 PMID: 18316146

150. Steptoe A, Deaton A, Stone AA. Subjective wellbeing, health, and ageing. Lancet. 2015 Feb 14;385(9968):640–8. doi: http://dx.doi.org/10.1016/S0140-6736(13)61489-0 PMID: 25468152

151. Lee C, Dobson AJ, Brown WJ, Bryson L, Byles J, Warner-Smith P, et al. Cohort Profile: the Australian Longitudinal Study on Women's Health. Int J Epidemiol. 2005 Oct;34(5):987–91. doi: http://dx.doi.org/10.1093/ije/dyi098 PMID:15894591 PMID: 15894591

152. Brooks-Wilson AR. Genetics of healthy aging and longevity. Hum Genet. 2013 Dec;132(12):1323–38. doi: http://dx.doi.org/10.1007/s00439-013-1342-z PMID: 23925498

153. Commission on Social Determinants of Health. Closing the gap in a generation: health equity through action on the social determinants of health. Final report of the Commission on Social Determinants of Health. Geneva: World Health Organization; 2008. (http://whqlibdoc.who.int/publications/2008/9789241563703_eng.pdf, accessed 5 June 2015).

154. WHO World Health Survey. In: World Health Organization, Health statistics and information systems [website]. Geneva: World Health Organization; 2015 (http://www.who.int/healthinfo/survey/en/, accessed 23 June 2015).

155. Plath D. International policy perspectives on independence in old age. J Aging Soc Policy. 2009 Apr-Jun;21(2):209–23. doi: http://dx.doi.org/10.1080/08959420902733173 PMID: 19333843

156. Kendig H, Hashimoto A, Coppard L. Family support for the elderly: the international experience. Oxford: Oxford University Press; 1992.

157. Aboderin I. Intergenerational support and old age in Africa. New Brunswick (New Jersey): Transaction Publishers; 2009.

158. Kunkel SR, Brown JS, Whittington FJ. Global aging: comparative perspectives on aging and the life course. New York: Springer; 2014. (http://USYD.eblib.com.au/patron/FullRecord.aspx?p=1611870, accessed 5 June 2015).

159. Phillips D, Cheng K. The impact of changing value systems on social inclusion: an Asia-Pacific perspective. In: Scharf T, Keating N, editors. From exclusion to inclusion in old age. Bristol: Policy Press; 2012. 109–24. doi: http://dx.doi.org/10.1332/policypress/9781847427731.003.0007

160. Michel JP, Newton JL, Kirkwood TB. Medical challenges of improving the quality of a longer life. JAMA. 2008 Feb 13;299(6):688–90. doi: http://dx.doi.org/10.1001/jama.299.6.688 PMID: 18270358

161. Haveman-Nies A, de Groot L, Burema J, Cruz JA, Osler M, van Staveren WA; SENECA Investigators. Dietary quality and lifestyle factors in relation to 10-year mortality in older Europeans: the SENECA study. Am J Epidemiol. 2002 Nov 15;156(10):962–8. doi: http://dx.doi.org/10.1093/aje/kwf144 PMID: 12419769

162. Hrobonova E, Breeze E, Fletcher AE. Higher levels and intensity of physical activity are associated with reduced mortality among community dwelling older people. J Aging Res. 2011;2011:651931. doi: http://dx.doi.org/10.4061/2011/651931 PMID: 21437004

163. Gupta PC, Mehta HC. Cohort study of all-cause mortality among tobacco users in Mumbai, India. Bull World Health Organ. 2000;78(7):877–83. PMID: 10994260

164. Musini VM, Tejani AM, Bassett K, Wright JM. Pharmacotherapy for hypertension in the elderly. Cochrane Database Syst Rev. 2009; (4):CD000028. PMID: 19821263

165. Estruch R, Ros E, Salas-Salvadó J, Covas MI, Corella D, Arós F, et al.; PREDIMED Study Investigators. Primary prevention of cardiovascular disease with a Mediterranean diet. N Engl J Med. 2013 Apr 4;368(14):1279–90. doi: http://dx.doi.org/10.1056/NEJMoa1200303 PMID: 23432189

166. Peto R, Darby S, Deo H, Silcocks P, Whitley E, Doll R. Smoking, smoking cessation, and lung cancer in the UK since 1950: combination of national statistics with two case-control studies. BMJ. 2000 Aug 5;321(7257):323–9. doi: http://dx.doi.org/10.1136/bmj.321.7257.323 PMID: 10926586

167. Andrieu S, Aboderin I, Baeyens JP, Beard J, Benetos A, Berrut G, et al. IAGG workshop: health promotion program on prevention of late onset dementia. J Nutr Health Aging. 2011 Aug;15(7):562–75. doi: http://dx.doi.org/10.1007/s12603-011-0142-1 PMID: 21808935

168. Lloyd-Sherlock P, Beard J, Minicuci N, Ebrahim S, Chatterji S. Hypertension among older adults in low- and middle-income countries: prevalence, awareness and control. Int J Epidemiol. 2014 Feb;43(1):116–28. doi: http://dx.doi.org/10.1093/ije/dyt215 PMID: 24505082

169. Arem H, Moore SC, Patel A, Hartge P, Berrington de Gonzalez A, Visvanathan K, et al. Leisure time physical activity and mortality: a detailed pooled analysis of the dose-response relationship. JAMA Intern Med. 2015 Jun;175(6):959–67. PMID: 25844730

170. Paterson DH, Warburton DE. Physical activity and functional limitations in older adults: a systematic review related to Canada's Physical Activity Guidelines. Int J Behav Nutr Phys Act. 2010;7(1):38. doi: http://dx.doi.org/10.1186/1479-5868-7-38 PMID: 20459782

171. Tak E, Kuiper R, Chorus A, Hopman-Rock M. Prevention of onset and progression of basic ADL disability by physical activity in community dwelling older adults: a meta-analysis. Ageing Res Rev. 2013 Jan;12(1):329–38. doi: http://dx.doi.org/10.1016/j.arr.2012.10.001 PMID: 23063488

172. Liu CJ, Latham NK. Progressive resistance strength training for improving physical function in older adults. Cochrane Database Syst Rev. 2009; (3):CD002759. PMID: 19588334

173. Jak AJ. The impact of physical and mental activity on cognitive aging. Curr Top Behav Neurosci. 2012;10:273–91. PMID: 21818703

174. Blondell SJ, Hammersley-Mather R, Veerman JL. Does physical activity prevent cognitive decline and dementia?: A systematic review and meta-analysis of longitudinal studies. BMC Public Health. 2014;14(1):510. doi: http://dx.doi.org/10.1186/1471-2458-14-510 PMID: 24885250

175. Norton S, Matthews FE, Barnes DE, Yaffe K, Brayne C. Potential for primary prevention of Alzheimer's disease: an analysis of population-based data. Lancet Neurol. 2014 Aug;13(8):788–94. doi: http://dx.doi.org/10.1016/S1474-4422(14)70136-X PMID: 25030513

176. Diep L, Kwagyan J, Kurantsin-Mills J, Weir R, Jayam-Trouth A. Association of physical activity level and stroke outcomes in men and women: a meta-analysis. J Womens Health (Larchmt). 2010 Oct;19(10):1815–22. doi: http://dx.doi.org/10.1089/jwh.2009.1708 PMID: 20929415

177. Bauman A, Singh M, Buchner D, Merom D, Bull F. Physical activity in older adults. Gerontologist. 2016 (In press.).

178. Saelens BE, Papadopoulos C. The importance of the built environment in older adults' physical activity: a review of the literature. Wash State J Public Health Pract. 2008;1(1):13–21.

179. Pollock ML, Franklin BA, Balady GJ, Chaitman BL, Fleg JL, Fletcher B, et al. AHA Science Advisory. Resistance exercise in individuals with and without cardiovascular disease: benefits, rationale, safety, and prescription: An advisory from the Committee on Exercise, Rehabilitation, and Prevention, Council on Clinical Cardiology, American Heart Association; Position paper endorsed by the American College of Sports Medicine. Circulation. 2000 Feb 22;101(7):828–33. doi: http://dx.doi.org/10.1161/01.CIR.101.7.828 PMID: 10683360

180. Howe TE, Rochester L, Neil F, Skelton DA, Ballinger C. Exercise for improving balance in older people. Cochrane Database Syst Rev. 2011; (11):CD004963. PMID: 22071817

181. Sherrington C, Whitney JC, Lord SR, Herbert RD, Cumming RG, Close JC. Effective exercise for the prevention of falls: a systematic review and meta-analysis. J Am Geriatr Soc. 2008 Dec;56(12):2234–43. doi: http://dx.doi.org/10.1111/j.1532-5415.2008.02014.x PMID: 19093923

182. Voukelatos A, Merom D, Sherrington C, Rissel C, Cumming RG, Lord SR. The impact of a home-based walking programme on falls in older people: the Easy Steps randomised controlled trial. Age Ageing. 2015 May;44(3):377–83. doi: http://dx.doi.org/10.1093/ageing/afu186 PMID: 25572426

183. Kshetrimayum N, Reddy CV, Siddhana S, Manjunath M, Rudraswamy S, Sulavai S. Oral health-related quality of life and nutritional status of institutionalized elderly population aged 60 years and above in Mysore City, India. Gerodontology. 2013 Jun;30(2):119–25. doi: http://dx.doi.org/10.1111/j.1741-2358.2012.00651.x PMID: 22364560

184. Petersen PE, Kandelman D, Arpin S, Ogawa H. Global oral health of older people–call for public health action. Community Dent Health. 2010 Dec;27(4) Suppl 2:257–67. PMID: 21313969

185. Elia M, Stratton RJ. Geographical inequalities in nutrient status and risk of malnutrition among English people aged 65 y and older. Nutrition. 2005 Nov-Dec;21(11-12):1100–6. doi: http://dx.doi.org/10.1016/j.nut.2005.03.005 PMID: 16308132

186. Risonar MG, Rayco-Solon P, Ribaya-Mercado JD, Solon JA, Cabalda AB, Tengco LW, et al. Physical activity, energy requirements, and adequacy of dietary intakes of older persons in a rural Filipino community. Nutr J. 2009;8(1):19. doi: http://dx.doi.org/10.1186/1475-2891-8-19 PMID: 19409110

187. Shahar S, Ibrahim Z, Fatah AR, Rahman SA, Yusoff NA, Arshad F, et al. A multidimensional assessment of nutritional and health status of rural elderly Malays. Asia Pac J Clin Nutr. 2007;16(2):346–53. PMID: 17468093

188. Morley JE, Silver AJ. Nutritional issues in nursing home care. Ann Intern Med. 1995 Dec 1;123(11):850–9. doi: http://dx.doi.org/10.7326/0003-4819-123-11-199512010-00008 PMID: 7486469

189. Pérez Llamas F, Moregó A, Tóbaruela M, García MD, Santo E, Zamora S. Prevalencia de desnutrición e influencia de la suplementación nutricional oral sobre el estado nutricional en ancianos institucionalizados [Prevalence of malnutrition and influence of oral nutritional supplementation on nutritional status in institutionalized elderly]. Nutr Hosp. 2011 Sep-Oct;26(5):1134–40. PMID: 22072365

190. Rodríguez N, Hernández R, Herrera H, Barbosa J, Hernández-Valera Y. Estado nutricional de adultos mayores institucionalizados venezolanos. [Nutritional status of institutionalized Venezuelan elderly.] Invest Clin. 2005 Sep;46(3):219–28. PMID: 16152778

191. Shabayek MM, Saleh SI. Nutritional status of institutionalized and free-living elderly in Alexandria. J Egypt Public Health Assoc. 2000;75(5-6):437–59. PMID: 17219883

192. Vellas B, Guigoz Y, Garry PJ, Nourhashemi F, Bennahum D, Lauque S, et al. The Mini Nutritional Assessment (MNA) and its use in grading the nutritional state of elderly patients. Nutrition. 1999 Feb;15(2):116–22. doi: http://dx.doi.org/10.1016/S0899-9007(98)00171-3 PMID: 9990575

193. Aliabadi M, Kimiagar M, Ghayour-Mobarhan M, Shakeri MT, Nematy M, Ilaty AA, et al. Prevalence of malnutrition in free living elderly people in Iran: a cross-sectional study. Asia Pac J Clin Nutr. 2008;17(2):285–9. PMID: 18586650

194. Beck AM, Kjær S, Hansen BS, Storm RL, Thal-Jantzen K, Bitz C. Follow-up home visits with registered dietitians have a positive effect on the functional and nutritional status of geriatric medical patients after discharge: a randomized controlled trial. Clin Rehabil. 2013 Jun;27(6):483–93. doi: http://dx.doi.org/10.1177/0269215512469384 PMID: 23258932

195. Tomata Y, Kakizaki M, Suzuki Y, Hashimoto S, Kawado M, Tsuji I. Impact of the 2011 Great East Japan Earthquake and Tsunami on functional disability among older people: a longitudinal comparison of disability prevalence among Japanese municipalities. J Epidemiol Community Health. 2014 Jun;68(6):530–3. doi: http://dx.doi.org/10.1136/jech-2013-203541 PMID: 24570399

196. Hirai H, Kondo N, Sasaki R, Iwamuro S, Masuno K, Ohtsuka R, et al. Distance to retail stores and risk of being homebound among older adults in a city severely affected by the 2011 Great East Japan Earthquake. Age Ageing. 2015 May;44(3):478–84. PMID: 25315229

197. Displacement and older people: the case of the Great East Japan Earthquake and Tsunami of 2011. Chiang Mai, Thailand: Help Age International; 2013 (http://www.helpage.org/silo/files/displacement-and-older-people-the-case-of-the-great-east-japan-earthquake-and-tsunami-of-2011.pdf, accessed 5 June 2015).

198. Elder abuse. Geneva: World Health Organization; 2014 (Fact Sheet No. 357; http://www.who.int/mediacentre/factsheets/fs357/en/, accessed 5 June 2015).

199. Krug E, Dahlberg LL, Mercy J, Zwi AB, Lozano R, editors. World report on violence and health. Geneva: World Health Organization; 2002. (http://whqlibdoc.who.int/publications/2002/9241545615_eng.pdf?ua=1, accessed 5 June 2015).

200. Dong X, Simon M, Mendes de Leon C, Fulmer T, Beck T, Hebert L, et al. Elder self-neglect and abuse and mortality risk in a community-dwelling population. JAMA. 2009 Aug 5;302(5):517–26. doi: http://dx.doi.org/10.1001/jama.2009.1109 PMID: 19654386

201. Schofield MJ, Powers JR, Loxton D. Mortality and disability outcomes of self-reported elder abuse: a 12-year prospective investigation. J Am Geriatr Soc. 2013 May;61(5):679–85. doi: http://dx.doi.org/10.1111/jgs.12212 PMID: 23590291

202. Dong X, Simon MA. Elder abuse as a risk factor for hospitalization in older persons. JAMA Intern Med. 2013 May 27;173(10):911–7. doi: http://dx.doi.org/10.1001/jamainternmed.2013.238 PMID: 23567991

203. Dong X, Chen R, Simon MA. Elder abuse and dementia: a review of the research and health policy. Health Aff (Millwood). 2014 Apr;33(4):642–9. doi: http://dx.doi.org/10.1377/hlthaff.2013.1261 PMID: 24711326

204. Lachs MS, Williams CS, O'Brien S, Pillemer KA. Adult protective service use and nursing home placement. Gerontologist. 2002 Dec;42(6):734–9. doi: http://dx.doi.org/10.1093/geront/42.6.734 PMID: 12451154

205. Pillemer KA, Burnes D, Riffin C, Lachs MS. Elder abuse. Gerontologist. 2016. Forthcoming.http://www.ncbi.nlm.nih.gov/entrez/query.fcgi?cmd=Retrieve&db=PubMed&list_uids=3342992&dopt=Abstract PMID: 3342992

206. Johannesen M, LoGiudice D. Elder abuse: a systematic review of risk factors in community-dwelling elders. Age Ageing. 2013 May;42(3):292–8. doi: http://dx.doi.org/10.1093/ageing/afs195 PMID: 23343837

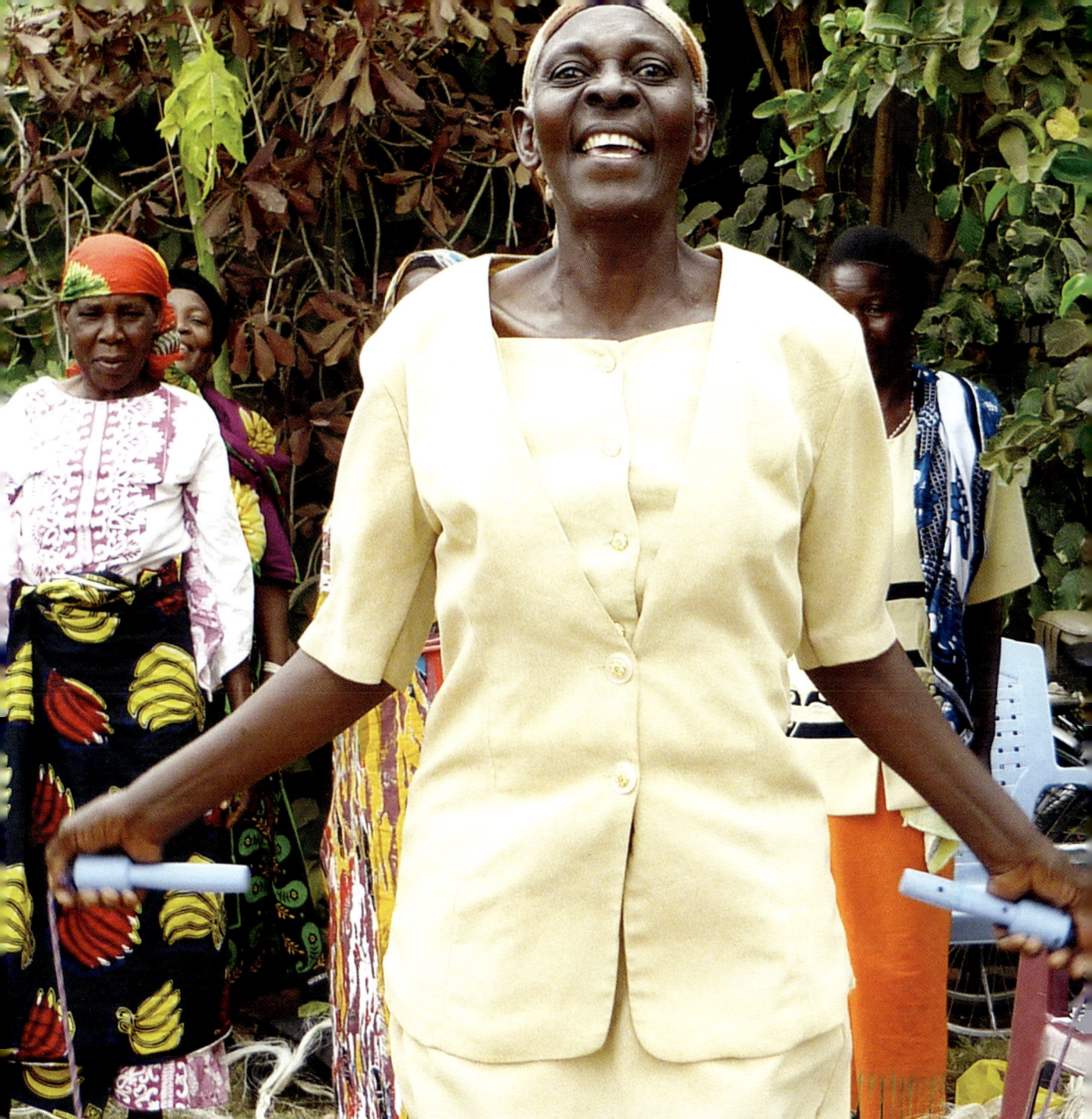

Chapter 4
Health systems

Margaret, 61, Tanzania

Margaret, is a retired law enforcement officer, and struggled to adapt to her financial and social status after retirement.

"I was married for 21 years until my husband died. I have four children, three boys and one girl. They live in Dar es Salaam. I take care of my three grandchildren on my own. It is very difficult. They have a lot of needs and I do not have the money to support them. I get only a little help from my children. Sometimes I skip meals so my grandchildren can go to school, it is better for me to eat, but they should go to school. Everything I have I direct to them.

When I was younger I had a good life with a monthly salary. I worked as a prison officer and then as a police officer. I was in the police force for 28 years. After I retired I had a lot of financial worries. I had to wait six months to get my police pension and it was only a small amount of money. I suffered from high blood pressure and depression because I did not have enough money to survive. I was finding life so difficult I stopped exercising because I was depressed and eating was a problem. When you don't work anymore people don't visit – their concern and attention goes away. I was very lonely and angry at everyone; I felt like I was dying before I joined the active ageing association.

When I was a police officer I used to be in the netball team. I was always physically fit. Now I am in a group I am exercising again. We do exercise classes, basket weaving and playing games like cards. I have learnt a lot of things about being healthy. …I am in much better health now; I do not have depression anymore or high blood pressure. I am also physically fit again. I find comfort in the group – I have company so I am no longer lonely. I also get information about my rights. Now I know that I should get free healthcare. I have learnt so much from the group it has given me the light – the way forward."

4

Health systems

Introduction

Chapter 3 outlines the complex health-related changes that occur in older age. Combined, these result in a general trend towards declining capacity with age and the increasing likelihood of having more than one clinical condition requiring ongoing monitoring or treatment. The marked heterogeneity in these trends emphasizes the potential for interventions to improve health, particularly for those with the most marked declines in capacity. Ensuring access to appropriate health services will be essential to overcoming these inequalities.

Yet today there are many barriers that limit the access of older people to health services, particularly in lower-income countries and among disadvantaged people in higher-income countries. Furthermore, when older people do have access, they are often faced with services that are not designed to meet their needs.

This chapter outlines the common gaps in current systems and explores the challenges to improving the quality of health care for older people. It then describes in detail the kind of health system that can deliver comprehensive and person-centred services to older populations, and the policy-level actions that can enhance this transformation.

Evidence from low- and middle-income countries is often lacking, so much of this discussion focuses on what is known from experiences in higher-income countries. However, the lessons learnt from high-income settings are pertinent to all countries.

Rising demand, barriers to use, poorly aligned services

Demand for health services

Because the health dynamics of older age are related to increased needs for health care, it might be expected that increasing age would be associated with increased health-care utilization. And given that the burden of disease and declines in capacity are greater in low- and middle-income countries, it might also be expected that this trend would be more marked in low-resource settings. However, evidence indicates there is a disconnect between health-care need and health-care utilization, both in these settings and in disadvantaged subgroups of older people in high-income settings. Fig. 4.1 uses data from the *WHO World Health Survey* to display the association between age and self-reported use of inpatient and outpatient services (*1*). In high-income countries, health-care utilization (particularly of inpatient care) appears to increase with age.

Yet this trend is not so marked in middle-income countries, and in low-income countries it disappears completely. This is consistent with research from sub-Saharan Africa showing that despite older people being in poorer health than those in younger age groups, older people use health services significantly less frequently (*2, 3*). This suggests there is significant unmet need and major service gaps in these settings. These patterns of utilization likely result from barriers to access, a lack of appropriate services and the prioritization of services towards the acute needs of younger people (and often it may be older people themselves who are responsible for making such decisions). These shortcomings are discussed in the section Barriers to use.

Even though a general trend towards an increase in demand for health (and long-term) care with age is present at the population level in high-income settings, the demand for health care may be quite variable within these populations and among individuals. This is not simply due to variations in health and functional status, although these do influence health-care use (*4*). Older people in high-income countries who have chronic health conditions tend to use more health care than those who do not have such conditions. Service use also rises with the number of multimorbid conditions (*5, 6*), and people who have both chronic conditions and functional limitations use services the most (*7*).

But another key determinant of this diversity in health-care utilization is socioeconomic status. Although the need for health care is likely to be higher among disadvantaged individuals, an analysis that included 12 European coun-

Fig. 4.1. **Percentage of respondents reporting use of health services, by age group and country income levels**

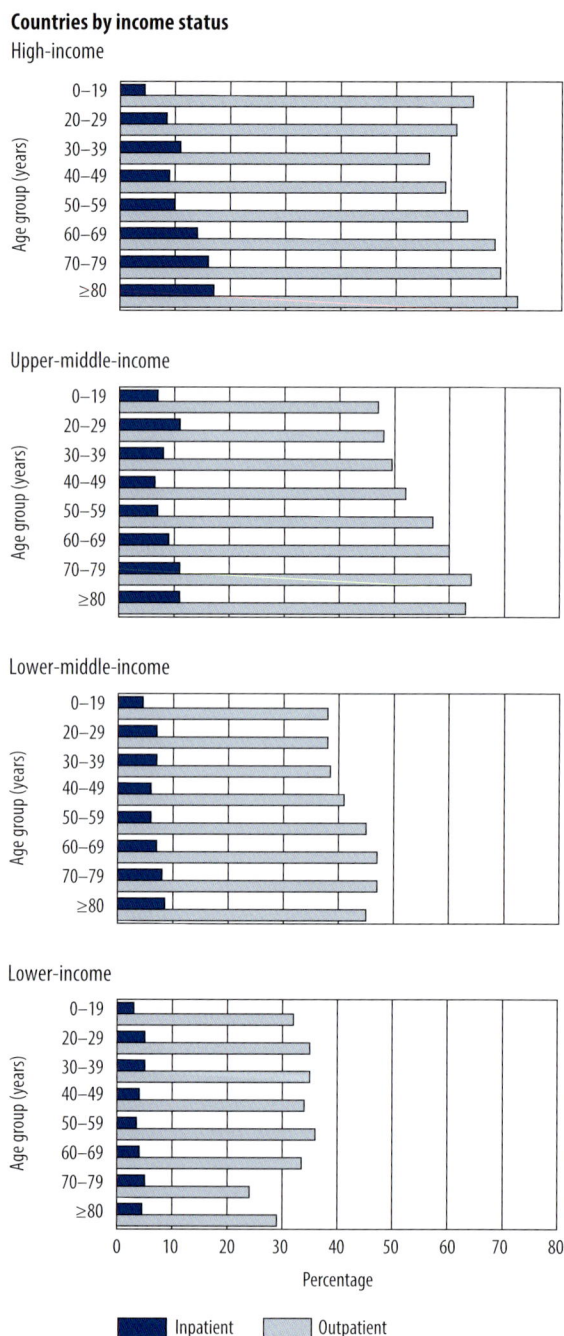

Source: (*1*).

tries found that among older adults with equal levels of need, lower socioeconomic status was associated with less frequent visits to medical specialists and dentists, but the trend was less apparent for hospitalizations and visits to general practitioners (8). Reduced access to health care among disadvantaged older people has also been observed in the United States (9). Even in high-income settings, those in greatest need may be those who use health services least.

Thus, although population ageing is likely to be associated with increasing health needs, particularly in low- and middle-income countries, the association with the demand for, and utilization of, health services is less clear-cut. Furthermore, both among and within nations, it is likely that disadvantaged older people are caught between their greater need for health care and having less access to, or less use of, appropriate services. In all countries, one key component of a health-systems response to population ageing must therefore be to breakdown the barriers that limit health-care utilization by the older people who need it.

Barriers to use

The barriers that many older people face in accessing health care are summarized in Table 4.1, which uses data from older people in the *WHO World Health Survey* (1). In low- and lower-middle-income countries, the greatest barriers appear to arise from the cost of the health-care visit and transportation. In total, more than 60% of older people in low-income countries did not access health care because of the cost of the visit, they did not have transportation, or they could not pay for transportation. Transportation may be a particularly important issue for older people who live in rural areas because services are often concentrated in large cities far from people's homes and communities (10). In contrast, in high-income countries the greatest barriers reported by older people appear to come from having been treated badly by health-care professionals in the past or older people perceiving themselves to be not sick enough to seek health care.

In countries where older people or their families must pay out of pocket for their care, wealth is

Table 4.1.   Reasons given by adults aged 60 years or older for not accessing health-care services, by countries' income category

Reason for not accessing health-care services	Country income category (% of respondents)			
	High-income	Upper-middle-income	Lower-middle-income	Low-income
Could not afford the visit	15.7	30.9[a]	60.9[a]	60.2[a]
No transport	12.1	19.3[a]	20.7[a]	29.1[a]
Could not afford transport	8.7	12.9[a]	28.1[a]	33.0[a]
Health-care provider's equipment inadequate	11.2	10.5	14.1[a]	16.7[a]
Health-care provider's skills inadequate	19.0	8.3	7.8	13.1[a]
Previously treated badly	23.8	8.7	7.9	8.3
Did not know where to go	12.2	9.7	9.8	7.8
Was not sick enough	21.5	31.8	27.3	25.8
Tried but was denied health care	20.0	16.2	8.3	8.5[a]
Other	43.8	22.5[a]	23.5[a]	13.9

[a] Results are significantly different (P < 0.05) from those reported by adults younger than 60 years.
Source: (1).

a strong determinant of health-care use (*4*). Data from SAGE, for example, showed that household wealth played an important part in determining health-care use among older Chinese and Ghanaians: the higher a person's wealth quintile, the more likely the person was to seek care (*11*). Of note, these were precisely the same countries in which respondents reported the greatest use of out-of-pocket payments, as shown in Fig. 4.2.

Affordability barriers also affect high-income countries, but can vary with the design of the health system. Research from the Commonwealth Fund (*6*), for example, shows that in the United States almost 20% of older adults miss health-care treatments due to cost-related issues, but in France only 3% of older adults report this problem (Fig. 4.3).

Other widespread barriers to access may arise from the failure of health services to account for the limitations in capacity common in older people. This occurs regardless of a country's income category and includes barriers such as a lack of accessible toilets, long queues for care, physical barriers to access, and communication barriers resulting from a lack of accessible infor-

Fig. 4.3. Percentage of adults aged 65 years or older who had problems accessing health-care services during the past year due to their cost, 11 countries, 2014

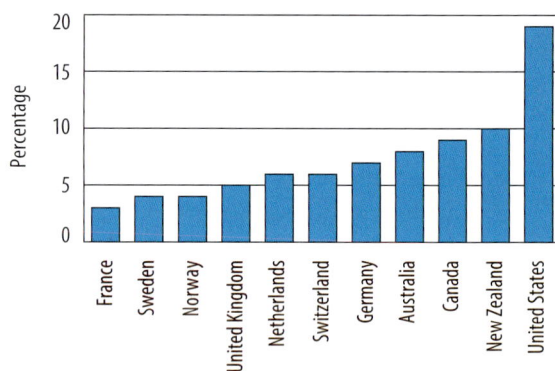

Note: Because of the cost, respondents with a medical problem did not visit a doctor, missed a medical test or treatment recommended by a doctor, did not fill out a prescription or missed a dose of medicine, or a combination of these.
Source: (*6*).

Fig. 4.2. Sources of payment for outpatient care (%), adults aged 50 years and older in six countries, 2007–2010

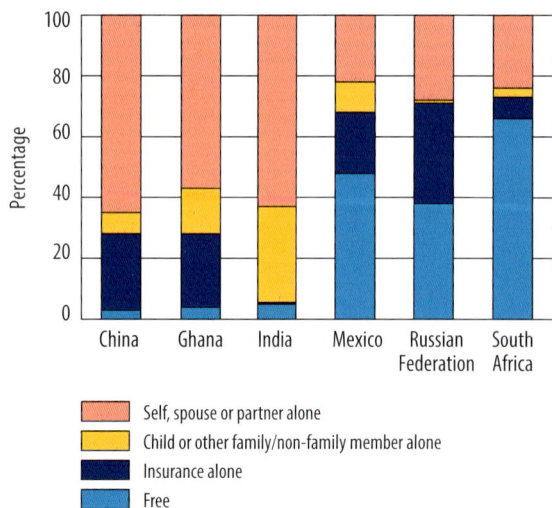

Self, spouse or partner alone
Child or other family/non-family member alone
Insurance alone
Free

Source: (*11*).

Box 4.1. A priority pass card helps older people access health services in Kuwait

In 2012, Kuwait implemented a simple but effective measure to improve the accessibility and delivery of health services to older people: it distributed a card granting priority access to older people to both general walk-in clinics and appointment-based chronic-disease management clinics. The Ministry of Health launched a media campaign to announce the introduction of the card, which was made available through local primary health-care centres. More than 31 000 cards have been distributed, corresponding to about 51% of the eligible population.

An initial survey revealed that card holders reported dramatically reduced waiting times and spending more time with their treating physicians. Some also said that they felt special when using their card and valued their preferential treatment as a sign of appreciation and respect.

mation for people with hearing loss or visual impairment, or both. Long waiting times and waiting in a queue can be particularly challenging for older people with physical disabilities or mobility restrictions, and for those with urinary incontinence (*12, 13*). Several countries in sub-Saharan Africa and elsewhere have taken steps to combat this problem, for example by reserving times at clinics only for older people (Box 4.1).

Systems designed for different problems

Those older people who are able to access health care will typically encounter a system that is not designed to address their needs. Instead, health services are often structured to diagnose and cure time-limited health issues using a biomedically based approach that emphasizes finding the problem and fixing it, which worked well when acute conditions or communicable diseases were the priority. Historically, paying attention to long-term health and functioning have been less of a priority.

In contrast, the health and social needs of ageing populations are typically complex and long-term, spanning a range of areas of functioning, and waxing and waning over time. As noted in Chapter 3, the risk of noncommunicable health conditions increases with age, and comorbidity becomes the norm rather than the exception. Chronic disease processes overlap and intersect with the underlying ageing process and ultimately impact on the intrinsic capacity of the older person. These complex dynamics require approaches that are different from those developed to address more acute problems.

Lack of coordination

It is not uncommon for numerous health professionals to be involved in the care of any given older person, especially in countries where there is a good availability of medical specialists. For example, in one survey of older adults across 11 high-income countries, 39% of respondents from

Germany had seen four or more doctors during the past year. Also, more than half of older adults in the United States and about 40% of older people in eight other high-income countries were taking four or more medications regularly (*6*).

To be safe and effective, the involvement of several health professionals and the use of multiple, potentially interacting interventions, necessitates a high degree of coordination over time, both between health professionals and across treatment levels and settings. Yet health systems often fall short in facilitating this coordination, leaving the burden on the older person or their family to communicate relevant health information when needed. Consequently, many older people suffer from gaps in the coordination of their care. In the survey described in the previous paragraph, up to 41% of respondents in Germany reported having problems with care coordination during the past 2 years (Fig. 4.4) (*6*).

Fig. 4.4.   Percentage of adults aged 65 years or older who experienced problems with the coordination of their care during the past 2 years, 11 countries, 2014

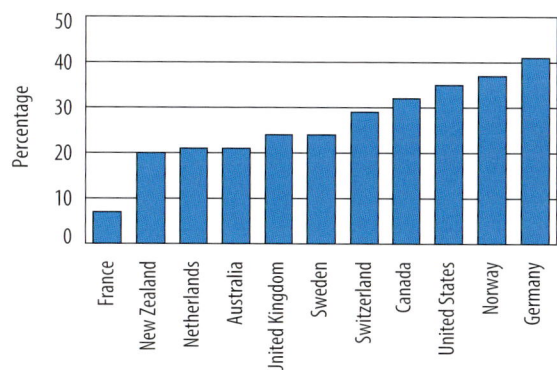

Note: Problems with care coordination included test results or records not being available at the time of an appointment, duplicate tests being ordered, receiving conflicting information from different doctors, a specialist lacking the patient's medical history or the regular doctor not being informed about specialist care, or a combination of these.
Source: (6).

Unprepared health workers

Health professionals are often unprepared to deal with the health-care needs of older adults. Many current training approaches were developed in the 20th century, when acute infectious diseases were the world's most prevalent health problems (14). As a result, health workers are trained primarily to identify and treat symptoms and conditions using an episodic approach to care.

This does not prepare them well for the holistic perspective that has been shown to be most effective when caring for older people, or to controlling and managing the consequences of chronic conditions in ways that fit with an older person's priorities (15–17). Health workers are often trained to respond to pressing health concerns, rather than to proactively anticipate and counter changes in function, and are rarely trained to work with older people to ensure they can increase control over their own health (14, 18, 19).

Furthermore, although most patients within health systems are older, curricula frequently overlook gerontological and geriatric knowledge and training, and may lack guidance on managing common problems, such as multimorbidity and frailty (20). For example, a survey of 36 countries found that 27% of medical schools did not conduct any training in geriatric medicine: this included 19% of schools in high-income countries, 43% of schools in economies in transition, and 38% of all schools in other countries (21). Moreover, medical trainees often fail to learn the sort of comprehensive biopsychosocial approaches necessary to treat older populations (22). Instead, their training is biomedical and often compartmentalized according to their disease specialty. These training deficiencies extend to other health workers (19, 23). This gap is particularly important in low- and middle-income countries, where these professionals are likely to form the front line in engaging with older people (Box 4.2).

Improving knowledge and skills in geriatric care is thus crucial for all health professions. This will require overcoming a widespread lack of faculty, lack of funding, lack of time in curricula that are already full, and the lack of recognition of the importance of geriatric training (19).

Furthermore, ensuring that health-care workers have skills and knowledge in geriatric care will probably not be sufficient on its own. Most health workers will also need competency in several nonmedical processes, including using shared decision-making, implementing team-based care, using information technology, and engaging in continual quality improvement (26). They will also need to be trained to overcome the ageist attitudes that are widespread in health-care settings.

> ### Box 4.2. Ghana: harnessing the potential of community health workers
>
> Ghana has undertaken reforms to better meet the needs of its rapidly ageing population (24). In 2010, it released its *National ageing policy: ageing with security and dignity* (25), and in 2011, it undertook a national assessment of the health situation and health-systems responses to ageing. The assessment identified significant treatment gaps and the need to better integrate the care of older people into existing health services. Specifically, stakeholders proposed using Ghana's well-established community health worker programme to meet the needs of its older population.
>
> Community health workers are the backbone of the Ghanaian health system, but before reform they would systematically exclude older people from their assessments of households' health needs. Successfully integrating an awareness of the issues associated with ageing into their work will require several components: training in *Healthy Ageing* issues; developing protocols and job aids on ageing and health; strengthening the links between communities and primary health-care providers; and defining performance targets and monitoring achievements within the overall programme. Efforts are underway to implement this strategy.

Ageism within health care

Ageism within health care can take several forms, including health-care workers having negative attitudes towards older people or the ageing process, engaging in patronizing behaviour, failing to consult older people about their preferences for care, and discouraging or restricting access to otherwise-indicated medical interventions.

Ageist attitudes are widespread in many societies and further reinforced during medical education. Medical students are rarely trained to handle the multiple and complex health issues and priorities of older adults, or to understand their priorities (22, 27). Textbooks often focus almost exclusively on the problems of ageing and underreport successes, which gives students narrow views of the ageing process.

Some health-care workers believe that their older clients are not capable of sharing in decision-making about their own care. Physicians in many countries fail to initiate discussions with older people about their care preferences (6), and doctors may be more responsive, egalitarian, patient, respectful and optimistic with younger clients than with older clients (27, 28).

Older people may also suffer from health-care rationing based on the notion that health services are a limited resource and must be allocated to achieve the greatest good for the greatest number of people (29). Proponents of this view argue that chronological age is an ethical, objective and cost-effective criterion for allocating health care because older people have already enjoyed life and have less future life to enjoy (29).

However, there are strong counter-arguments to these approaches, ranging from equity-based and rights-based perspectives to arguments emphasizing that at any point in time older people have made the greatest contributions to the socioeconomic development that allowed the services to be created, so they should at least be entitled to some of the benefits. But perhaps the greatest argument against the age-based rationing of health care is the lack of a clear association between chronological age and health. Prioritizing services for someone aged 55 years who has multimorbidities and a limited life expectancy over services for someone aged 70 years who is in good health and has a longer life expectancy is not consistent with the argument used to justify the age-based rationing of services. The rationing of health care based on chronological age is simply an example of discrimination against older people (30, 31).

Economic impact of population ageing on health systems

This report argues that investments in health systems can yield significant dividends in the health and well-being of older people. Key questions arise for policy-makers. Will the benefits of these investments be outweighed by the health-care costs of a longer life? What overall impact will population ageing have on health-care expenditures?

For many reasons it is extremely difficult to predict the impact that population ageing will have on health-care expenditures. First, although older age is generally associated with an increased need for care, the link between the need for care and utilization is weak. For example, despite the high burden of disease in low-income settings, older people tend to use health services significantly less often than younger adults (2, 3). Even in high-income countries, poorer older people, who generally have greater needs, tend to use services less often than their more financially secure peers (8, 9).

Even if these inequalities in demands for care were overcome and overall demand increased to better match needs, the link between age and health-care expenditures is not linear. Indeed, there is growing evidence from high-income countries that starting at around age 70, health-care expenditure per person falls significantly, and expenditures made outside the traditional health system increase (32–34).

For example, a recent analysis of expenditures by the Torbay Care Trust in England found that expenditures increased across all services as age increased, but beyond a peak at ages 65–74 years, expenditures fell for acute and elective admissions to hospital as well as for outpatient visits (Fig. 4.5) (32). Although it is important to rule

Fig. 4.5. **Annual cost of health-care services, by age group and type of service, Torbay (population, 145 000), England, 2010–2011**

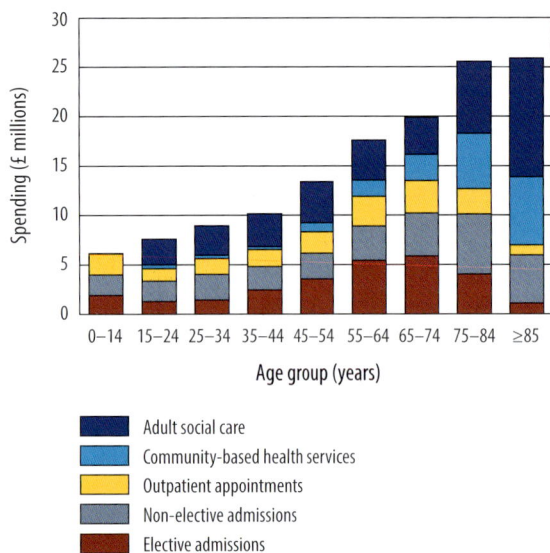

Source: (*32*).

out aged-based discrimination and rationing of health services as the major factors underlying these findings, they suggest the possibility that as population distributions move towards increasingly older ages health-care expenditures might actually fall. The findings also emphasize the need for health care and long-term care systems to work in an integrated fashion to ensure the delivery of efficient and effective care.

Furthermore, the link between age and health-care costs is strongly influenced by the health system itself. For example, one study of OECD countries suggested that age-related increases in cost are much higher in Canada and the United States than in Spain and Sweden, with costs in Australia, Japan and the United Kingdom lying somewhere between (*35*). This is likely to reflect different provider systems, incentives, approaches to interventions in frail older people, and cultural norms, particularly near the time of death.

Indeed, there is considerable evidence that the time to death is a better predictor of health-

care expenditure than chronological age (*36, 37*). For example, research from Australia and the Netherlands estimated that around 10% of all health-care expenditures reflect the cost of caring for people during their last year of life, and that these costs fall with increasing age (*38, 39*). In the United States, around 22% of all medical costs may be spent on patients during the last year of life (*40*). The impact of time to death on expenditure is partly driven by the complexity of health states during this period, but it is also likely to reflect cultural and medical norms. For example, costs are likely to be higher when death in hospital is the norm, although hospital admission may have little impact on clinical course and is unlikely to have benefits in terms of the well-being of those using more intensive services (*41*).

Starting from the perspective of time to death can lead to different predictive models for the possible impact of future demographic changes on health-care costs. For example, and somewhat counterintuitively, although the population in the United Kingdom has experienced significant ageing that will continue for several years, the proportion of the population with less than 15 years to live is actually falling and will continue to fall for the foreseeable future (*42*). Because it is these last years of life that are by far the greatest driver of increasing health-care expenditures, the economic modelling of future costs needs to consider these trends alongside changes in the proportion of older people in a population. Doing so suggests that the demographic changes being experienced in the United Kingdom may have much more modest influences on health care spending than are commonly assumed.

Furthermore, rising life expectancy means that the last years of life will increasingly occur in advanced old age. Because this is an age group among which health-service expenditures tend to fall, enabling people to live long and healthy lives may actually ease pressures on the inflation of health-care costs (*43*).

One concern may be that interventions in midlife might merely postpone expenditures to

Table 4.2.   Lessons learnt from countries' experiences with care integration and coordination

Country	Key features of integration	Results
Australia: coordinated care trials (*48, 49*)	Whole-of-population approach encompassed improvements made to the access and delivery of primary health-care services and improvements in care coordination for the community – Care coordination organized for those with chronic and complex needs – Expanded use of information management and technology – Creation of robust mechanisms to resolve conflicts	– Clients felt supported and less anxious – General practitioners had high satisfaction – Emergency room visits were reduced as were lengths of stay after interventions – Reduced referrals to community health services
Brazil: case study, incorporating topic of ageing into the national family health programme (Box 4.9)	– Home visits undertaken by a multidisciplinary team composed of a doctor, a nurse and social worker – Health workers were trained to assess frailty and functioning – Strong referral links established with primary health-care clinics	– Results have not yet been documented
Canada (Quebec): Program of Research to Integrate Services for the Maintenance of Autonomy (PRISMA) (*50*)	Coordination established between decision-makers and managers – System had a single entry point – Used a case-management process – Developed individualized service plans and a single assessment – Focused on clients' functional autonomy – A computerized clinical chart was used for communicating among institutions to monitor clients	– Increase in client satisfaction and empowerment – Lower incidence of functional decline – Lower prevalence of unmet needs – Reduced number of emergency room visits and hospitalizations – No increase in the number of consultations with health professionals or use of home-care services – Improved the performance of the system at no additional cost
Thailand: Friends Help Friends project (*Source*: Ekachai Piensriwatchara and Puangpen Chanprasert, Department of Health, Ministry of Public Health, Thailand, personal communication, January 2015)	Long-term care led by the Ministry of Health – Supported informal caregivers who were providing long-term care – Informal caregivers and community volunteers were formally engaged with the system and provided home visits and assessments of function – A health professional affiliated with a nearby health centre provided supervision and logistical support	– Results have not yet been documented
England: case studies (*49, 51*)	– Implemented real integration: vertical (hospital to home) and horizontal (multidisciplinary teams) – Programme targeted people in the community who had complex needs – Multidisciplinary teams composed of care coordinators, community nurses, occupational therapists, physiotherapists and social workers – Funds were pooled rom National Health Service clinical commissioning groups and local authorities	– Increased staff motivation and received positive evaluations from general practitioners – Decreased waiting times for support for long-term care – Reduced emergency admissions, bed days and lengths of stay – There were fewer placements in residential homes – Improved the performance of the system at no additional cost

a later period in life and result in greater cumulative costs across an individual's life course. Although there is only limited research in this field, this does not appear to be the case, with the immediate benefits and the delayed costs appearing to balance out over time (*44*, *45*). Furthermore, one study from the Netherlands (a country with a comprehensive system of long-term care) mirrors the trend noted above, with better health in early older age resulting in lower hospital expenditures during the remaining lifetime but in higher expenditures for long-term care (*46*).

Combined, this patchy body of research in high-income countries suggests that predicting increases in health-care costs on the basis of population ageing is simplistic and unlikely to lead to good policy decisions. This is reinforced by historical analyses, which suggest that ageing may be a much smaller influence on growth in health-care expenditures than several other factors. For example, research in the United States between 1940 and 1990 (a period of significantly faster growth in the proportion of older people in the population than has occurred since) found that ageing contributed to only around 2% of the increase in health expenditures observed during that period (*33*). In comparison, technology-related changes in practice were responsible for between 38% and 65% of growth, increasing prices were responsible for between 11% and 22%, and growth in personal income was responsible for between 5% and 23% (*33*). Similarly, research on expenditures in France between 1992 and 2000 found the contribution of ageing to be relatively small, with the impact of changes in clinical practice being almost four times as large (*47*).

In many low- and middle-income countries (and in some higher-income countries) where utilization is much lower than should be the case, given the health needs of older people, services will be required to expand to meet the needs of this segment of the population. However, the associated pressures on expenditures are not associated with ageing so much as they are with ensuring that the right to health of all segments of the population is equitably met.

Therefore, it seems reasonable to conclude that having an increasing proportion of older people in the population does not present a major economic barrier to redesigning health systems in the ways suggested in this report. Indeed, given the likelihood that the approaches proposed are both more effective and more equitable, and that the coordination of care that lies at their core has been shown to be no more expensive (Table 4.2), it seems reasonable to argue for these changes from an economic perspective as well as a *Healthy Ageing* perspective.

Box 4.3. In Karnataka state, India, oral health is a priority

The oral health of older people is frequently overlooked, despite its importance to nutrition and to declines in capacity. The Indian state of Karnataka has taken important steps to address this issue: for the first time in the country, in March 2014 oral health was integrated into its national health policies. This reform is of particular importance in India because most of its older population is economically vulnerable and has poor access to oral care, frequently resulting in the loss of teeth.

Karnataka has taken additional state-level action to capitalize on this reform. The state government has proposed providing dentures free of charge through its 42 dental colleges; these services will be funded by the Karnataka state government. The dental colleges will be reimbursed for every denture that is delivered. Community outreach to local villages will help identify older adults who need dentures, and aim at encouraging them to seek care at one of the dental colleges.

The results of this intervention still need to be determined, but this strategy highlights how all aspects of older people's health can be addressed by *Healthy Ageing* policies, including the frequently forgotten area of oral health. This also demonstrates how older people's right to health – especially that of the most vulnerable in society – can be met through concerted action.

Responses

The previous section illustrated that although the world is experiencing a rapid transition towards ageing populations, health systems generally have not kept pace. Most health services around the world have been designed around acute care models that are poorly aligned with the dominant health issues of older age. This failure in care is exacerbated by age-

Box 4.4. What are *Healthy Ageing* assessments and comprehensive care plans?

A *Healthy Ageing* assessment considers multiple domains of intrinsic capacity and the environments in which people live. This assessment is completed as soon as possible after people enter into contact with health services. The likelihood of multiple health issues occurring among older people frequently necessitates the involvement of several generalist and specialist health workers, and the social service sector. As such, the assessment can be completed as a multistep process, if needed, to ensure that all relevant parties are brought into the conversation (*52, 53*).

Care plans are developed as part of this comprehensive assessment. The plan includes the older person's goals, how they will be addressed, the roles that different sectors of the health and social system will have, and a plan for follow-up and reassessment. Once the care plan has been developed, it serves as a roadmap for unifying actions and a ruler for measuring progress against the older person's goals and objectives.

Comprehensive care plans are collaborative. The initial assessment and discussion involve the older person, key family members, other decision-makers and the health workers in charge of planning care. This discussion should identify and clarify the needs and objectives of the older person, as well as the health and social services that might help them achieve their goals (*54*).

Comprehensive care plans are a key tool for reorienting health systems towards care that is integrated and centred on older people. When used to their full potential, they enhance integration between health-care and social-care services, and facilitate coordination among a range of different health services. Research has shown that comprehensive care plans can improve both the quality of care and health outcomes (*17, 55*).

based discrimination and by ignorance of the priorities and needs of older people. New approaches are needed to foster *Healthy Ageing*.

Evidence suggests that the best way to design systems to better meet the needs of older people is by placing them at the centre of service delivery. Practically, this means that health care is organized around their needs and preferences, and designed for integration across service levels and types. This can overcome the disjointedness and inefficiencies of many health systems and ensure care is driven by an older person's changing and diverse needs rather than by the service structure.

Achieving these changes will require a shift that extends well beyond clinic walls, and will necessitate a re-evaluation of all aspects of the health system (Box 4.3 and Box 4.4). The following sections describe how such systems can be developed around the shared goal of optimizing trajectories of intrinsic capacity (Fig. 4.6).

Fig. 4.6.   Designing health systems to encourage *Healthy Ageing*

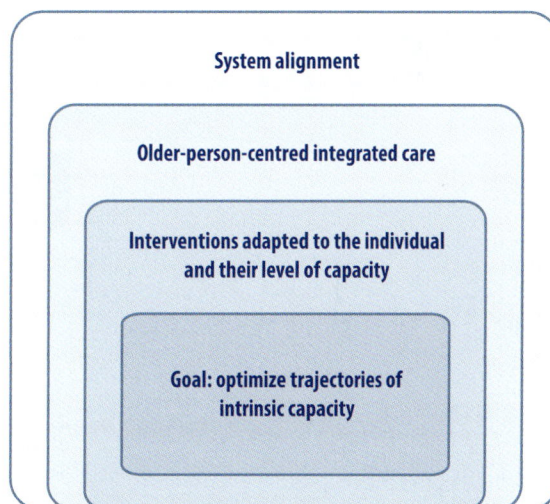

The goal: optimize trajectories of intrinsic capacity

Health systems are needed that share the *Healthy Ageing* goals of building and maintaining functional ability. However, within these goals, the main role of health systems will be to optimize trajectories of intrinsic capacity.

Evidence suggests that focusing primarily on older people's intrinsic capacity is more effective than prioritizing the management of specific chronic diseases (*15–17*). This is not to reject the worth of disease management, but rather to underscore that it is an older person's physical and mental capacities that should be the targets of, and entry points for, health interventions. Approaching older people through the lens of intrinsic capacity and the environments in which they live helps ensure that health services are oriented towards the outcomes that are most relevant to their daily lives. It can also help avoid unnecessary treatments, polypharmacy and their side-effects (*10, 56, 57*).

Adapt interventions to individuals and their levels of capacity

The second half of life is characterized by great heterogeneity in trajectories of intrinsic capacity. Yet within any population of older people, many individuals will experience periods of high and stable capacity, declining capacity, and a significant loss of capacity. Each of these three periods requires different responses to be emphasized, and these are summarized in Fig. 4.7.

Fig. 4.7. **Three common periods of intrinsic capacity in older age; risks and challenges, goals and key responses of a health system**

Period	High and stable capacity	Declining capacity	Significant loss of capacity
Risks and challenges	Risk behaviours, emerging NCDs	Falling mobility, sarcopaenia, frailty, cognitive impairment or dementia, sensory impairments	Difficulty performing basic tasks, pain and suffering caused by advanced chronic conditions
Goals	Build and maintain capacity and resilience	Reverse, stop or slow the loss of capacity	Compensate for loss of capacity
Responses	Reduce risk factors and encourage healthy behaviours; Early detection and management of chronic diseases; Build resilience through capacity-enhancing behaviours, strengthening personal skills and building relationships	Implement multicomponent programmes delivered at primary health-care level; Treat the underlining causes of declines in capacity; Maintain muscle mass and bone density through exercise and nutrition	Interventions to recover and maintain intrinsic capacity; Care and support to compensate for losses in capacity and ensure dignity; Rapid access to acute care; Palliative and end-of-life care

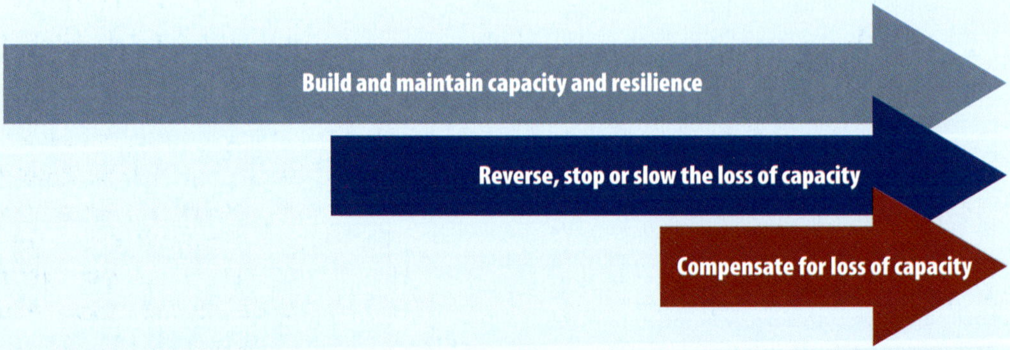

NCDs: noncommunicable diseases.

People with high and stable capacity

For older people with high and stable levels of capacity, the goal is to continue to build and maintain these levels for as long as possible. The emphasis will be on preventing disease and reducing risk, promoting capacity-enhancing behaviours, ensuring that acute problems are adequately addressed, and detecting and managing chronic noncommunicable diseases at an early stage.

Behaviours such as maintaining an unhealthy diet, having a sedentary lifestyle, and using tobacco increase the risk of a range of noncommunicable diseases well into older age, and strategies to reduce their impact continue to be effective (58–66). Behavioural interventions for older people on this trajectory therefore focus upon reducing these risks.

The early detection and treatment of noncommunicable diseases is another area in which action can be taken during this period. The effective management of care for people with, or at high risk for, cardiovascular disease, cancer, chronic respiratory disease, diabetes and other noncommunicable diseases can prevent the accumulation of functional deficits, reduce the need for hospitalization and costly high-technology interventions, and reduce premature deaths (64, 65, 67). There is a range of effective interventions for preventing and controlling noncommunicable diseases, and many countries – mostly high-income countries – have already achieved major reductions in deaths from chronic disease by implementing these interventions (68). Yet more focused action and political commitments are needed in many parts of the world, especially in low-income and middle-income countries, to close the gap for older people in the treatment of chronic diseases (69). Guidance is available for implementing interventions in low-resource primary-care settings (70).

Particular attention needs to be paid to hypertension, which is responsible for a significant proportion of cardiovascular disease, associated declines in intrinsic capacity, and premature death. Yet it is possible to minimize these risks if hypertension is detected and treated at an early stage. People with hypertension should have an assessment of their total cardiovascular risk, including tests for diabetes mellitus and other risk factors. Hypertension and diabetes are closely associated, and one cannot be properly managed without giving attention to the other (71). Evidence indicates that this total-risk approach to treatment decision-making, as opposed to decision-making based on the presence of any single risk factor, helps prevent the use of unnecessary medications and, thus, their side-effects (72).

People with declining capacity

As the underlying changes of ageing advance and chronic diseases arise, intrinsic capacity starts to decline. This process is complex and dynamic: it may occur slowly as part of the ageing process or rapidly, particularly as a consequence of a specific health condition or trauma. Intervening at this stage is essential because the process of becoming frail or care-dependent can be delayed, slowed or even partly reversed by interventions targeted early in the process of functional decline (73–75).

Ensuring that people engage in healthy behaviours remains crucial, but the focus broadens from reducing risk factors to encompassing actions that can directly help maintain and reverse losses in intrinsic capacity. For example, aerobic exercise is important for preventing cardiovascular disease (76), but exercise that can help build muscle mass, increase strength and improve balance becomes increasingly important as people grow older (Chapter 3), especially among middle-aged women who are at heightened risk for osteoporosis (77, 78). Nutritional advice also changes, with the focus shifting to nutrient density, particularly to vitamins and micronutrients, although calorie and protein intakes are also important targets (Chapter 3) (79).

Effective interventions start with a comprehensive assessment of the intrinsic capacity of the older person and its trajectory; the specific conditions, behaviours and risks that may influence this capacity in the future; and the person's environments. This *Healthy Ageing* assessment provides the information needed to prioritize and tailor interventions (Box 4.4). These can inform multicomponent programmes, which have been shown in primary health-care settings to be effective in improving intrinsic capacity, maintaining independent living and preventing care dependency (*80–83*).

Box 4.5. Brain health across the life course in Indonesia

The Indonesian Ministry of Health's Centre of Health and Intelligence, has recently implemented an initiative aimed at building cognitive resilience and functioning across the life course. The activities start early in life and include:

- ensuring brain stimulation of and adequate nutrition to the fetus during pregnancy;
- ensuring sensory–motor stimulation in infants, and using games and learning tools for cognitive stimulation in toddlers;
- optimizing the learning environment for school-age children and teens;
- providing health promotion activities for adults that are targeted at encouraging healthy lifestyles, physical exercise, social activities and the development of stress-management skills;
- ensuring early detection of cognitive decline or related degenerative or vascular disorders in older adults.

The central tool used in this initiative is known as the executive brain assessment. The tool assesses different competencies, emotional intelligence and cognitive function, and indicates which activities should be offered to the person enrolled in the programme.

This initiative is notable in that it demonstrates a life-course approach to building cognitive resilience and resources, which are important in preventing and delaying cognitive declines later in life. The Ministry of Health has implemented the programme nationally.

Source: Trisa Wahyuni Putri, Centre of Health and Intelligence, Ministry of Health, Indonesia, personal communication, 24 September 2014.

Because of their central importance, interventions to improve nutrition and encourage physical exercise are likely to be included in most multicomponent programmes (*66*). In particular, highly intensive strength training is the key intervention necessary to prevent and reverse frailty and sarcopenia; it also indirectly protects the brain against depression and cognitive decline (Box 4.5) (*84, 85*). One systematic review reported a 50% reduction in the relative risk of developing functional limitations among people aged 65–85 years who engaged in regular physical activity of at least moderate intensity (*86*). Because a lack of strength is a major cause of falls in people who are frail (*87–89*), strength training can empower older people to maintain or regain autonomy and independence.

People with a significant loss of capacity

Many people reach a point in older age where they are no longer able to perform the basic tasks necessary for day-to-day life without the assistance of others. This stage is characterized by care dependency, which is primarily addressed through long-term care systems (Chapter 5). Nonetheless, health systems maintain important roles for people who have significant losses in capacity, including providing ongoing management of disease, rehabilitation, and palliative and end-of-life care. Health systems also need to ensure that people have timely access to primary, specialty and acute care when needed. There is good evidence that specialist acute-care geriatric wards deliver higher-quality care with shorter lengths of stay and lower costs than general hospital care (*54, 90, 91*).

The integration of health-care and long-term care services will be crucial to maintaining the functional ability and dignity of older people at this stage of life. Care coordination has been shown to be beneficial, and care plans help prevent unnecessary hospital admissions, ensure there are links with long-term care services, and support people to remain at home (*92*).

One option for delivering services for people with a significant loss of capacity is through hospital-at-home services. These services involve a team of health-care and long-term care professionals who provide treatment at home for people who would otherwise be admitted to an acute care hospital. Evidence has shown that these services have high client and caregiver satisfaction, reduce deaths and reduce readmission rates (93, 94).

Rehabilitation services are another crucial component of health care at this stage. They can help prevent permanent disability and care dependency, and have been shown to reduce avoidable hospital admissions and delayed discharges (92). Acute hospitals must play their part in ensuring adequate inpatient rehabilitation, but most rehabilitation services can be provided outside hospital settings, in communities or at home (85).

Palliative and end-of-life care strive to ensure that people with advanced illness are treated with dignity and respect, and according to their needs and wishes (Box 5.8). Key health-care functions for these types of care are communicating accurate information about treatment and prognosis, initiating advanced care planning, and managing pain and symptoms. The availability and use of analgesics – opioid and nonopioid – is important to minimize suffering. However, social support is also crucial during this last stage of life, and health systems need to encourage and enable this, even within hospital settings.

Implement older-person-centred and integrated care

Evidence suggests that older-person-centred and integrated care is the best approach for implementing this complex spectrum of interventions across older people's lives (95–98). Care that is centred on older people is grounded in the perspective that older people are more than vessels of their disorders or health conditions. They are individuals with unique experiences, needs and preferences. Also, they are seen in the context of their daily lives, as part of a family and a community. In contrast to ageist attitudes, their dignity and autonomy are respected and embraced in a culture of shared decision-making.

At the level of clinical care, integrated care refers to services that span the care continuum, are integrated within and among the different levels and sites of care within the health-care and long-term care systems (including within the home), and are offered according to people's needs throughout the life course (99). From the perspective of the client, integrated care is seamless across diseases, settings and time. Important clinical-level elements of designing care for older people with chronic and multiple conditions include using *Healthy Ageing* assessments, engaging in care planning and providing a single point of entry (Table 4.3) (48, 50, 51, 100).

The importance of integration is emphasized by the *WHO global strategy on people-centred*

Table 4.3.   Conventional care versus older-person-centred and integrated care

Conventional care	Older-person-centred and integrated care
Focuses on a health condition (or conditions)	Focuses on people and their goals
Goal is disease management or cure	Goal is maximizing intrinsic capacity
Older person is regarded as a passive recipient of care	Older person is an active participant in care planning and self-management
Care is fragmented across conditions, health workers, settings and life course	Care is integrated across conditions, health workers, settings and life course
Links with health care and long-term care are limited or non-existent	Links with health care and long-term care exist and are strong
Ageing is considered to be a pathological state	Ageing is considered to be a normal and valued part of the life course

and integrated health services (99). The strategy calls for shifting the way health services are funded, managed and delivered, and proposes five interdependent strategic directions that need to be adopted for health services to become more people-centred and integrated. However, for each specific context, the exact mix of strategies that will be used needs to be designed and developed, taking into account local contexts, values and preferences (*99*).

This section presents the key elements of the strategy that are most relevant to older people's health. Integration can occur at the level of the health-care organization and the community, and at the broader levels of policies, financing mechanisms and shared governance structures (*101*). But integration between primary health care and all other levels and settings of care is crucial (*102*).

Only a few countries have implemented integrated care for older people and evaluated its use in their health systems. The limited amount of documented research suggests a diverse range of approaches can have benefits in terms of satisfaction, intrinsic capacity and reduced hospitalizations (Table 4.2).

Because systems around the world are so different, no single organizational model can be applied universally to integrate care (*49*). However, evidence suggests that integration can be best achieved by bringing services together to meet the needs of older people using a person-centred approach and by placing strong emphasis on case management, support for self-management and support for ageing in place (by providing community-based care). These approaches are outlined below.

Implement case management: one goal, one assessment, one care plan

A strong case-management system is one in which individual needs are assessed, a comprehensive care plan is developed (Box 4.4), and services are managed and driven towards the single goal of maintaining functional ability (*103*). Case man-

Box 4.6. Individualized care plans for older people living in slum areas in Rio de Janeiro, Brazil

In 2012, the Centre for Study and Research on Ageing in Brazil piloted a new project in the Rio de Janeiro neighbourhood of Rocinha, Brazil's largest slum, with a simple yet ambitious goal: to provide adequate health care to frail older people. From the beginning, the centre's interdisciplinary team collaborated closely with three family health clinics in Rocinha. The clinics' staff received initial training in geriatrics, and started referring older people to the centre using standardized selection criteria and screening questions. People who were referred to the centre were offered a comprehensive multidimensional geriatric assessment, resulting in an individualized care plan. This plan was sent to the person's health clinic, which could contact the centre at any time for discussion or clarification. After 4–5 months, the older person returned to the centre for a follow-up evaluation.

During the 1-year pilot phase, almost 3000 appointments resulted in more than 350 older people receiving individual care plans. An initial evaluation of the programme demonstrated high levels of adherence by clients in the areas of medication and nutrition; recommendations regarding physical exercise and environmental changes were followed by about half of those who had an individual care plan. Over the course of the pilot phase, additional clinics joined the programme, and the centre now accepts referrals from public-health clinics throughout the whole state of Rio de Janeiro.

Since 2014, the centre has offered a broader range of support services to health clinics and their patients, including referrals to various specialists (dentists, nutritionists, speech therapists, occupational therapists and physiotherapists), cognitive assessments, support groups for family caregivers, and workshops about issues such as preventing falls and ensuring adequate nutrition.

agement generally translates into a single point of entry and coordination via a case manager who helps with assessment, shares information, and coordinates services across multiple health workers and care settings (*49*).

Systematic reviews have reported that case management improves intrinsic capacity, different aspects of medication management and the use of community services (*16*). It also improves health outcomes for frail older people (*16, 17*) and has clinical benefits for several chronic illnesses (*104*). Box 4.6 also shows that it is achievable in resource-poor settings.

Healthy Ageing assessments and care plans can be particularly effective in three situations. For people with multimorbidity, they can facilitate clinical management across different providers and unite them around one goal (*105*). For people admitted to inpatient hospital care, they can help to reduce the risks and prevent the harms of hospitalization and can facilitate successful discharge back home (*54*). And for people discharged from hospitals to long-term care programmes, they can ensure that the necessary follow-up occurs and links are made between health care and social care services (*105*).

Regular and sustained follow-up of older people is part of most case-management approaches. It promotes early detection of complications or changes in functional status, thus preventing unnecessary emergencies and related inefficiencies. It also provides a forum for monitoring progress against the care plan and a means for providing additional support as needed.

Provide systematic support for self-management

Offering support for self-management is another tool for providing person-centred and integrated care to older adults (*106, 107*). It consists of providing them with the information, skills and tools that they need to manage their health conditions, prevent complications, maximize their intrinsic capacity and maintain their quality of life. This does not imply that older adults will be expected to "go it alone" or that unreasonable or excessive demands will be placed on them. It does, however, recognize their autonomy and abilities to direct their own care in consultation

and partnership with health-care professionals, their own families and other caregivers.

The Chronic Disease Self-Management Program (*108*) is the most extensively researched programme for providing self-management support to older people. Working with groups of older people, laypeople provide training in management of cognitive symptoms, advice on methods for managing negative emotions, and they also discuss topics such as medications, diet, fatigue and how to interact productively with health-care workers. Lay-leaders teach the courses in an interactive manner designed to enhance participants' confidence in their abilities to execute specific self-care tasks. The goal is not to provide disease-specific content, but rather to use interactive exercises to build self-efficacy and other skills that will help participants live actively. A vital element is exchange and discussion among participants and with peer leaders.

Chronic disease self-management programmes have been shown to improve a wide range of outcomes among older adults. Improvements have been observed in levels of physical activity (*109–111*), self-care (*109*), chronic pain (*112*), and self-efficacy (*109–112*). Nonetheless, the magnitude of measured improvements is generally small, and longer-term outcomes have not been well documented (*113*). In addition, most of the research has not taken into account older people who leave the programmes (*113*).

Older people's participation in community-based self-management programmes is generally low, and those who do participate tend to be in better physical health (*114*). These findings point to the need for proactive outreach to community-dwelling older people, as well as the need for additional formats to support self-management that have fewer physical barriers to participation.

Although not as extensively researched, routine health-care visits provide excellent opportunities to build and reinforce self-management skills. In this context, successful self-management is not a standalone activity, but rather an ongoing opportunity to encourage older people and their caregivers to take part in shared decision-making and to share responsibility for the older person's health and well-being. Various clinical models have been developed to guide these interactions (*115–117*). Telephone or Internet-based self-management programmes offer other options.

Support ageing in place

Older people often identify a preference for growing old in their own homes or at least within the communities where they live (*118–120*). This allows them to maintain the relationships and community networks that can foster well-being and act as resources in times of adversity. Although the focus of ageing in place has frequently been on ensuring appropriate and affordable housing and age-friendly built environments, as well as providing instrumental support, health services also have an important role to play by providing care that reaches people where they live. Thus, models of care will need to be reoriented towards prioritizing primary care and community-based care. This encompasses a shift from inpatient care to ambulatory and outpatient care, to more home-based interventions, community engagement and a fully integrated referral system (*99*).

Several approaches may be effective. For example, home visits delivered by health professionals in the context of community-based programmes have been shown to have positive effects (*80, 121*), although the measured benefits have been variable across studies and outcome indicators. In 2014, a review of 64 randomized trials found that home-based visits were effective when they included multidimensional assessments and five or more visits (*122*). The greatest overall effects were made in reducing the number of visits to emergency departments, hospital admissions, the length of stay, the number of falls, and improving physical functioning (*122*). To be maximally effective, home-based services must be complemented by strong links with primary health-care services, include scheduled follow-up, and target people at low risk of death (*123*).

Box 4.7. Ageing in place: the role of community health workers

Evidence and experience suggest that community health workers in low- and middle-income countries could be important resources for promoting *Healthy Ageing* in place.

In WHO's African Region, community health programmes are the backbone of the health systems. Community health workers have become key to ensuring that primary health-care services meet the needs of the community, particularly with regard to maternal and child health, and their effectiveness is reflected in reductions in mortality among mothers and children.

Interest has grown in potentially developing the roles of community health workers to help control chronic noncommunicable diseases. As the sole primary-care provider offering community outreach, these health workers are ideally situated to implement age-appropriate care for older people, case-finding (that is, identifying frail or dependent older people in the community who have not sought help at the health facility) and home-based assessment and intervention (*127, 128*).

Home visits delivered in the context of community-based programmes for older people are included in national policies in several high-income countries, including Australia, Denmark and the United Kingdom. These programmes aim to delay or prevent functional decline, care dependence and subsequent nursing home admissions by providing primary preventive measures (for example, immunizations and exercise), secondary measures (for example, detecting untreated problems) and tertiary prevention (for example, improving medication use). Although evaluations have suggested that some of these programmes have been effective, uncertainty remains about whether they can prevent functional decline, which programme components are effective, and which populations are most likely to benefit (*127, 129*).

Home-based physical-activity interventions for older people have also shown some promising results (*124*). Providing physical-activity interventions in people's homes addresses barriers to exercise that older adults commonly face: it removes the transportation barrier and makes it easier to integrate physical activity into daily life (*125*, *126*). Home-based physical-activity interventions are most accessible when they do not require a physician's referral.

Community outreach and case-finding are other important aspects that facilitate ageing in place. These services can reach older people who do not present to health centres, and can facilitate the identification, monitoring and support of older people who need health services. Community health workers hold promise for fulfilling many of these functions in low- and middle-income countries (Box 4.7).

At the population level, the health sector can also be involved in designing and implementing other programmes to foster *Healthy Ageing*, for example by advising on the design of physical-activity programmes that are appropriate for older people.

Align health systems

Well-aligned health systems can enable the provision of older-person-centred and integrated care. WHO has identified areas that need to be focused on to build strong (or well-aligned) health systems (*121*); they include service delivery; human resources; health infrastructure, including products, vaccines and appropriate technologies; information and data services; leadership and governance; and financing. This section will explore the actions that can be taken in these areas to promote integrated and person-centred care for ageing populations (*130*).

Service delivery: creating age-friendly health infrastructure

In addition to creating systems that deliver the interventions that are important for older people, primary health services should be located close to where they live, and priority for services should be given to vulnerable groups and underserved areas (*131*). This is important generally, but especially for older people. Distances to health cen-

tres that might be reasonable for the general population can be insurmountable for older people with significant impairments; accessible and affordable public transportation is a related consideration (Chapter 6) (*132*). Specialist health services are likely to be more centrally located, and thus may entail longer travel distances. In these cases, it is essential that age-friendly and affordable transportation options are available.

Across all service settings, the physical infrastructure of health centres and hospitals can be designed in an age-friendly manner. This might include elevators, escalators, ramps, doorways and passages that are accessible to an individual with significant loss of physical capacity or who uses a wheelchair, suitable stairs (not too high or steep) with hand railings, nonslip flooring, rest areas with comfortable seating, and signs that are large, clear and well lit (*132*). Age-friendly procedures could be put in place (for example, clinics could offer times specifically tailored to older people, or preferential queuing) (Box 4.1), and all staff, including porters and office staff, could receive training in how to help make services more age-friendly.

Human resources: transforming the workforce

WHO defines the health workforce as, "all people engaged in actions whose primary intent is to enhance health" (*133*). This includes various health professionals from the public and private sectors, as well as all other support workers whose main function relates to delivering or supporting the provision of health promotion activities, and preventive, curative, rehabilitative and palliative care.

Transforming the workforce to respond to the priorities of the 21st century requires a broad coalition of health-care and long-term care workers to collaborate with community partners, older people and their families. The services they provide should be responsive to the future needs and expectations of older people.

To achieve this, health professionals of all types must have the right competencies, but they also must operate in environments that make the best use of these talents. This will require that they be organized into multidisciplinary teams and have access to tools to help them provide good-quality integrated care that extends beyond the realm of health facilities to include home care (Box 7.1).

To fill the roles needed, health workers will require several key competencies. They need to be able to perform basic screening to assess functioning, including vision, hearing, cognition, nutritional status and oral health (Box 4.3), and they need to be able to manage health conditions that are common in older people, such as frailty, osteoporosis and arthritis. They should understand how depression, dementia and harmful alcohol use typically manifest in older people, and they should know how to identify neglect or abuse. Additionally, health workers should be able to conduct *Healthy Ageing* assessments and plan care because these are key tools for implementing older-person-centred and integrated care. Beyond these specific competencies, health workers need more general competencies in communication, teamwork, information technology and public health.

Equivalent changes will need to be made to preservice training models for the workforce; these models have generally not kept pace with the rapid epidemiological and demographic transitions that are underway. Changes to preservice training might include adopting competency-based curricula that include the competencies mentioned above, promoting interprofessional education, and expanding training from academic centres into primary-care settings and communities (*14*). The capacity of educational institutions might need to be developed to make it possible for them to reach established standards (*134*). WHO's guidelines on transforming and scaling-up health professionals' education and training present key recommendations for expanding and reforming education and training to increase the quantity, quality and relevance of health professionals (*135*). It is equally important to foster skills that allow closer integration of health and social services.

For existing staff, in-service training and continuing professional development are essential for consolidating knowledge and upgrading skills. Proven approaches for consolidating new skills include providing ongoing support and supervision for staff, and ensuring that generalists and geriatric specialists engage in joint consultations.

Beyond training, health workers need to be deployed in a manner that is consistent with the objective of delivering older-person-centred and integrated care, and multidisciplinary teams are an essential part of this process. Multidisciplinary teams share responsibility and accountability for clinical processes and care outcomes both for individuals and across defined populations. To succeed, teams must meet regularly, share information, explicitly define clinical roles and perform complementary yet coordinated functions for the same people and populations (*136*). Teams may be found within the same clinic or setting, but may also be formed across multiple settings; they may be connected by information and communication technologies (ICT) and supported by occasional face-to-face meetings.

The specific mix of skills needed on multidisciplinary teams depends on the staff within the health system and their defined scopes of practice. That being said, nurses have been shown to be central to providing integrated care. The involvement of, or leadership by, appropriately trained nurses or other health workers who may complement physicians in key functions (such as assessment, treatment management, self-management support and follow-up) has been shown repeatedly to improve health workers' adherence to guidelines and patients' satisfaction, clinical and health status, and use of health services (*137–139*).

Other core team members ideally would include a general practitioner, a social worker, a community-based worker and a geriatrician for consultation and support. Further team members could include pharmacists, dietitians, rehabilitation therapists and psychologists, to name only some of the possible professionals who might be involved. Finally, lay health workers, sometimes known as expert patients, can share knowledge and experience with other patients who share a common illness.

In anticipating future demand, innovations are needed in defining the educational requirements, competencies and career pathways for the new types of health workers necessary to respond to future needs. For example, designated care coordinators, who might be from one of the professional groups listed above or from another professional background, could oversee the comprehensive care plan. In many low- and middle-income settings, associate clinicians (for example, clinical officers, health officers or medical assistants) have emerged as a new category in response to shortages in health workforces and challenges in retaining staff in rural and underserved areas (*137, 140–142*).

Finally, although this report emphasizes that the needs of older people will be best met if all professionals receive adequate training in geriatrics, this cannot be achieved without a critical mass of specialist geriatric expertise or the availability of geriatricians to see and treat complex cases. In many countries, there are startlingly low numbers of geriatricians, and many more will be needed merely to meet current needs. Furthermore, a much stronger academic base will be required to identify the most effective interventions and services. Although not all health services will need academic geriatric units and specialists, these will be crucial in building evidence and in raising the status of a field that is often perceived as unattractive.

Health information systems and eHealth: investments are key

Using ICT in health care, or eHealth, will be a critical tool for transforming health systems and services to deliver person-centred and integrated care that is appropriate to older people and aligned with the *Healthy Ageing* agenda. The strategic use of ICT will be essential to improv-

ing the functional ability of future generations, integrating and managing the care of older persons, assessing the impact of interventions and ensuring accountability for services provided.

Advances in ICT are being used worldwide to improve access to, and the quality and safety of, health care, as well as to ensure the cost effectiveness of health-service delivery (*143*). In the European Union, for example, the introduction of ICT and telemedicine is estimated to have improved the efficiency of health care by 20% (*144*). In many countries today, eHealth is changing how health care is delivered and how health systems work.

Electronic health records and related health-information systems can capture, organize and share information about individual clients and clinical populations to help identify older people's needs, plan their care over time, monitor responses to treatment and assess health outcomes. They can also facilitate collaboration between health workers and between health-care teams and their clients, who may be located in diverse settings or geographical locations. Health services such as telemedicine and remote consultation allow clients to have access to diagnostic and therapeutic expertise that might otherwise not be available locally. In many ways, ICT has become fundamental to the effective management of chronic diseases and the implementation of care by multidisciplinary teams.

ICT is also used in a range of settings to make up-to-date knowledge more easily accessible and help health workers provide safe evidence-based care. For example, automated reminders, prompts and warnings incorporated into clinical health-records systems can assist personnel in meeting quality standards and systematically documenting the results of diagnostic tests and the care delivered.

Increasingly, eHealth is employed to improve the quality of life of older people. For example, it is used to link older people living at home with their health-care team, as well as with community and social services, to combat their loneliness and isolation, support independence and facilitate the self-management of their conditions.

Research is underway on the use of ICT by older people to monitor their health. For example, wearable devices could be used to collect information on their physical activity, diet and measures of capacity, such as gait speed.

Research on the genetic determinants of capacity in older people and biomarkers of early decline aims to allow personalized advice to be given to people at a much earlier stage than is now possible. Information systems need to be developed in ways that can fully utilize the benefits of these innovations.

The usefulness of health information systems also extends more broadly to include monitoring, evaluation and planning at the policy level, and to improve the care of older people, ideally across health-care and long-term care systems. However, for these uses to be realized, common indicators must be broadly agreed and consistently used. Indicators of underlying causes and domains of functional capacity – such as undernutrition, mobility impairment, cognitive impairment and sensory impairments – must be defined and operationalized, and routinely assessed in older age groups. Various instruments for capturing functional capacity may provide useful starting points for developing indicators across health-care and social-care systems (145–147).

Medical products, vaccines and technologies: ensuring access

Medical products, essential medicines and health technologies are indispensable to helping older people remain healthy, active and independent as long as possible.

Medications for older people need to be safe, properly prescribed, available and accessible; yet achieving these goals is a significant challenge for most health systems. Older people take more medications than younger people, and they often take several medications at the same time (known as polypharmacy). In addition, as the body ages, the effects of medications also change, and medication mismanagement can increase with age. Therefore, improving the use of medicines in older people, including implementing appropriate prescribing, is an area that requires urgent attention (Box 4.8).

Countries can consider taking action on several fronts. For example, guidelines for appropriate prescribing might be needed, and programmes to ensure free access to essential medicines for older people may be of additional benefit. Brazil, for example, improved access to medications by offering a free supply of five essen-

---

Box 4.8. Australia: involving pharmacists in integrated care to tackle medication-related problems

In Australia, older people at heightened risk for medication-related problems are helped by a Home Medicines Review service that uses pharmacists to prevent, detect and resolve issues. The service consists of the following steps.

1. General practitioners identify at-risk older people using standard criteria, for example those who take five or more medications or those who take a medication with a narrow therapeutic window, which must be administered with great care and control to avoid adverse effects. These older people are referred to their preferred community pharmacy.

2. A pharmacist interviews the older person, usually at home, to obtain a comprehensive medication profile.

3. The pharmacist prepares a written report documenting the findings and recommendations; this is sent to the person's general practitioner.

4. The general practitioner and the older person agree on a medication management plan based on the report.

This service represents a key component of Australia's National Medicines Policy, which aims to ensure that medicines are used safely and effectively. Since 2001, more than 620 000 medication reviews have been conducted across the country. The results of an evaluation indicate that the reviews optimize prescribing for older people and thereby prevent unnecessary adverse effects (148).

tial medicines to older adults receiving treatment through its public-health system; medicines for chronic diseases are freely distributed to older people through the public-health services and the national family health programme (*149*).

Essential medicines lists likely need to be reoriented to the health dynamics of older people. For example, food supplements, vitamins and micronutrients are not normally included in these lists, yet they deserve consideration for inclusion due to their impact on older people's functioning. Other conditions, such as dementia and sarcopenia, do not yet have a strong evidence base for pharmacological management, and so more research is needed before including medications to manage these disorders (*150*).

Ensuring access to assistive health technologies is another important area where action can be taken within this domain. These technologies can help older people maintain their ability in the face of declines in capacity; they can improve well-being and quality of life; they can reduce falls and hospitalizations; and they can lessen worries for older people and their families (*151*). Integrating health-technology products and services into national health and ageing policies would help ensure equity and provide the necessary policy and regulatory environments that are conducive to increasing access to these technologies. Financial schemes for purchasing these technologies would also need to be considered.

Near-term solutions do not need to focus on new technologies but can be drawn from existing technologies or the convergence between them. Surveys of the assistive devices used by older people suggest that it is the basic items that are most widely used, including vision and hearing aids, basic mobility devices (such as canes and walking frames), toileting equipment, and cushions or other means of adjusting furniture or beds (*152*). It should be a priority to make these more widely available and affordable.

Future technologies should address the needs and preferences of older people in addition to targeting specific physical impairments

and noncommunicable diseases. Although these traditional domains of health technology will continue to be important, there is a need to extend the scope of technologies and devices. In an era when social isolation and loneliness dramatically affect older adults' mental and physical health, health technologies can play an important part in reducing the physical and emotional distance among family members, and between older people and their caregivers and other members of the community. Supporting home-based care, a rising domain of health technology, will continue to be important. Wearable devices will create opportunities for the closer monitoring of function and tailoring personalized care. At the same time, there is a need to extend the scope of technologies and devices to address issues such as cognitive decline and frailty, where specialized human resources are scarce and training is insufficient. However, computer interfaces, robotic assistance and virtual social networks can only complement basic human needs for physical, emotional and social contact.

Leadership and governance: making *Healthy Ageing* central to policies and plans

Policy reforms are the linchpin for developing and implementing integrated health-service responses to ageing populations. Fundamental to the success of these responses are commitments from governments, and formal policies, legislation, regulations and financing that concretize these commitments.

For person-centred and integrated care for older people to occur, health-care policies and plans must consider the needs of ageing populations first (Box 4.9). All too often, older people are rendered invisible in policies and plans. A first step would be to review policies and plans with this caveat in mind. Revisions of plans and policies can address issues important to ageing populations, such as care coordination, self-management support, ageing in place and functional outcomes. Where relevant, policies and

Box 4.9. Integrating ageing into Brazil's national family health strategy

In 2006, Brazil's national ageing and health policy called attention to the needs of the country's ageing population, which previously had been overlooked in the country's policies and health strategies. The new policy has facilitated better care for older people by using Brazil's commitment to universal health coverage and its robust national family health programme as the main vehicles for improvement.

A key feature of the family health programme is the use of multidisciplinary teams, composed not only of doctors and nurses but also physiotherapists, psychologists, physical educators, nutritionists and occupational therapists, among others. These teams work together in a family-health support hub, which provides health and social services, community outreach, case-finding and home visits to a defined geographical area.

All health professionals have learnt how to assess older people's functional status, including frailty, in conjunction with conducting a psychosocial evaluation. This comprehensive assessment has become the key tool for integrating care from diverse services and providers. The development of a new guideline on comprehensive primary health care for older people has complemented this training.

Ageing considerations were then integrated into a range of clinical-care procedures; in addition, new interventions targeted especially to older people were introduced. Some of these interventions are delivered in the communities where older people live through self-help groups, classes to encourage healthy behaviours, and physical exercise and dance classes. A strength of the programme has been the engagement and participation of communities. For example older people and volunteers are responsible for many of the social-care initiatives delivered by the centre.

Source: Eduardo Augusto Duque Bezerra, City Public Health Manager, Pernambuco, Brazil, personal communication, March 2015.

care and long-term care systems. Developing joint budgeting, monitoring and accountability systems can solidify integration.

Ageist policies and procedures need to be identified and changed. These changes might include, for example, adapting national health indicators to include measurements of health issues important to older people (for example, dementia or sensory impairments), extending the collection of health data to all ages, disaggregating data by age and sex in groupings of 5 years or 10 years rather than including older people in a category of "over 70", and mandating that new medications brought to market for particular diseases be evaluated within the frame of common multimorbidities.

Furthermore, attention is needed to address health-care inequities among older people. Poor and marginalized older people typically have greater exposures to health risks, more health problems and more difficulty accessing services. Looking at differences between the richest and poorest 20% of households provides insights on 40% of the population. Yet capacity and functioning, as well as risk factors, diseases and access to services, differ across the entire spectrum of society, from the poorest to the richest, and often by other social characteristics.

Health systems can contribute to reducing the huge and remediable differences within countries, although doing so requires commitment and a clear understanding of the situation (*153*). Those systems that successfully address equity tend to share several broad features. They aim at providing universal health coverage and offer particular benefits to children and older people, socially disadvantaged and marginalized groups, and others who are often not adequately covered. They use a comprehensive approach to understand the broader determinants of health and understand the differential exposures and vulnerabilities of individuals and groups, and they incorporate concerns about health equity into public-health programmes (*154*). Both total inequalities and social gradients are measured,

plans should reflect integration across care levels (for example, across primary health-care and hospital-based services) and also across health-

and from that information inequities in health can be identified and monitored. Systems that successfully address equity involve population groups and civil society organizations that advocate for older adults in decision-making, particularly those working with socially disadvantaged and marginalized groups. And finally, they possess leadership, processes and mechanisms that encourage intersectoral action to promote *Healthy Ageing*.

In some countries, ageing issues will be incorporated within a general health policy and plan, while in others it will appear as a separate document. The ideal situation may be one in which *Healthy Ageing* is incorporated within the national health policy and plan, with a supplementary, more comprehensive plan on ageing and health policy providing more details (*24*).

Health financing: alignment with *Healthy Ageing* goals

Health services for ageing populations can be supported by health-financing policies. An important starting point is to ensure that good information is available, which will allow both the tracking of overall levels of spending as well as a detailed analysis of how money is spent and the outputs or outcomes it generates. As this report has emphasized, expenditures on the health of older people are investments in their ability to do the things that matter. Ways of measuring the economic benefit of this action are urgently needed.

Health-financing policies should be aligned with goals for universal health coverage of ageing populations, which is defined by WHO as ensuring that all people have access to needed health services – such as prevention, health promotion, and treatment and rehabilitation – without the risk of financial hardship associated with accessing services (*155*). Aligning health-financing policies with the goals of universal health coverage would protect older people from foregoing essential health care because of the financial costs or from facing severe financial hardship and even impoverishment due to their needs for care.

Practically speaking, health-financing policies encompass raising revenues, pooling and allocating funds, and determining the way in which services are purchased. In terms of raising revenues, ensuring that there are adequate levels of public funding is critical to limit reliance on user fees for essential services and, hence, to ensure financial protection. Pooling resources across population groups ensures efficient risk sharing, and is particularly important for ageing populations.

The goal of purchasing in person-centred and integrated care aimed at older people is to provide services that are affordable and accessible to all. Health-financing policies need to ensure that systemic incentives lead to these comprehensive services and do not encourage ad hoc responses to be made to separate issues in isolation. For example, health providers should have a financial incentive to undertake comprehensive assessments, provide preventive interventions to delay or revert declines in capacity, and support long-term care (including rehabilitation, and palliative and hospice care). Home-based care also should be included in the package of covered services.

Particular attention will be needed to ensure not only adequate remuneration for health workers providing care to ageing populations but also to ensure there are appropriate incentives, especially for those working in community-based and primary health-care settings. Financial incentives can support efforts to encourage health workers to practise in underserved areas, and are increasingly used in the health sector in conjunction with salaried and fee-for-service arrangements.

Reframing medical research

Much medical research is focused on disease. This prevents a better understanding of the subtle changes in intrinsic function that occur both before and after the onset of disease and the factors that influence these changes.

Underlying changes in capacity and body functions, and the frequent presence of comorbidities, mean that older people have physiological responses that can be quite different from those of other age groups. Yet clinical trials routinely exclude older participants or those with comorbidities, meaning that findings may not be directly applicable to older populations (*156, 157*).

The design of clinical trials needs to be revisited to better identify how older people respond to various medications and combinations of medications (*158*). Specifically, more research is needed that looks at how commonly prescribed medications affect people with multimorbidity, which is a departure from the typical default assumption that the optimal treatment of someone with more than one health issue is to add together different interventions (*158*). And outcomes need to be considered not only in terms of disease markers but also in terms of intrinsic capacity. Improved postmarketing surveillance can help fill this gap until new approaches to clinical trials that are more relevant to older age have been developed.

Translational research into ageing and longevity will need to include more social science if it is to produce interventions for slowing declines in capacity. For example, understanding why some older people do not take their medication could boost adherence and, therefore, the effectiveness of medicines (*159*). Moreover, messaging and other strategies to encourage positive health-related behaviours may need to be different for older age groups (*160, 161*).

Finally, for health systems to be sustainable, it will be important to ensure that the strategies adopted are cost effective. However, it would be wrong to assume that cost-effectiveness findings from analyses of younger age groups can simply be extrapolated to older people, where risks may be more prevalent and adverse consequences more common (*162*). One outcome may be that both screening and treatment are more cost effective in older adults.

However, perhaps the most important change will need to be in the mindset of grant-makers and researchers. Not only will they need to focus more concretely on trajectories of intrinsic capacity and functional ability as outcomes but they will also need to overcome ageist attitudes and change their policies and procedures to be more inclusive of older people in research designs. This will require the reallocation of budgets, which are currently relatively small in ageing-related research (*163*).

Conclusion

To meet the needs of ageing populations, significant changes are required in the way health systems are structured and health care is delivered. In many places, particularly in low- and middle-income countries, access and affordability are key barriers to care. New services and approaches will need to be developed in these settings.

But globally, the services that are available are often a poor fit with the health needs of older people. They will have to be redesigned to deliver the comprehensive and coordinated care that has been shown to be more appropriate and more effective. The starting point will need to be to put older people at the centre of health care. This will require focusing on their unique needs and preferences, and including them as active participants in care planning and in managing their health states.

But changes are needed to the systems too. Health services have to be better integrated between levels and across specialist groupings. Much better coordination is needed with long-term care systems, and possibly formal integration as well. Case management, support for self-management, and support for ageing in place need to be woven into the fabric of health care for older people.

These changes appear to be both affordable and sustainable. Although much of the debate on population ageing assumes it will be associated with an unmanageable increase in the demand for services, the evidence suggests it will be a much less significant driver of inflation in health-care costs than factors such as new technologies and changes in clinical practice. Indeed, the integrated and person-centred approaches outlined in this chapter have been shown to not only have better outcomes for older people but also to be no more expensive than traditional services.

Although transforming health systems requires action on several fronts, three key themes emerge as priorities:

- shifting the clinical focus from disease to intrinsic capacity;
- rebuilding health systems to provide more person-centred and integrated care to older people;
- transforming the health workforce so that it can better provide the care that these new systems will require.

Key actions related to each of these themes are discussed in Chapter 7.

References

1. WHO World Health Survey: 2002–2004. In: World Health Organization, Health statistics and information systems [website]. Geneva: World Health Organization; 2015 (http://www.who.int/healthinfo/survey/en/, accessed 23 June 2015).

2. McIntyre D. Health policy and older people in Africa. In: Lloyd-Sherlock P, editor. Living longer: ageing, development and social protection. London: Zed Books; 2004:160–83 (http://zedbooks.co.uk/node/21198, accessed 9 June 2015).

3. Aboderin I, Kizito P. Dimensions and determinants of health in old age in Kenya. Nairobi: National Coordinating Agency for Population and Development; 2010.

4. He W, Muenchrath MN, Kowal P. Shades of gray: a cross-country study of health and well-being of the older populations in SAGE countries, 2007–2010. Washington (DC): United States Government Printing Office; 2012 (http://www.census.gov/prod/2012pubs/p95-12-01.pdf, accessed 9 June 2015).

5. Bähler C, Huber CA, Brüngger B, Reich O. Multimorbidity, health care utilization and costs in an elderly community-dwelling population: a claims data based observational study. BMC Health Serv Res. 2015;15(1):23. doi: http://dx.doi.org/10.1186/s12913-015-0698-2 PMID: 25609174

6. Osborn R, Moulds D, Squires D, Doty MM, Anderson C. International survey of older adults finds shortcomings in access, coordination, and patient-centered care. Health Aff (Millwood). 2014 Dec;33(12):2247–55. doi: http://dx.doi.org/10.1377/hlthaff.2014.0947 PMID: 25410260

7. Alecxih L, Shen S, Chan I, Taylor D, Drabek J. Individuals living in the community with chronic conditions and functional limitations: a closer look. Washington (DC): Office of the Assistant Secretary for Planning and Evaluation, Office of Disability, Aging and Long-Term Care Policy, United States Department of Health and Human Services; 2010 (http://www.aspe.hhs.gov/daltcp/reports/2010/closerlook.pdf, accessed 9 June 2015).

8. Terraneo M. Inequities in health care utilization by people aged 50+: evidence from 12 European countries. Soc Sci Med. 2015 Feb;126:154–63. doi: http://dx.doi.org/10.1016/j.socscimed.2014.12.028 PMID: 25562311

9. Fitzpatrick AL, Powe NR, Cooper LS, Ives DG, Robbins JA. Barriers to health care access among the elderly and who perceives them. Am J Public Health. 2004 Oct;94(10):1788–94. doi: http://dx.doi.org/10.2105/AJPH.94.10.1788 PMID: 15451751

10. Balarajan Y, Selvaraj S, Subramanian SV. Health care and equity in India. Lancet. 2011 Feb 5;377(9764):505–15. doi: http://dx.doi.org/10.1016/S0140-6736(10)61894-6 PMID: 21227492

11. WHO Study on global AGEing and adult health (SAGE). In: World Health Organization, Health statistics and information systems [website]. Geneva: World Health Organization; 2015 (http://www.who.int/healthinfo/sage/en/, accessed 23 June 2015).

12. Dey S, Nambiar D, Lakshmi JK, Sheikh K, Srinath Reddy K.Health of the elderly in India: challenges of access and affordability. In: Smith JP, Majmundar M, editors. Aging in Asia: findings from new and emerging data initiatives. Washington (DC): National Academies Press; 2012 (http://www.nap.edu/catalog/13361/aging-in-asia-findings-from-new-and-emerging-data-initiatives, accessed 9 June 2015).

13. Albanese E, Liu Z, Acosta D, Guerra M, Huang Y, Jacob KS, et al. Equity in the delivery of community healthcare to older people: findings from 10/66 Dementia Research Group cross-sectional surveys in Latin America, China, India and Nigeria. BMC Health Serv Res. 2011;11(1):153. doi: http://dx.doi.org/10.1186/1472-6963-11-153 PMID: 21711546

14. Frenk J, Chen L, Bhutta ZA, Cohen J, Crisp N, Evans T, et al. Health professionals for a new century: transforming education to strengthen health systems in an interdependent world. Lancet. 2010 Dec 4;376(9756):1923–58. doi: http://dx.doi.org/10.1016/S0140-6736(10)61854-5 PMID: 21112623

15. Ham C. The ten characteristics of the high-performing chronic care system. Health Econ Policy Law. 2010 Jan;5(Pt. 1):71–90. doi: http://dx.doi.org/10.1017/S1744133109990120 PMID: 19732475

16. Low LF, Yap M, Brodaty H. A systematic review of different models of home and community care services for older persons. BMC Health Serv Res. 2011;11(1):93. doi: http://dx.doi.org/10.1186/1472-6963-11-93 PMID: 21549010

17. Eklund K, Wilhelmson K. Outcomes of coordinated and integrated interventions targeting frail elderly people: a systematic review of randomised controlled trials. Health Soc Care Community. 2009 Sep;17(5):447–58. doi: http://dx.doi.org/10.1111/j.1365-2524.2009.00844.x PMID: 19245421

18. Pruitt SD, Epping-Jordan JE. Preparing the 21st century global healthcare workforce. BMJ. 2005 Mar 19;330(7492):637–9. doi: http://dx.doi.org/10.1136/bmj.330.7492.637 PMID: 15774994

19. Committee on the Future Health Care Workforce for Older Americans; Board on Health Care Services; Institute of Medicine of the National Academies Press. Retooling for an aging America: building the health care workforce. Washington (DC): National Academies Press; 2008 (http://books.nap.edu/openbook.php?record_id=12089, accessed 9 June 2015).

20. Mateos-Nozal J, Beard JR. Global approaches to geriatrics in medical education. Eur Geriatr Med. 2011;2(2):87–92. doi: http://dx.doi.org/10.1016/j.eurger.2011.01.001

21. Keller I, Makipaa A, Kalenscher T, Kalache A. Global survey on geriatrics in the medical curriculum. Geneva: World Health Organization; 2002 (http://www.who.int/ageing/projects/en/alc_global_survey_tegeme.pdf, accessed 9 June 2015).

22. Stall N. Time to end ageism in medical education. CMAJ. 2012 Apr 3;184(6):728. doi: http://dx.doi.org/10.1503/cmaj.112179 PMID: 22410378

23. Center for Health Workforce Studies. The Impact of the aging population on the health workforce in the United States. Rensselaer (NY): University at Albany, School of Public Health; 2006 (http://www.albany.edu/news/pdf_files/impact_of_aging_full.pdf, accessed 9 June 2015).

24. Araujo de Carvalho I, Byles J, Aquah C, Amofah G, Biritwum R, Panisset U, et al. Informing evidence-based policies for ageing and health in Ghana. Bull World Health Organ. 2015 Jan 1;93(1):47–51. doi: http://dx.doi.org/10.2471/BLT.14.136242 PMID: 25558107

25. National ageing policy: ageing with security and dignity. Accra: Government of Ghana; 2010 (http://www.ghanaweb.com/GhanaHomePage/blogs/blog.article.php?blog=3442&ID=1000008901, accessed 23 June 2015).

26. Boult C, Counsell SR, Leipzig RM, Berenson RA. The urgency of preparing primary care physicians to care for older people with chronic illnesses. Health Aff (Millwood). 2010 May;29(5):811–8. doi: http://dx.doi.org/10.1377/hlthaff.2010.0095 PMID: 20439866

27. Adelman RD, Capello CF, LoFaso V, Greene MG, Konopasek L, Marzuk PM. Introduction to the older patient: a "first exposure" to geriatrics for medical students. J Am Geriatr Soc. 2007 Sep;55(9):1445–50. doi: http://dx.doi.org/10.1111/j.1532-5415.2007.01301.x PMID: 17767689

28. Band-Winterstein T. Health care provision for older persons: the interplay between ageism and elder neglect. J Appl Gerontol. 2013 PMID: 24652870

29. Reese PP, Caplan AL, Bloom RD, Abt PL, Karlawish JH. How should we use age to ration health care? Lessons from the case of kidney transplantation. J Am Geriatr Soc. 2010 Oct;58(10):1980–6. doi: http://dx.doi.org/10.1111/j.1532-5415.2010.03031.x PMID: 20831719

30. Galea S, Vlahov D, Tracy M, Hoover DR, Resnick H, Kilpatrick D. Hispanic ethnicity and post-traumatic stress disorder after a disaster: evidence from a general population survey after September 11, 2001. Ann Epidemiol. 2004 Sep;14(8):520–31. doi: http://dx.doi.org/10.1016/j.annepidem.2004.01.006 PMID: 15350950

31. Making fair choices on the path to universal health coverage. Final report of the WHO Consultative Group on Equity and Universal Health Coverage. Geneva: World Health Organization; 2014 (http://apps.who.int/iris/bitstream/10665/112671/1/9789241507158_eng.pdf, accessed 9 June 2015).

32. Oliver D, Foot C, Humphries R. Making our health and care systems fit for an ageing population. London: The King's Fund; 2014 (http://www.kingsfund.org.uk/sites/files/kf/field/field_publication_file/making-health-care-systems-fit-ageing-population-oliver-foot-humphries-mar14.pdf, accessed 9 June 2015).

33. Kingsley DE. Aging and health care costs: narrative versus reality. Poverty Public Policy. 2015;7(1):3–21. doi: http://dx.doi.org/10.1002/pop4.89

34. Rolden HJA, van Bodegom D, Westendorp RGJ. Variation in the costs of dying and the role of different health services, socio-demographic characteristics, and preceding health care expenses. Soc Sci Med. 2014 Nov;120(0):110–7. doi: http://dx.doi.org/10.1016/j.socscimed.2014.09.020 PMID: 25238558

35. Hagist C, Kotlikoff L. Who's going broke? Comparing healthcare costs in ten OECD countries. Cambridge (MA): National Bureau of Economic Research; 2005 (Working Paper 11833; http://www.nber.org/papers/w11833.pdf, accessed 9 June 2015).

36. Wong A, van Baal PH, Boshuizen HC, Polder JJ. Exploring the influence of proximity to death on disease-specific hospital expenditures: a carpaccio of red herrings. Health Econ. 2011 Apr;20(4):379–400. doi: http://dx.doi.org/10.1002/hec.1597 PMID: 20232289

37. Hoover DR, Crystal S, Kumar R, Sambamoorthi U, Cantor JC. Medical expenditures during the last year of life: findings from the 1992–1996 Medicare current beneficiary survey. Health Serv Res. 2002 Dec;37(6):1625–42. doi: http://dx.doi.org/10.1111/1475-6773.01113 PMID: 12546289

38. Kardamanidis K, Lim K, Da Cunha C, Taylor LK, Jorm LR. Hospital costs of older people in New South Wales in the last year of life. Med J Aust. 2007 Oct 1;187(7):383–6. PMID: 17907999

39. Polder JJ, Barendregt JJ, van Oers H. Health care costs in the last year of life–the Dutch experience. Soc Sci Med. 2006 Oct;63(7):1720–31. doi: http://dx.doi.org/10.1016/j.socscimed.2006.04.018 PMID: 16781037

40. Hoover DR, Crystal S, Kumar R, Sambamoorthi U, Cantor JC. Medical expenditures during the last year of life: findings from the 1992–1996 Medicare current beneficiary survey. Health Serv Res. 2002 Dec;37(6):1625–42. doi: http://dx.doi.org/10.1111/1475-6773.01113 PMID: 12546289

41. Marik PE. The cost of inappropriate care at the end of life: implications for an aging population. Am J Hosp Palliat Care. 2014;pii:1049909114537399. http://ajh.sagepub.com/content/early/2014/06/05/1049909114537399.abstract?rss=1 PMID: 24907121

42. Spijker J, MacInnes J. Population ageing: the timebomb that isn't? BMJ. 2013;347 Nov 12:f6598. doi: http://dx.doi.org/10.1136/bmj.f6598 PMID: 24222481

43. Rechel B, Doyle Y, Grundy E, McKee M. How can health systems respond to population aging? Copenhagen: World Health Organization; 2009. (http://www.euro.who.int/__data/assets/pdf_file/0004/64966/E92560.pdf, accessed 9 June 2015).

44. Lubitz J, Cai L, Kramarow E, Lentzner H. Health, life expectancy, and health care spending among the elderly. N Engl J Med. 2003 Sep 11;349(11):1048–55. doi: http://dx.doi.org/10.1056/NEJMsa020614 PMID: 12968089

45. Gandjour A. Health care expenditures from living longer–how much do they matter. Int J Health Plann Manage. 2014 Jan;29(1):43–51. doi: http://dx.doi.org/10.1002/hpm.2164 PMID: 23418021

46. Wouterse B, Huisman M, Meijboom BR, Deeg DJ, Polder JJ. Modeling the relationship between health and health care expenditures using a latent Markov model. J Health Econ. 2013 Mar;32(2):423–39. doi: http://dx.doi.org/10.1016/j.jhealeco.2012.11.005 PMID: 23353134

47. Dormont B, Grignon M, Huber H. Health expenditure growth: reassessing the threat of ageing. Health Econ. 2006 Sep;15(9):947–63. doi: http://dx.doi.org/10.1002/hec.1165 PMID: 16958079

48. Esterman AJ, Ben-Tovim DI. The Australian coordinated care trials: success or failure? The second round of trials may provide more answers. Med J Aust. 2002 Nov 4;177(9):469–70. PMID: 12405885

49. Goodwin N, Dixon A, Anderson G, Wodchis W. Providing integrated care for older people with complex needs: lessons from seven international case studies. London: The King's Fund; 2014 (http://cdn.basw.co.uk/upload/basw_102418-7.pdf, accessed 9 June 2015).

50. Hébert R, Raîche M, Dubois MF, Gueye NR, Dubuc N, Tousignant M; PRISMA Group. Impact of PRISMA, a coordination-type integrated service delivery system for frail older people in Quebec (Canada): a quasi-experimental study. J Gerontol B Psychol Sci Soc Sci. 2010 Jan;65B(1):107–18. doi: http://dx.doi.org/10.1093/geronb/gbp027 PMID: 19414866

51. Goodwin N, Sonola L, Thiel V, Kodner DL. Co-ordinated care for people with complex chronic conditions. London: The King's Fund; 2013 (http://www.kingsfund.org.uk/sites/files/kf/field/field_publication_file/co-ordinated-care-for-people-with-complex-chronic-conditions-kingsfund-oct13.pdf, accessed 9 June 2015).

52. Bernabei R, Landi F, Onder G, Liperoti R, Gambassi G. Second and third generation assessment instruments: the birth of standardization in geriatric care. J Gerontol A Biol Sci Med Sci. 2008;63(3):308–13.

53. Conroy SP, Stevens T, Parker SG, Gladman JR. A systematic review of comprehensive geriatric assessment to improve outcomes for frail older people being rapidly discharged from acute hospital: 'interface geriatrics'. Age Ageing. 2011;40(4):436–43.

54. Ellis G, Whitehead MA, Robinson D, O'Neill D, Langhorne P. Comprehensive geriatric assessment for older adults admitted to hospital: meta-analysis of randomised controlled trials. BMJ. 2011 Oct 27;343:d6553. doi: http://dx.doi.org/10.1136/bmj.d6553 PMID: 22034146

55. Rubenstein LZ, Stuck AE, Siu AL, Wieland D. Impacts of geriatric evaluation and management programs on defined outcomes: overview of the evidence. J Am Geriatr Soc. 1991 Sep;39(9 Pt. 2):8S–16S; discussion 17S–18S. doi: http://dx.doi.org/10.1111/j.1532-5415.1991.tb05927.x PMID: 1832179

56. Odden MC, Peralta CA, Haan MN, Covinsky KE. Rethinking the association of high blood pressure with mortality in elderly adults: the impact of frailty. Arch Intern Med. 2012 Aug 13;172(15):1162–8. doi: http://dx.doi.org/10.1001/archinternmed.2012.2555 PMID: 22801930

57. Managing older people with type 2 diabetes: global guideline. Brussels: International Diabetes Federation; 2013 (http://www.ifa-fiv.org/wp-content/uploads/2014/02/IDF-Guideline-for-Older-People.pdf, accessed 9 June 2015).

58. Musini VM, Tejani AM, Bassett K, Wright JM. Pharmacotherapy for hypertension in the elderly. Cochrane Database Syst. Rev. 2009;(4):CD000028.http://www.ncbi.nlm.nih.gov/entrez/query.fcgi?cmd=Retrieve&db=PubMed&list_uids=19821263&dopt=Abstract PMID: 19821263

59. Estruch R, Ros E, Salas-Salvadó J, Covas MI, Corella D, Arós F, et al.; PREDIMED Study Investigators. Primary prevention of cardiovascular disease with a Mediterranean diet. N Engl J Med. 2013 Apr 4;368(14):1279–90. doi: http://dx.doi.org/10.1056/NEJMoa1200303 PMID: 23432189

60. Michel JP, Newton JL, Kirkwood TB. Medical challenges of improving the quality of a longer life. JAMA. 2008 Feb 13;299(6):688–90. doi: http://dx.doi.org/10.1001/jama.299.6.688 PMID: 18270358

61. Peto R, Darby S, Deo H, Silcocks P, Whitley E, Doll R. Smoking, smoking cessation, and lung cancer in the UK since 1950: combination of national statistics with two case-control studies. BMJ. 2000 Aug 5;321(7257):323–9. doi: http://dx.doi.org/10.1136/bmj.321.7257.323 PMID: 10926586

62. Preventing chronic diseases: a vital investment. Geneva: World Health Organization; 2005 (http://whqlibdoc.who.int/publications/2005/9241563001_eng.pdf, accessed 9 June 2015).

63. Elwood P, Galante J, Pickering J, Palmer S, Bayer A, Ben-Shlomo Y, et al. Healthy lifestyles reduce the incidence of chronic diseases and dementia: evidence from the Caerphilly cohort study. PLOS ONE. 2013;8(12):e81877. doi: http://dx.doi.org/10.1371/journal.pone.0081877 PMID: 24349147

64. Fulop T, Larbi A, Witkowski JM, McElhaney J, Loeb M, Mitnitski A, et al. Aging, frailty and age-related diseases. Biogerontology. 2010 Oct;11(5):547–63. doi: http://dx.doi.org/10.1007/s10522-010-9287-2 PMID: 20559726

65. Beck AM, Kjær S, Hansen BS, Storm RL, Thal-Jantzen K, Bitz C. Follow-up home visits with registered dietitians have a positive effect on the functional and nutritional status of geriatric medical patients after discharge: a randomized controlled trial. Clin Rehabil. 2013 Jun;27(6):483–93. doi: http://dx.doi.org/10.1177/0269215512469384 PMID: 23258932

66. Dorner TE, Lackinger C, Haider S, Luger E, Kapan A, Luger M, et al. Nutritional intervention and physical training in malnourished frail community-dwelling elderly persons carried out by trained lay "buddies": study protocol of a randomized controlled trial. BMC Public Health. 2013;13(1):1232. doi: http://dx.doi.org/10.1186/1471-2458-13-1232 PMID: 24369785

67. Global action plan for the prevention and control of noncommunicable diseases 2013–2020. Geneva: World Health Organization; 2013 (http://www.who.int/global-coordination-mechanism/publications/global-action-plan-ncds-eng.pdf?ua=1, accessed 9 June 2015).

68. Epping-Jordan JE, Galea G, Tukuitonga C, Beaglehole R. Preventing chronic diseases: taking stepwise action. Lancet. 2005 Nov 5;366(9497):1667–71. doi: http://dx.doi.org/10.1016/S0140-6736(05)67342-4 PMID: 16271649

69. Lloyd-Sherlock P, Beard J, Minicuci N, Ebrahim S, Chatterji S. Hypertension among older adults in low- and middle-income countries: prevalence, awareness and control. Int J Epidemiol. 2014 Feb;43(1):116–28. doi: http://dx.doi.org/10.1093/ije/dyt215 PMID: 24505082

70. Prevention and control of noncommunicable diseases: guidelines for primary health care in low-resource settings. Geneva: World Health Organization; 2012 (http://apps.who.int/iris/bitstream/10665/76173/1/9789241548397_eng.pdf, accessed 9 June 2015).

71. A global brief on hypertension: silent killer, global public health crisis. Geneva: World Health Organization; 2013 (WHO/DCO/WHD/2013.2; http://apps.who.int/iris/bitstream/10665/79059/1/WHO_DCO_WHD_2013.2_eng.pdf, accessed 9 June 2015).

72. Prevention of cardiovascular disease: guidelines for assessment and management of total cardiovascular risk. Geneva: World Health Organization; 2007 (http://www.who.int/cardiovascular_diseases/guidelines/Full%20text.pdf, accessed 9 June 2015).

73. Daniels R, van Rossum E, de Witte L, Kempen GI, van den Heuvel W. Interventions to prevent disability in frail community-dwelling elderly: a systematic review. BMC Health Serv Res. 2008;8(1):278. doi: http://dx.doi.org/10.1186/1472-6963-8-278 PMID: 19115992

74. Daniels R, van Rossum E, Metzelthin S, Sipers W, Habets H, Hobma S, et al. A disability prevention programme for community-dwelling frail older persons. Clin Rehabil. 2011 Nov;25(11):963–74. doi: http://dx.doi.org/10.1177/0269215511410728 PMID: 21849375

75. Clegg A, Young J, Iliffe S, Rikkert MO, Rockwood K. Frailty in elderly people. Lancet. 2013 Mar 2;381(9868):752–62. doi: http://dx.doi.org/10.1016/S0140-6736(12)62167-9 PMID: 23395245

76. Murtagh EM, Murphy MH, Boone-Heinonen J. Walking: the first steps in cardiovascular disease prevention. Curr Opin Cardiol. 2010 Sep;25(5):490–6. doi: http://dx.doi.org/10.1097/HCO.0b013e32833ce972 PMID: 20625280

77. Edwards MH, Dennison EM, Aihie Sayer A, Fielding R, Cooper C. Osteoporosis and sarcopenia in older age. Bone. 2015 Apr 14; doi: http://dx.doi.org/10.1016/j.bone.2015.04.016 PMID: 25886902

78. Giangregorio LM, Papaioannou A, MacIntyre NJ, Ashe MC, Heinonen A, Shipp K, et al. Too fit to fracture: outcomes of a Delphi consensus process on physical activity and exercise recommendations for adults with osteoporosis with or without vertebral fractures. Osteoporos Int. 2014;25(3):821–35. doi: http://dx.doi.org/10.1007/s00198-013-2523-2 PMID: 25510579

79. Levine ME, Suarez JA, Brandhorst S, Balasubramanian P, Cheng CW, Madia F, et al. Low protein intake is associated with a major reduction in IGF-1, cancer, and overall mortality in the 65 and younger but not older population. Cell Metab. 2014 Mar 4;19(3):407–17. doi: http://dx.doi.org/10.1016/j.cmet.2014.02.006 PMID: 24606898

80. Beswick AD, Rees K, Dieppe P, Ayis S, Gooberman-Hill R, Horwood J, et al. Complex interventions to improve physical function and maintain independent living in elderly people: a systematic review and meta-analysis. Lancet. 2008 Mar 1;371(9614):725–35. doi: http://dx.doi.org/10.1016/S0140-6736(08)60342-6 PMID: 18313501

81. Gill TM, Baker DI, Gottschalk M, Peduzzi PN, Allore H, Byers A. A program to prevent functional decline in physically frail, elderly persons who live at home. N Engl J Med. 2002 Oct 3;347(14):1068–74. doi: http://dx.doi.org/10.1056/NEJMoa020423 PMID: 12362007

82. Ferrucci L, Guralnik JM, Studenski S, Fried LP, Cutler GB Jr, Walston JD; Interventions on Frailty Working Group. Designing randomized, controlled trials aimed at preventing or delaying functional decline and disability in frail, older persons: a consensus report. J Am Geriatr Soc. 2004 Apr;52(4):625–34. doi: http://dx.doi.org/10.1111/j.1532-5415.2004.52174.x PMID: 15066083

83. Pel-Littel RE, Schuurmans MJ, Emmelot-Vonk MH, Verhaar HJ. Frailty: defining and measuring of a concept. J Nutr Health Aging. 2009 Apr;13(4):390–4. doi: http://dx.doi.org/10.1007/s12603-009-0051-8 PMID: 19300888

84. Wendel-Vos GC, Schuit AJ, Tijhuis MA, Kromhout D. Leisure time physical activity and health-related quality of life: cross-sectional and longitudinal associations. Qual Life Res. 2004 Apr;13(3):667–77. doi: http://dx.doi.org/10.1023/B:QURE.0000021313.51397.33 PMID: 15130029

85. Chodzko-Zajko WJ, Proctor DN, Fiatarone Singh MA, Minson CT, Nigg CR, Salem GJ, et al.; American College of Sports Medicine. American College of Sports Medicine position stand. Exercise and physical activity for older adults. Med Sci Sports Exerc. 2009 Jul;41(7):1510–30. doi: http://dx.doi.org/10.1249/MSS.0b013e3181a0c95c PMID: 19516148

86. Paterson DH, Warburton DE. Physical activity and functional limitations in older adults: a systematic review related to Canada's Physical Activity Guidelines. Int J Behav Nutr Phys Act. 2010;7(1):38. doi: http://dx.doi.org/10.1186/1479-5868-7-38 PMID: 20459782

87. Wolfson L, Judge J, Whipple R, King M. Strength is a major factor in balance, gait, and the occurrence of falls. J Gerontol A Biol Sci Med Sci. 1995 Nov;50(Spec. No.):64–7. PMID: 7493221

88. Gomes GA, Cintra FA, Batista FS, Neri AL, Guariento ME, Sousa ML, et al. Elderly outpatient profile and predictors of falls. Sao Paulo Med J. 2013;131(1):13–8. doi: http://dx.doi.org/10.1590/S1516-31802013000100003 PMID: 23538590

89. Landi F, Liperoti R, Russo A, Giovannini S, Tosato M, Capoluongo E, et al. Sarcopenia as a risk factor for falls in elderly individuals: results from the ilSIRENTE study. Clin Nutr. 2012 Oct;31(5):652–8. doi: http://dx.doi.org/10.1016/j.clnu.2012.02.007 PMID: 22414775

90. Baztán JJ, Suárez-García FM, López-Arrieta J, Rodríguez-Mañas L, Rodríguez-Artalejo F. Effectiveness of acute geriatric units on functional decline, living at home, and case fatality among older patients admitted to hospital for acute medical disorders: meta-analysis. BMJ. 2009 Jan 22;338:b50. doi: http://dx.doi.org/10.1136/bmj.b50 PMID: 19164393

91. González Montalvo JI, Gotor Pérez P, Martín Vega A, Alarcón Alarcón T, Álvarez de Linera JL, Gil Garay E, et al. La unidad de ortogeriatría de agudos. Evaluación de su efecto en el curso clínico de los pacientes con fractura de cadera y estimación de su impacto económico. [The acute orthogeriatric unit. Assessment of its effect on the clinical course of patients with hip fractures and an estimate of its financial impact]. Rev Esp Geriatr Gerontol. 2011 Jul-Aug;46(4):193–9. (in Spanish). PMID: 21507529

92. Patterson L. Making our health and care systems fit for an ageing population: David Oliver, Catherine Foot, Richard Humphries. King's Fund March 2014. Age Ageing. 2014 Sep;43(5):731. doi: http://dx.doi.org/10.1093/ageing/afu105 PMID: 25074536

93. Shepperd S, Wee B, Straus SE. Hospital at home: home-based end of life care. Cochrane Database Syst. Rev. 2011;(7):CD009231. PMID: 21735440

94. Caplan GA, Sulaiman NS, Mangin DA, Aimonino Ricauda N, Wilson AD, Barclay L. A meta-analysis of "hospital in the home". Med J Aust. 2012 Nov 5;197(9):512–9. doi: http://dx.doi.org/10.5694/mja12.10480 PMID: 23121588

95. McDonald KM, Schultz EM, Chang C. Evaluating the state of quality-improvement science through evidence synthesis: insights from the closing the quality gap series. Perm J. 2013 Fall;17(4):52–61. doi: http://dx.doi.org/10.7812/TPP/13-010 PMID: 24079357

96. Ouwens M, Wollersheim H, Hermens R, Hulscher M, Grol R. Integrated care programmes for chronically ill patients: a review of systematic reviews. Int J Qual Health Care. 2005 Apr;17(2):141–6. doi: http://dx.doi.org/10.1093/intqhc/mzi016 PMID: 15665066

97. Nolte E, Pitchforth E. What is the evidence on the economic impacts of integrated care? Copenhagen: World Health Organization; 2014 (http://www.euro.who.int/__data/assets/pdf_file/0019/251434/What-is-the-evidence-on-the-economic-impacts-of-integrated-care.pdf, accessed 9 June 2015).

98. Johri M, Beland F, Bergman H. International experiments in integrated care for the elderly: a synthesis of the evidence. Int J Geriatr Psychiatry. 2003 Mar;18(3):222–35. doi: http://dx.doi.org/10.1002/gps.819 PMID: 12642892

99. WHO global strategy on people-centred and integrated health services. Geneva: World Health Organization; 2015 (WHO/HIS/SDS/2015.6; http://www.who.int/servicedeliverysafety/areas/people-centred-care/global-strategy/en/, accessed 9 June 2015).

100. Chernichovsky D, Leibowitz AA. Integrating public health and personal care in a reformed US health care system. Am J Public Health. 2010 Feb;100(2):205–11. doi: http://dx.doi.org/10.2105/AJPH.2008.156588 PMID: 20019310

101. Valentijn PP, Schepman SM, Opheij W, Bruijnzeels MA. Understanding integrated care: a comprehensive conceptual framework based on the integrative functions of primary care. Int J Integr Care. 2013 Jan-Mar;13:e010. PMID: 23687482

102. The world health report 2008. Primary health care: now more than ever. Geneva: World Health Organization; 2008 (http://www.who.int/whr/2008/en/, accessed 9 June 2015).

103. Goodwin N, Sonola L, Thiel V, Kodner DL. Co-ordinated care for people with complex chronic conditions: key lessons and markers for success. London: The King's Fund; 2013 (http://www.kingsfund.org.uk/sites/files/kf/field/field_publication_file/co-ordinated-care-for-people-with-complex-chronic-conditions-kingsfund-oct13.pdf, accessed 9 June 2015).

104. Norris SL, Nichols PJ, Caspersen CJ, Glasgow RE, Engelgau MM, Jack L Jr, et al. The effectiveness of disease and case management for people with diabetes. A systematic review. Am J Prev Med. 2002 May;22(4) (Suppl.):15–38. doi: http://dx.doi.org/10.1016/S0749-3797(02)00423-3 PMID: 11985933

105. Conroy S, Dowsing T. What should we do about hospital readmissions? Age Ageing. 2012 Nov;41(6):702–4. doi: http://dx.doi.org/10.1093/ageing/afs154 PMID: 23045361

106. Nuñez DE, Keller C, Ananian CD. A review of the efficacy of the self-management model on health outcomes in community-residing older adults with arthritis. Worldviews Evid Based Nurs. 2009;6(3):130–48. doi: http://dx.doi.org/10.1111/j.1741-6787.2009.00157.x PMID: 19656354

107. Sherifali D, Bai JW, Kenny M, Warren R, Ali MU. Diabetes self-management programmes in older adults: a systematic review and meta-analysis. Diabet Med. 2015 Apr 10. doi: http://dx.doi.org/10.1111/dme.12780 PMID: 25865179

108. Lorig KR, Ritter P, Stewart AL, Sobel DS, William Brown B, Bandura A, et al. Chronic disease self-management program: 2-year health status and health care utilization outcomes. Med Care. 2001 Nov;39(11):1217–23. doi: http://dx.doi.org/10.1097/00005650-200111000-00008 PMID: 11606875

109. Jonker AA, Comijs HC, Knipscheer KC, Deeg DJ. Promotion of self-management in vulnerable older people: a narrative literature review of outcomes of the Chronic Disease Self-Management Program (CDSMP). Eur J Ageing. 2009 Dec;6(4):303–14. doi: http://dx.doi.org/10.1007/s10433-009-0131-y PMID: 19920862

110. Kim SH, Youn CH. Efficacy of chronic disease self-management program in older Korean adults with low and high health literacy. Asian Nurs Res (Korean Soc Nurs Sci). 2015 Mar;9(1):42–6. doi: http://dx.doi.org/10.1016/j.anr.2014.10.008 PMID: 25829209

111. Melchior MA, Seff LR, Bastida E, Albatineh AN, Page TF, Palmer RC. Intermediate outcomes of a chronic disease self-management program for Spanish-speaking older adults in South Florida, 2008–2010. Prev Chronic Dis. 2013;10:E146. doi: http://dx.doi.org/10.5888/pcd10.130016 PMID: 23987252

112. Reid MC, Papaleontiou M, Ong A, Breckman R, Wethington E, Pillemer K. Self-management strategies to reduce pain and improve function among older adults in community settings: a review of the evidence. Pain Med. 2008 May-Jun;9(4):409–24. doi: http://dx.doi.org/10.1111/j.1526-4637.2008.00428.x PMID: 18346056

113. Franek J. Self-management support interventions for persons with chronic disease: an evidence-based analysis. Ont Health Technol Assess Ser. 2013;13(9):1–60. PMID: 24194800

114. Dattalo M, Giovannetti ER, Scharfstein D, Boult C, Wegener S, Wolff JL, et al. Who participates in chronic disease self-management (CDSM) programs? Differences between participants and nonparticipants in a population of multimorbid older adults. Med Care. 2012 Dec;50(12):1071–5. doi: http://dx.doi.org/10.1097/MLR.0b013e318268abe7 PMID: 22892650

115. Rubak S, Sandbaek A, Lauritzen T, Christensen B. Motivational interviewing: a systematic review and meta-analysis. Br J Gen Pract. 2005 Apr;55(513):305–12. PMID: 15826439

116. Emmons KM, Rollnick S. Motivational interviewing in health care settings. Opportunities and limitations. Am J Prev Med. 2001 Jan;20(1):68–74. doi: http://dx.doi.org/10.1016/S0749-3797(00)00254-3 PMID: 11137778

117. Whitlock EP, Orleans CT, Pender N, Allan J. Evaluating primary care behavioral counseling interventions: an evidence-based approach. Am J Prev Med. 2002 May;22(4):267–84. doi: http://dx.doi.org/10.1016/S0749-3797(02)00415-4 PMID: 11988383

118. Public housing in Singapore: residents' profile, housing satisfaction and preferences. HDB Sample Household Survey 2013. Singapore: Housing and Development Board, Singapore Government; 2014.

119. Keenan TA. Home and community preferences of the 45+ Population. Washington (DC): AARP; 2010 (http://assets.aarp.org/rgcenter/general/home-community-services-10.pdf, accessed 9 June 2015).

120. Costa-Font J, Elvira D, Mascarilla-Miró O. `Ageing in Place'? Exploring Elderly people's housing preferences in Spain. Urban Stud. 2009;46(2):295–316. doi: http://dx.doi.org/10.1177/0042098008099356

121. Huss A, Stuck AE, Rubenstein LZ, Egger M, Clough-Gorr KM. Multidimensional preventive home visit programs for community-dwelling older adults: a systematic review and meta-analysis of randomized controlled trials. J Gerontol A Biol Sci Med Sci. 2008 Mar;63(3):298–307. doi: http://dx.doi.org/10.1093/gerona/63.3.298 PMID: 18375879

122. Mayo-Wilson E, Grant S, Burton J, Parsons A, Underhill K, Montgomery P. Preventive home visits for mortality, morbidity, and institutionalization in older adults: a systematic review and meta-analysis. PLOS ONE. 2014;9(3):e89257. doi: http://dx.doi.org/10.1371/journal.pone.0089257 PMID: 24622676

123. Stuck AE, Egger M, Hammer A, Minder CE, Beck JC. Home visits to prevent nursing home admission and functional decline in elderly people: systematic review and meta-regression analysis. JAMA. 2002 Feb 27;287(8):1022–8. doi: http://dx.doi.org/10.1001/jama.287.8.1022 PMID: 11866651

124. Ashworth NL, Chad KE, Harrison EL, Reeder BA, Marshall SC. Home versus center based physical activity programs in older adults. Cochrane Database Syst. Rev. 2005;(1):CD004017. PMID: 15674925

125. Geraedts H, Zijlstra A, Bulstra SK, Stevens M, Zijlstra W. Effects of remote feedback in home-based physical activity interventions for older adults: a systematic review. Patient Educ Couns. 2013 Apr;91(1):14–24. doi: http://dx.doi.org/10.1016/j.pec.2012.10.018 PMID: 23194823

126. Opdenacker J, Delecluse C, Boen F. A 2-year follow-up of a lifestyle physical activity versus a structured exercise intervention in older adults. J Am Geriatr Soc. 2011 Sep;59(9):1602–11. doi: http://dx.doi.org/10.1111/j.1532-5415.2011.03551.x PMID: 21883103

127. Elkan R, Kendrick D, Dewey M, Hewitt M, Robinson J, Blair R, et al. Effectiveness of home based support for older people: systematic review and meta-analysis. BMJ. 2001;323(7315):719–25.

128. van Haastregt JC, Diederiks JP, van Rossum E, de Witte LP, Crebolder HF. Effects of preventive home visits to elderly people living in the community: systematic review. BMJ. 2000;320(7237):754–8.

129. Bouman A, van Rossum E, Nelemans P, Kempen GI, Knipschild P. Effects of intensive home visiting programs for older people with poor health status: a systematic review. BMC Health Serv Res. 2008;8:74.

130. Everybody's business: strengthening health systems to improve health outcomes. WHO's framework for action. Geneva: World Health Organization; 2007 (http://www.who.int/healthsystems/strategy/everybodys_business.pdf, accessed 9 June 2015).

131. Montenegro H, Holder R, Ramagem C, Urrutia S, Fabrega R, Tasca R, et al. Combating health care fragmentation through integrated health service delivery networks in the Americas: lessons learned. J Integr Care. 2011;19(5):5–16. doi: http://dx.doi.org/10.1108/14769011111176707

132. Global age-friendly cities: a guide. Geneva: World Health Organization; 2007 (http://www.who.int/ageing/publications/Global_age_friendly_cities_Guide_English.pdf, accessed 9 June 2015).

133. The world health report 2006: working for health. Geneva: World Health Organization; 2006 (http://www.who.int/whr/2006/en/, accessed 9 June 2015).

134. Global consensus for social accountability of medical schools. In: Global consensus for social accountability [website]. Global consensus for social accountability; 2010 (http://healthsocialaccountability.org/, accessed 9 June 2015).

135. Transforming and scaling up health professionals' education and training: World Health Organization guidelines 2013. Geneva: World Health Organization; 2013 (http://apps.who.int/iris/bitstream/10665/93635/1/9789241506502_eng.pdf, accessed 9 June 2015).

136. Wagner EH. The role of patient care teams in chronic disease management. BMJ. 2000 Feb 26;320(7234):569–72. doi: http://dx.doi.org/10.1136/bmj.320.7234.569 PMID: 10688568

137. Abegunde DO, Shengelia B, Luyten A, Cameron A, Celletti F, Nishtar S, et al. Can non-physician health-care workers assess and manage cardiovascular risk in primary care? Bull World Health Organ. 2007 Jun;85(6):432–40. doi: http://dx.doi.org/10.2471/BLT.06.032177 PMID: 17639240

138. Wilson IB, Landon BE, Hirschhorn LR, McInnes K, Ding L, Marsden PV, et al. Quality of HIV care provided by nurse practitioners, physician assistants, and physicians. Ann Intern Med. 2005 Nov 15;143(10):729–36. doi: http://dx.doi.org/10.7326/0003-4819-143-10-200511150-00010 PMID: 16287794

139. Aubert RE, Herman WH, Waters J, Moore W, Sutton D, Peterson BL, et al. Nurse case management to improve glycemic control in diabetic patients in a health maintenance organization: a randomized, controlled trial. Ann Intern Med. 1998 Oct 15;129(8):605–12. doi: http://dx.doi.org/10.7326/0003-4819-129-8-199810150-00004 PMID: 9786807

140. Epping-Jordan JE, van Ommeren M, Ashour HN, Maramis A, Marini A, Mohanraj A, et al. Beyond the crisis: building back better mental health care in 10 emergency-affected areas using a longer-term perspective. Int J Ment Health Syst. 2015;9(1):15. doi: http://dx.doi.org/10.1186/s13033-015-0007-9 PMID: 25904981

141. Samb B, Celletti F, Holloway J, Van Damme W, De Cock KM, Dybul M. Rapid expansion of the health workforce in response to the HIV epidemic. N Engl J Med. 2007 Dec 13;357(24):2510–14. doi: http://dx.doi.org/10.1056/NEJMsb071889 PMID: 18077816

142. Buchan J, Dal Poz MR. Skill mix in the health care workforce: reviewing the evidence. Bull World Health Organ. 2002;80(7):575–80. PMID: 12163922

143. Beard JR, Bloom DE. Towards a comprehensive public health response to population ageing. Lancet. 2015 Feb 14;385(9968):658–61. doi: http://dx.doi.org/10.1016/S0140-6736(14)61461-6 PMID: 25468151

144. eHealth and ageing. In: Digital Agenda for Europe: a Europe 2020 initiative [website]. Brussels: European Commission; 2015 (http://ec.europa.eu/digital-agenda/en/ehealth-and-ageing, accessed 9 June 2015).

145. Üstün TB, Chatterji S, Kostanjsek N, Rehm J, Kennedy C, Epping-Jordan J, et al.; WHO/NIH Joint Project. Developing the World Health Organization Disability Assessment Schedule 2.0. Bull World Health Organ. 2010 Nov 1;88(11):815–23. doi: http://dx.doi.org/10.2471/BLT.09.067231 PMID: 21076562

146. The International classification of functioning, disability and health. Geneva: World Health Organization; 2001.

147. McHorney CA, Ware JE Jr, Raczek AE. The MOS 36-Item Short-Form Health Survey (SF-36): II. Psychometric and clinical tests of validity in measuring physical and mental health constructs. Med Care. 1993 Mar;31(3):247–63. doi: http://dx.doi.org/10.1097/00005650-199303000-00006 PMID: 8450681

148. Castelino RL, Bajorek BV, Chen TF. Retrospective evaluation of home medicines review by pharmacists in older Australian patients using the medication appropriateness index. Ann Pharmacother. 2010;44(12):1922–9.

149. Paniz VMV, Fassa AG, Facchini LA, Piccini RX, Tomasi E, Thumé E, et al. Free access to hypertension and diabetes medicines among the elderly: a reality yet to be constructed. Cad Saude Publica. 2010 Jun;26(6):1163–74. doi: http://dx.doi.org/10.1590/S0102-311X2010000600010 PMID: 20657981

150. Qaseem A, Snow V, Cross JT Jr, Forciea MA, Hopkins R Jr, Shekelle P, et al; American College of Physicians/American Academy of Family Physicians Panel on Dementia. Current pharmacologic treatment of dementia: a clinical practice guideline from the American College of Physicians and the American Academy of Family Physicians. Ann Intern Med. 2008 Mar 4;148(5):370–8. doi: http://dx.doi.org/10.7326/0003-4819-148-5-200803040-00008 PMID: 18316755

151. Assistive devices background paper: prepared for the World report on ageing and health. Geneva: World Health Organization; 2015.

152. Spillman BC. Assistive device use among the elderly: trends, characteristics of users, and implications for modeling. Washington (DC): Office of Disability, Aging and Long-Term Care Policy, Office of the Assistant Secretary for Planning and Evaluation, US Department of Health and Human Services; 2005 (http://aspe.hhs.gov/daltcp/reports/astdev.htm, accessed 9 June 2015).

153. Gilson L, Doherty J, Loewenson R, Francis V. Challenging inequity through health systems: final report of the Knowledge Network on Health Systems. Geneva: WHO Commission on the Social Determinants of Health; 2007. (http://www.who.int/social_determinants/resources/csdh_media/hskn_final_2007_en.pdf, accessed 9 June 2015).

154. Sadana R, Blas E. What can public health programs do to improve health equity? Public Health Rep. 2013 Nov;128(Suppl. 3):12–20. PMID: 24179274

155. World health report 2010. Health systems financing: the path to universal coverage. Geneva: World Health Organization; 2010 (http://www.who.int/whr/2010/en/, accessed 29 June 2015).

156. Gurwitz JH, Goldberg RJ. Age-based exclusions from cardiovascular clinical trials: implications for elderly individuals (and for all of us). Comment on "the persistent exclusion of older patients from ongoing clinical trials regarding heart failure". Arch Intern Med. 2011 Mar 28;171(6):557–8. doi: http://dx.doi.org/10.1001/archinternmed.2011.33 PMID: 21444845

157. Boyd CM, Vollenweider D, Puhan MA. Informing evidence-based decision-making for patients with comorbidity: availability of necessary information in clinical trials for chronic diseases. PLOS ONE. 2012;7(8):e41601. doi: http://dx.doi.org/10.1371/journal.pone.0041601 PMID: 22870234

158. Banerjee S. Multimorbidity—older adults need health care that can count past one. Lancet. 2015 Feb 14;385(9968):587-9. PMID: 25468155

159. de Souto Barreto P. Ageing: research needs social science. Nature. 2014 Aug 21;512(7514):253. doi: http://dx.doi.org/10.1038/512253e PMID: 25143106

160. Carstensen L, Hartel C. Motivation and behavioral change. In: When I'm 64.. Washington (DC): National Academies Press; 2006: 34–54 (http://www.nap.edu/catalog/11474/when-im-64, accessed 9 June 2015).

161. Notthoff N, Carstensen LL. Positive messaging promotes walking in older adults. Psychol Aging. 2014 Jun;29(2):329–41. doi: http://dx.doi.org/10.1037/a0036748 PMID: 24956001

162. Aedoand C, Walker D. Methodological issues in assessing the cost-effectiveness of interventions to improve the health of older people. In: Dangour AD, Grundy EMD, Fletcher AE, editors. Ageing well: nutrition, health, and social interventions. Boca Raton (FL): CRC Press; 2007:127–37. doi: http://dx.doi.org/10.1201/9781420007565.ch11

163. Fontana L, Kennedy BK, Longo VD, Seals D, Melov S. Medical research: treat ageing. Nature. 2014 Jul 24;511(7510):405–7. doi: http://dx.doi.org/10.1038/511405a PMID: 25056047

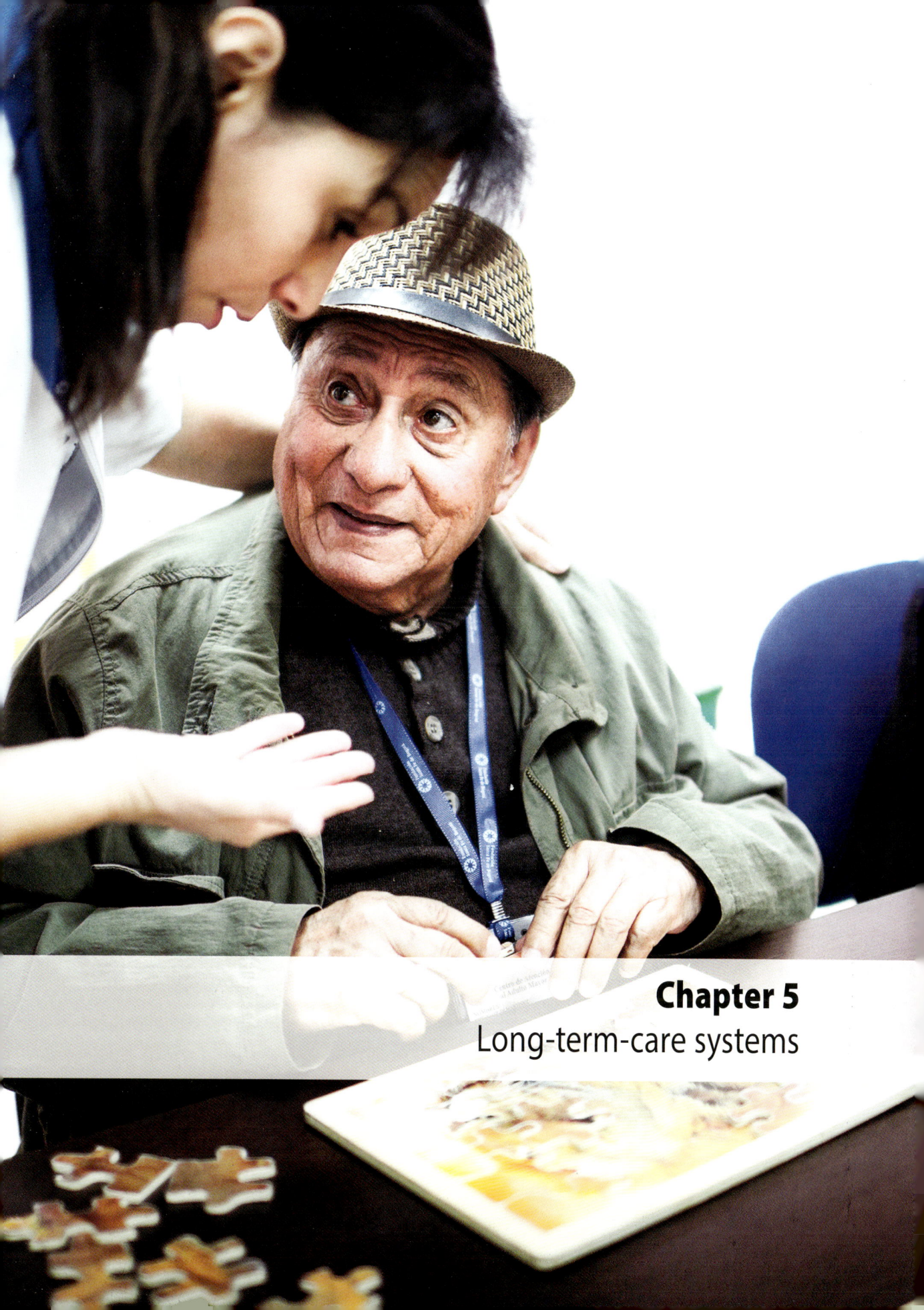

Chapter 5
Long-term-care systems

Joaquin, 80, Colombia

Thirteen years ago Joaquin was diagnosed with Alzheimer's disease. His wife Mara Leonor, aged 70, is taking care of him. Married for over fifty years they have six children and seven grandchildren. Mara Leonor says:

"The hardest thing has been to understand the disease. Once we understood the illness everything became easier. We cannot fight against the disease and less against Joaquín, he cannot be blamed and it is the family that must understand and be trained to live with this new situation. One of the doctors who attended Joaquin recommended the Fundación Acción Familiar Alzheimer (Foundation for Family Action on Alzheimer), and then I started taking training courses for caregivers, and we learned together in this way."

"Twice a week Joaquin goes to a daycare center. It's a break for me to have that support, because there are things I must attend to. Pay bills, request appointments etc. It also gives me time to visit families that I have met in the foundation. Thanks to all that I have learned I can help other families to learn to live with this disease, there are many people who call me to organize some workshops. I have been trained myself every day because it became a personal challenge. I have learned about a disease that I had never heard of and now I feel that the roles are reversed. Joaquín took care of me his whole life and now it's my turn."

5

Long-term-care systems

Introduction

Regardless of their age or level of intrinsic capacity, older people have a right to a dignified and meaningful life. For people with significant losses of intrinsic capacity, this is often possible only with the care, support and assistance of others.

The form that this long-term care takes varies markedly among, and even within, countries. Responsibility often falls on families, and can present them with significant psychological, social and economic costs. But governments, particularly in high-income countries, are playing an increasing role. This has led to lively debates in many countries on how care can be delivered in a sustainable manner and on what is the appropriate balance between families and the government in providing care and support. Yet there is less discussion about the nature and quality of the care and support provided, and little thought is given to quantifying the benefits that might accrue from these investments. In addition, older people receiving care are frequently stereotyped and marginalized as being burdens.

This chapter outlines an alternative way of dealing with this crucial challenge to *Healthy Ageing*. Although there are numerous definitions of long-term care, this report uses the term to refer to:

> the activities undertaken by others to ensure that people with or at risk of a significant ongoing loss of intrinsic capacity can maintain a level of functional ability consistent with their basic rights, fundamental freedoms and human dignity.

In other words, long-term care is simply a means to ensure that older people with a significant loss of capacity can still experience *Healthy Ageing*. As with all stages in the life course, this can be achieved through two mechanisms:
- optimizing the recipient's trajectory of intrinsic capacity;
- compensating for a loss of capacity by providing the environmental support and care necessary to maintain functional ability at a level that ensures well-being.

Two key principles underpin the definition of long-term care.

First, even in circumstances in which older people have a significant loss of functioning, they still "have a life". They have the right and deserve the freedom to realize their continuing aspirations to well-being, meaning and respect.

Second, as with other phases of life, intrinsic capacity during a period of significant loss is not static, but rather declines in capacity are part of a continuum and in some cases may be preventable or reversible. Fully meeting the needs of someone at this stage of life therefore demands that efforts be made to optimize these trajectories of capacity, thus reducing the deficits that will need to be compensated for through other mechanisms of care.

Framing the purpose of long-term care in this way has several important implications. For example, potential recipients of long-term care include not just those who are already care-dependent but also those with significant losses of capacity and at high risk of deteriorating to this state. Implementing simple interventions may avoid the need for more intensive interventions later.

Furthermore, care dependence is not considered as a fixed, all or nothing, state. For example, rehabilitation, good nutrition or physical activity might improve an older person's capacity to the point that the need for long-term care diminishes or even disappears.

Finally, making functional ability the ultimate goal of long-term care, rather than focusing simply on meeting older people's basic needs for survival, requires caregivers to focus on other domains. These include older people's abilities to move around; to build and maintain relationships; to learn, grow and decide; and to contribute to their communities (Chapter 6). For older people with significant losses of capacity to achieve these things, caregivers will need appropriate knowledge, training, and support.

Achieving these goals is likely to involve a variety of caregivers working in a wide range of settings. This report uses the term long-term-care system to refer to all these caregivers and the settings they may operate in, as well as the governance and support services that can help them in their roles. The long-term-care system thus spans family members, friends, volunteers who provide care and support, the workforce of paid and unpaid caregivers, care coordination, community-based services and institutional care, as well as services that support caregivers and ensure the quality of the care they provide (for example by offering respite care, and providing information, education, accreditation, financing and training). This system significantly overlaps with the health system and those who provide health care.

This report argues that in the 21st century, no country can afford not to develop a coordinated system for long-term care. However, this does not imply that there is one system that is appropriate for all settings. Rather, each country needs to take stock of its unique situation to identify the best system for its context.

The growing need for long-term care

Most estimates of the number of older people in need of long-term care are gross underrepresentations because they assume that need arises only when losses of capacity have occurred to the point that people face difficulty performing basic tasks, such as eating, bathing, dressing, getting in and out of bed, or using a toilet. As described in Chapter 3, this report uses the term care-dependent to describe these very limited states of functioning. So these estimates do not include older people who have less significant losses but who may still benefit from care and support. They also serve to reinforce threshold perspectives on declining functioning, which may be useful as mechanisms for identifying those eligible for services, but fail to account for the continuum of trajectories of *Healthy Ageing* and the opportunities to influence them. Yet often there is no stark shift between when an older person does not need care and support and when they do.

Nonetheless, survey data have revealed that a significant proportion of older people are care-dependent, and the prevalence increases with age (Chapter 3). However, there is marked variation among countries, ranging from less than 5% of the population aged 65–74 years in Switzerland being care-dependent to around 50% of people of the same age in many low- and middle-income countries (depending on how it is measured). Among people older than 74 years, the prevalence is even higher.

This higher prevalence of care dependence in low- and middle-income countries than in high-income countries is important because these are generally the settings with the least infrastructure in place to meet this significant need. It is also noteworthy that care dependence is more prevalent among women than men of the same age (1). This might be due to gender-based differences in specific health conditions and social relations (Chapter 3) (2).

Global population ageing will significantly increase the absolute number of older people who are care-dependent.

Many low- and middle-income countries will experience sharper increases due to the more rapid pace of population ageing, with some seeing a doubling in the absolute number of older people who are care-dependent by 2050 (3). Indeed, this trend may be an underestimate, given the higher prevalence of significant losses of capacity among older people in these countries (Fig. 3.17). Sub-Saharan Africa may be confronted with particularly high increases (4).

Current approaches to long-term care

Long-term care is provided in settings that range from the recipient's home to community centres, assisted living facilities, nursing homes, hospitals and other health facilities. The scope and intensity of the care and support provided can differ in any of these settings.

In this report community-based care refers to all forms of care that do not require an older person to reside permanently in an institutional care setting. This type of care can be provided in older people's homes, or in community or day centres. Community-based care can facilitate ageing in place and has the potential to delay admission to a nursing home, reduce the number of days spent in hospital, and improve quality of life (5, 6).

Residential care is delivered in assisted-living facilities and nursing homes, among other locations. In the second half of the 20th century, residential care was often based on a medical model of service delivery, thus looking and operating more like a hospital than a home. More recently, alternative residential care concepts have been receiving increasing attention. In countries such as Germany, Japan, the Netherlands, Sweden and the United States, some hospital-like institutional care settings are being redesigned into smaller group homes that provide a more home-like atmosphere and offer around-the-clock care. These innovative approaches aim to treat residents as people first, not patients (7). Overall, these new care concepts hold promise for older people, family members and volunteers who provide care and support, and other care workers, and for improving the quality of care (8–13).

Furthermore, many high-income countries are in the process of shifting the emphasis of long-term care services from residential care to community-based care (14). In many OECD countries, between one half and three quarters of older people receive long-term care at home (15).

The long-term-care workforce: often undervalued and lacking support and training

The workforce providing long-term care comprises a diverse spectrum of people and skills. At one end of the spectrum are unpaid, untrained informal caregivers who receive no outside support; they include family members, friends and neighbours. At the other end of the spectrum lie highly trained care professionals. Between these two extremes are individuals who have diverse training, expertise, status and remuneration levels. For example, large differences exist between a caregiver who has no formal training but is paid by relatives to look after a care-dependent older person at home and a caregiver who has completed advanced, accredited training and is licenced by the government and participates in regular continuing education activities. Furthermore, the distinction between paid care workers and family caregivers is not always simple. Family caregivers can be highly skilled and experienced, and in some countries they may receive cash benefits from the government or insurance schemes (14).

One common element across this diverse spectrum is that women make up the majority of caregivers, be they family members, neighbours or friends who provide care and support, or paid care workers (16). As can be seen in Table 5.1, daughters and daughters-in-law provide a large

proportion of care for their family members, although spouses, most of whom are likely to be older people, also provide a substantial degree of support. In some settings, such as urban China and urban Peru, a substantial amount of care provided in the home comes from paid caregivers, most of whom are untrained. This reliance on paid home-care workers is made possible by women with little formal education, who may have migrated from rural to urban areas, and are paid relatively little to provide care.

As people have fewer children and live longer, and as countries develop economically and women increasingly enter the paid workforce, relying on unpaid informal caregivers without providing additional support is unlikely to be sustainable. This is true not only for high-income countries (14) but also for low- and middle-income countries, where changes are happening even more rapidly (18, 19).

Due to the ageing of the population and the expected decline in the availability of unpaid informal caregivers, the demand for paid care workers in the labour force is expected to at least

Table 5.1. **Characteristics of caregivers and care arrangements (%) for community-based care-dependent older people, China, Mexico, Nigeria and Peru, 2003–2008**

Characteristics	China		Mexico		Nigeria[a] (n = 228)	Peru	
	Urban (n = 183)	Rural (n = 54)	Urban (n = 114)	Rural (n = 82)		Urban (n = 135)	Rural (n = 26)
Caregiver							
Spouse	38.8	38.9	16.7	15.9	13.7	18.5	26.9
Child or child-in-law	43.2	59.3	73.7	65.8	68.0	40.0	50.0
Non-relative	16.4	1.9	3.6	0.0	1.4	25.2	3.8
Female caregiver	67.2	50.0	83.3	81.7	63.2	85.9	88.5
Care arrangements							
Caregiver has reduced work to provide care	3.8	48.1	25.4	36.6	39.2	16.3	23.1
Additional informal caregiver(s) provide help	7.1	22.2	55.3	58.5	66.5	45.9	57.7
Paid care worker helps with care	45.4	1.9	3.5	1.2	2.1	33.3	7.7

[a] Data collection for Nigeria was not complete.
Source: (17).

double by 2050 (*15*). However, many paid care workers are unprepared for the demands placed upon them, and lack adequate training (*20–22*). Furthermore, health care and social-care students as well as faculty often have negative perceptions and beliefs about older people, together with the persistent but incorrect belief that caring for older people is simple (*23*). Moreover, negative attitudes about providing long-term care make it difficult to recruit paid care workers in many countries. This may reflect ageism in the broader culture, the tendency to equate long-term care with poor-quality working conditions, or the low status accorded to caregiving (*24*).

Financing long-term care: it always has a cost

In many countries, discussions about long-term care focus on the sustainability of current financing arrangements in the face of rapidly growing demand. And these concerns are not unjustified: across the countries that are members of the OECD, government spending on long-term care grew by an average of 4.8% annually from 2005 to 2011 (*15*). European Union projections foresee at least a doubling of current expenditure levels by 2060 (*25*).

Despite these broad similarities, government expenditures in the OECD are highly variable: in 2011, spending ranged from more than 3.5% of gross domestic product (GDP) in the Netherlands and Sweden to less than 0.3% in Estonia, Greece, Hungary and Portugal (*15*). The main cause of this variability is the comprehensiveness of government support for long-term care, both in terms of the range of services included and the proportion of the total cost that older people are required to pay (*14*). In addition, access to services is sometimes means-tested.

Moreover, informal care is rarely included in estimates of the costs of long-term care. These nongovernment costs can be substantial and include the costs of unpaid labour and forgone educational and income-earning opportunities for family caregivers and cash payments made by older people or their families for private care (*26*). Family members who adopt unpaid caregiving roles often experience significant challenges to maintaining their employment or other income-earning activities. Caregiving can be incompatible with a full-time job and can constrain the usual career progression. For those of working age, informal caring is associated with a higher risk of poverty and it can reduce or totally remove later pension entitlements (*27*).

Many countries rely on out-of-pocket payments to fund at least a portion of long-term care. These payments often have a significant adverse impact on the disposable income of older people and their families. In many low-income countries, where governments do not finance long-term care, the entire financial burden falls directly on older people or their families. But even in Europe, older people's out-of-pocket payments account for 9.6% of their household income on average, and can account for as much as 25% (*28*). The poor, women and the very old are particularly affected by these costs (*29*).

Finally, as described in Chapter 4, in high-income countries health-care utilization tends to fall among people over the age of around 75 years, provided long-term care is available for support. Where long-term care is not available, other costs are likely to arise from the inappropriate use of acute health-care services. Thus, although government expenditures on long-term care may appear to be low, these are likely to have been shifted, at least in part, to the health sector.

Hence, all long-term care – even that provided free by family members – has a cost. Someone inevitably pays for this care in one way or another. A core policy issue is how these costs can be equitably shared across societies.

Where it exists, public funding for long-term care is generally derived from general taxation, compulsory saving schemes, or a combination of the two. Most schemes and systems also involve copayments from both public and private sources. As with health-financing schemes, long-term care that is financed via universal pre-payment, risk-pooling and strategic purchasing enables the financial burden to be spread among all participants, and helps ensure access for poorer older people (Box 5.1).

Regardless of the funding source, several strategies have been used in higher-income settings to lessen the burdens on and costs to informal caregivers. In some countries, payments are made directly to caregivers, both to support their caregiving functions and to compensate them for potential lost earnings. For example, the high-income Nordic countries (Denmark, Finland, Norway and Sweden) employ family caregivers via their municipalities (14); in Canada, tax credits are available for caregivers (14). These schemes remain limited, however, and policy-makers have expressed understandable concerns that the fiscal demands of extending these benefits to all informal caregivers would be high. Several middle-income countries are considering similar schemes, again on a limited basis. For example, Chile has introduced payments for caregivers of highly-dependent older people, although the total number of paid caregivers is capped.

To help carers maintain a role in the workforce, some governments have passed legislation that requires employers to provide leave from work for family members so that they can care for older relatives. There are variations, however, in the preconditions for and length of leave, and in whether employers or employment insurance policies are required to pay workers during their leave. In 2004, two thirds of OECD members required that employers offer care leave unless there were strong commercial reasons to deny requests. However, survey data for the same year showed that only 37% of European employers offered this benefit (14). In low- and middle-income countries, where much paid work is in informal small-scale activities, and where the state regulation of employers is often limited, the challenges of implementing paid care leave will be particularly great and could lead to discrimination against women in recruitment.

Box 5.1. Financing long-term care in Japan

In Japan before the 1990s, the state provision of long-term care was limited and mainly funded at the level of local government. Access was usually means-tested, resulting in older people who were not considered to be poor paying fully for their care (30). In 2000, Japan's government recognized that unmet demand was escalating; in response, it introduced an insurance system for long-term care with the objectives of reducing the burden on family caregivers and integrating health care and welfare services into a comprehensive plan for insured populations.

Since 2000, individuals' benefits have been determined based on a needs assessment. Those using long-term care services contribute 10% towards the cost of care (although there is a ceiling for low-income insured people), with the remaining benefits being funded equally by insurance contributions and tax revenues. The system provides a generous set of services, including community-based and residential care, as well as free choice of services and providers (31).

This new insurance scheme prompted a substantial increase in access to professional long-term care, with the proportion of people aged 65 and older using community services rising from 39% in 1999 to 61% in 2001.

Because local governments are responsible for managing the system, disparities have emerged among different areas of the country. This has prompted debate about how to encourage uniformity of access to services across the entire country (32).

Increases in providing access to care homes has been more modest because the government controls the supply and older people are still required to pay a portion of the associated costs. Concerns have been raised that these payments may pose a significant access barrier to older people from poor families.

In addition to leave from work, options for part-time or flexible working arrangements have been legislated in some countries. In many of these countries, however, employers can deny workers' requests for flexibility on operational or business grounds (14).

Other countries pay care-dependent older people in cash or vouchers to enable them to meet their own long-term care costs. In Spain, for example, an allowance is paid directly to the person receiving care to help organize home care from family members (*14*). A positive feature of this approach is that it can potentially empower older people and enhance their autonomy. In practice, however, this approach can be quite challenging, particularly for older people with cognitive impairments or low levels of education. As with making payments to caregivers, policy-makers are wary of the fiscal implications of providing these benefits on a large scale.

Care provision: outdated and fragmented

The quality of long-term care often leaves much room for improvement, even in high-income countries (*33*, *34*). Quality is undermined by two major factors: the type of care that is provided, which is often at odds with the major objectives of long-term care, and in some cases may even be abusive, and the lack of integration with health-care services. The lack of effective regulations and standards, and the low priority given to long-term care, further undermine its quality.

Although there are outstanding exceptions, significant threats to the quality of care come from outdated ideas and ways of working, which often focus on keeping older people alive rather than on supporting dignified living and maintaining their intrinsic capacity. Within this paradigm, older people may be regarded as passive recipients of care, and services may be built around the needs of service providers rather than the needs and preferences of the older person. Care may focus on meeting people's basic needs, such as bathing or dressing, at the expense of the broader objectives of ensuring their well-being, that their lives have meaning and that they feel respected (*34*). Fragmentation and the inflexibility of responsibilities for care within residential settings can further exacerbate these problems (*35–37*). For example, care workers who are responsible for discrete tasks, such as cooking or giving medications, may not be aware of an older person's needs and wishes.

In some cases, long-term care is outright harmful to older people's safety and dignity. For example, although the prevalence of elder abuse has been estimated at around 10% in the general community, the physical abuse of older people with dementia has been estimated to affect up to 23% (Chapter 3). Human rights violations can occur in both community and residential settings. Examples include the use of physical restraints to deal with challenging behaviours or to prevent people from falling (*38–40*) and the inappropriate prescribing of antipsychotic medications to control behaviour (*41*). Often, family members and paid care workers may be unaware of alternatives to these measures (*42*, *43*). Thus, elder abuse can further compromise the autonomy, dignity and safety of already vulnerable older people. Moreover, in some circumstances, the older person may not be the only victim because abuse may be a consequence of burnout in caregivers who feel overloaded (*44*).

A lack of integration between long-term care and mainstream health care, both administratively and at the points of use, is another factor undermining care quality. The strict separation of social care and support and mainstream health services can result in fragmented coverage, gaps in the provision of long-term care and the inappropriate use of acute health-care services. More and better coordination is required at a systems level.

Responding to the challenge of long-term care

Globally, long-term care will have to evolve in radical ways if growing needs are to be sustainably met. This transformation will require a coordinated and multisectoral response that involves a wide range of stakeholders, both within and outside governments. More fundamentally, mindsets about what long-term care might comprise must be completely reset. Entirely new ways of thinking about long-term care – and the systems for delivering it – need to be developed.

Without a major reorientation of policies, many countries will fall even further behind in providing what is needed. Formal services for long-term care will continue to be in short supply, and where they are available, outdated models of residential care are likely to be perpetuated. Care-dependent older people will continue to be vulnerable to elder abuse. Long-term care and mainstream health care will remain disconnected. And the mainly female care workforce will continue to be exploited in inequitable and unjust ways.

Moving towards an integrated system: a revolutionary agenda

Changes need to encompass two broad areas. First, long-term care must be recognized as a public good both societally and politically. The enormous social and economic costs of neglecting this challenge also need to be acknowledged.

Second, long-term care must be redefined. Instead of thinking about long-term care as a minimal and basic safety net that provides rudimentary support to older people who can no longer look after themselves, perceptions must shift towards a more positive and proactive agenda. Within this new framework, long-term care must be oriented towards both optimizing intrinsic capacity and compensating for a lack of capacity at a level that maintains an older person's functional ability and ensures dignity and well-being. More broadly, long-term care must promote social cohesion and gender justice, and ensure an acceptable level of well-being for all members of society, including not only dependent older people but also those who care for them (Box 5.2). Furthermore, as with health care,

Box 5.2. Community-based interventions to support caregivers of older people with dementia in Goa, India

In Goa, as across India as a whole, formal long-term care services are generally lacking. Nursing homes do not admit people with dementia, and as of 2008, specialized dementia homes did not exist. The responsibility for people with dementia is placed largely on family members, who experience high burdens and high levels of psychological distress.

In response, a community-based intervention has been developed to offer support and education to families of people with dementia by making use of locally available health and human resources. It provides basic information about dementia, the associated challenging behaviours and how to manage them, and the availability of government services. Information is also provided about how older caregivers can help with activities of daily living (ADLs), how to obtain referrals to doctors or psychiatrists for severe symptoms, and informal support groups.

This intervention has improved caregivers' mental health and reduced stress; in addition, limited evidence indicates that it may have enhanced the functional status of people with dementia and reduced the challenging behaviours associated with the condition (45).

The same intervention package has produced similar effects in Peru and in the Russian Federation (46, 47), indicating that this relatively simple and affordable intervention could potentially be extended across many low- and middle-income countries where resources and infrastructure are limited.

wherever possible long-term care should be framed in a way that maximizes the role of the older person and enables their self-management.

Achieving these goals in an equitable, sustainable and socially just manner is likely to require fundamental shifts in models of national development. These need to reflect the crucial role of long-term care in maintaining social cohesion, the opportunities and economic growth that can accompany reform, and the rights of vulnerable older people.

General principles of an integrated system of long-term care

All countries need a fully integrated system of long-term care, regardless of their level of economic development or the proportion of care-dependent older people within their populations. Governments should take overall responsibility for ensuring that the system works, but this does not mean that governments must fund or provide all services.

Long-term care systems will necessarily vary considerably among countries, reflecting the available resources; the current infrastructure, including health-care services; and cultural preferences. In developing a comprehensive system, countries need to take these differences into account, as well as considering the current and future numbers of older people and their needs for long-term care; existing models of service delivery; and the availability and skills of informal caregivers and paid care workers. Other factors that will need to be considered include the presence and nature of information and data systems, the existing infrastructure, the availability of assistive technologies, the resources that are available nationally, and care policies.

Despite this diversity, some general principles apply.

- Long-term care must be affordable and accessible. Special attention should be given to ensuring that poor and marginalized people are able to access services.
- Long-term care must uphold the human rights of care-dependent older people. Care must be provided in a manner that enhances older people's dignity, and enables their self-expression and, where possible, their ability to make choices.
- Wherever possible, long-term care should enhance older people's intrinsic capacities.
- Long-term care should be person-centred. It should be oriented around the needs of the older person rather than the structure of the service.
- The long-term care workforce, paid and unpaid, should be treated fairly, and it should receive the social status and recognition it deserves.
- National governments must take overall responsibility for the stewardship of long-term care systems.

Fig. 5.1 shows the main elements of an older-person-centred system of long-term care. These include the caregivers and settings that allow care to be provided to the older person. But almost as important are the support services that can be provided to ease the burden of care (for example, through offering respite care) and to ensure the appropriateness and quality of the care that is provided (for example, by providing information, training and accreditation to caregivers), and the stewardship that will generate resources for the system and allow it to function in a coordinated and focused way. All countries already have at least some elements of this system, but in many cases these elements have been poorly articulated, do not comprise an integrated whole or do not reflect the guiding principles outlined above.

Fig. 5.1.   Elements of an older-person-centred system of long-term care

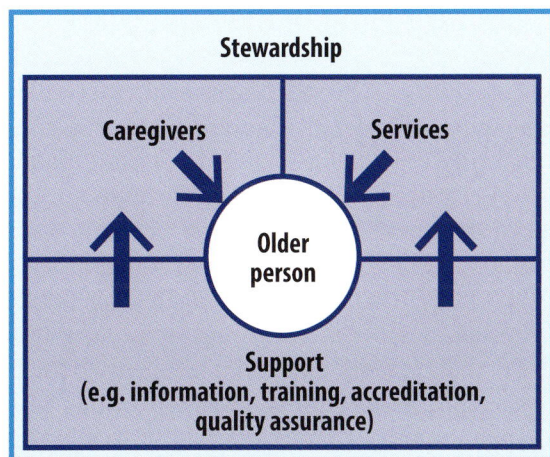

Countries have considerable scope for diversity, innovation and flexibility in terms of how to apply these elements. In all cases, however, effective and integrated partnerships among governments, families, volunteers, nongovernmental organizations, health and social care professionals and the private sector are essential. Who actually provides which services will vary across countries.

Flowing from the general principles outlined above, specific strategies can be identified to guide the development of an effective system of long-term care, whatever form that system takes. These strategies include:

- enabling older people to remain in or maintain connections with their community and social networks – that is, enabling ageing in place;
- supporting and building the capacities of paid and unpaid caregivers;
- promoting integrated care through the use of case management strategies and broader collaborations;
- establishing equitable and sustainable financing for long-term care.

Underpinning all these strategies is a need for more knowledge about what works in settings that have different resource constraints and different challenges in order to ensure equitable access across low-, middle- and high-income countries.

Enabling ageing in the right place

As described in Chapter 2, ageing in place refers to a common preference among older people for remaining in their local community and maintaining their social networks throughout the ageing process. There are many ways for older people to age in place. Sometimes it means staying in place: that is, continuing to live in the same home. For others, it means moving to a home that is safer and more adapted to their needs while maintaining vital connections with their community, friends and family. In all cases

the focus should be on the older person ageing in a place that is right for them.

Ageing in the right place may require a wide array of services and a family of caregivers (48). Together, these can broaden the options for an older person from an all-or-nothing choice between permanent residential care and living at home without support. Innovative assistive health technologies (Box 5.3) also hold promise for helping to meet this aim.

One example of these principles being applied in practice is the Republic of Korea's insurance scheme for long-term care, which was established in 2008 (52, 53). The scheme includes individual needs assessments, and offers a range of services including home care, domestic help, public-health nurses, day-care and short-term stay centres.

Building workforce capacity and supporting caregivers

There are multiple challenges to developing and supporting the paid and unpaid workforce that provides long-term care. These include a need to ensure a sufficient supply of caregivers, whether paid or unpaid, as well as ensuring that they are adequately trained and support, and treated fairly in the workplace.

Ensuring supply

Supply can be optimized by taking action in several areas. Increasing the pay and benefits could help with recruiting and retaining paid care workers. Another important step would be to improve their working conditions, whether by providing training, career opportunities, appropriate workloads, flexible work hours and giving care workers meaningful authority to make decisions (54, 55). Care workers whose work is valued and appreciated, and who feel part of a clinical team, have higher levels of job satisfaction and are more likely to stay in their jobs (14).

Beyond this, the image and status of caregiving needs to improve. Modernizing the image of

Box 5.3.   Innovative assistive health technologies can enable ageing in place

Innovative assistive health technologies for long-term care – such as remote monitoring and robotic carers – have received a great deal of attention. They are often presented as highly promising means for enhancing the functional ability of older people who have declines in their intrinsic capacity, for improving their quality of life as well as that of their caregivers, and for potentially reducing individual and societal costs and enabling ageing in place (*49*).

The reality of innovative assistive health technologies is more nuanced. Solid research on the impact of various devices and interventions is scarce, and new technologies can present threats to older people's privacy and autonomy if they are not deployed in a considered and person-centred manner.

Notwithstanding the need for more research, the use of particular types of innovative technologies should be based on the needs and preferences of the older person or their caregiver. For example, using tracking and tracing technology might be a good solution for someone with early dementia who wants to walk independently in their neighbourhood. During the later stages of dementia, however, this technology might not offer the same advantages and a different approach would need to be used (*50*).

Several additional ethical issues related to the use of innovative assistive health technologies bear consideration. The impact of innovative technologies on older people's privacy, autonomy and social participation must always be taken into account. Certain forms of innovative technologies might have the unintended effect of isolating older people or restricting their freedom of movement. These potential harms must be weighed against the benefits on a case-by-case basis. Nonetheless, research indicates that older people have few ethical objections to using innovative technologies and often view them as an acceptable alternative to a lack of care or institutionalization (*51*).

Multiple stakeholders should be involved in developing sound policies for the use of innovative assistive health technologies. Policy-makers, care providers, members of industry and academia, and, importantly, older people must be involved in policy development. Technologies need to be developed that reflect the needs and preferences of their end-users; and training for caregivers, health professionals and others is crucial. Finally, developing financing mechanisms for research and development, and to ensure equitable implementation requires careful attention, especially in lower-income countries.

long-term care and reducing negative stereotypes about caregivers' roles would help attract more people to this area of work. Providing opportunities for continuing education and career progression could further help change perceptions that caregiving is a dead-end job. Providing academic opportunities for caregivers and establishing a serious research agenda may also shift perceptions and the value placed on caregiving, as well as fostering the rigorous identification of effective practices and care models.

The overall pool of potential care workers would be increased if more men could be attracted to this role. In several European countries, the share of male caregivers increases with age, showing that men, most likely spouses, already comprise the majority of informal caregivers aged 75 years or older; although in other age groups and among non-spouse informal caregivers, they are much less well represented (*56*). This suggests, however, that men may be more willing to fill a caregiving role than is widely believed. Collecting further information on how and why men are engaged in caregiving would help society tap into this resource (*57*).

Immigrants provide another potential employment pool, but the practice of relying on foreign-born workers to fill these positions is fraught with legal and ethical considerations. In countries with a high proportion of migrant workers who provide care, efforts must be made to ensure that the immigration of care workers does not drain skilled workers from lower-income countries (*58*). WHO has put together a global code of ethics that provides some guidance in how issues on recruitment can be approached

Box 5.4.   Older people's associations: harnessing the power of older age

Older people's associations are an innovative approach to taking community-based action. These organizations empower people in later life, using their skills, capacities and willingness to actively engage with and serve their communities. Their importance in promoting the well-being of older people, including those who are poor and disadvantaged, has been recognized by the Association of Southeast Asian Nations, the United Nations, WHO and governments throughout Asia (*61*). For example, China recently issued a policy promoting the improvement and expansion of their 490 000 associations to align them better with their development goals.

Older people's associations are multifunctional and conduct a wide range of activities, the most common of which focus on improving incomes through microcredit and income-generating activities; providing health and care for older people, including through community-care programmes aimed at care-dependent older people; providing social and cultural activities as well as disaster preparedness; and enabling social participation. The associations may also provide social assistance in the form of money, food and labour for those in the community who are most in need of them. The associations work closely with public authorities not only to ensure that their community members are receiving the services they are entitled to, such as social pensions and health insurance, but also to advocate for the development and expansion of the services and resources provided by the local authorities. The associations also work to ensure their own financial sustainability, and in Viet Nam, associations have demonstrated their capacity to fundraise.

Older people's associations have great potential for fostering *Healthy Ageing*. For their members, they organize regular health check-ups, carry out health-education activities and regular physical exercise sessions, as well as conveying knowledge about healthy living and preventing and managing noncommunicable diseases. In South East Asia the associations are developing a holistic community-care approach to support the increasing numbers of older people who are highly dependent and need help with ADLs, have a limited income or lack adequate care from their families. These activities include recruiting, training and managing home-care volunteers from the community to provide personal-care assistance to older people who need it. The associations can also help pay for transportation to health stations when required, and offer links to complementary services, such as those that provide assistive devices or rehabilitation. Some associations also mobilize resources and labour to modify and repair homes, and in disaster-prone areas they ensure that all at-risk older people have a designated emergency buddy to support them in times of danger. Older people's associations have been effectively drawing on the resources inherent in older populations to mobilize entire communities.

(*59*). Furthermore, it will be crucial to ensure that these care workers have adequate skills and knowledge to fulfil the expectations of their roles.

There may also be an opportunity to involve communities and neighbourhoods more directly in supporting long-term care, particularly by encouraging local volunteering (*60*) and enabling the contribution of older community members. Older people's associations are one mechanism by which this can happen (Box 5.4).

Training and accreditation

Ensuring that all care workers have skills and knowledge commensurate with their roles is another essential factor in building overall capacity. Specific training requirements will vary according to where the caregiver lies on the spectrum between unpaid family caregiver and highly trained professional caregiver. For example, unpaid family caregivers or volunteers might be encouraged but not required to participate in basic skills courses or offered information through the Internet (Box 5.5). All paid care workers, regardless of their roles, might need to demonstrate knowledge of basic information and skills, such as exercise routines or the monitoring of chronic conditions, or participate in continuing education courses either in person or via the Internet. Professional care workers (that is, those with formal qualifications in care-related disciplines) require much more extensive and lengthy training, and might

Box 5.5.   An Internet-based intervention for informal caregivers of people with dementia

The Internet is a powerful tool for supporting family caregivers, especially those who face barriers to accessing in-person support. This group includes caregivers in remote or rural areas, in low- and middle-income countries, with time constraints, or without access to transportation. Internet interventions have been shown to reduce caregivers' depression, increase their confidence and improve their self-efficacy (62).

One example is a guided self-help Internet intervention called *Mastery over Dementia* (63).

This programme was developed for caregivers of people with dementia, and consists of eight core lessons and one booster lesson summarizing what has been taught. After each lesson, caregivers are asked to do homework and to send it to their coach, who has three working days to provide feedback. Caregivers can proceed to the next lesson only after they have opened and read their coach's feedback. Caregivers are also asked to keep a diary describing daily events and their related thoughts and feelings. A randomized controlled trial of this intervention found that it decreased symptoms of depression and anxiety among caregivers (64). Being older than 75 years was not a barrier to participation; however, more than half (55.7%) of all participants did not complete all lessons, indicating there is room for improvement in the intervention (65).

Given the promise of this approach, WHO is working with international partners to develop a comprehensive online support tool called iSupport http://www.who.int/mental_health/neurology/dementia/isupport/en. The portal aims at relieving burdens and improving self-efficacy and mental health by emphasizing self-help, skills training and support for caregivers of people with dementia. This tool will be available via personal computers, tablets and smartphones through a secured Internet connection. Providing access via smartphones is key to ensuring access for caregivers in parts of the world (such as Asia) where there are high rates of smartphone use.

be regulated via professional licencing boards. All professional education programmes should

be allied to robust and effectively implemented accreditation mechanisms.

Education should cover not only specific conditions or health states but also ageist attitudes. It should instil the necessary information, attitudes and skills to enable care workers to practise older-person-centred care. (See Box 5.6 for an example of education for caregivers of people with dementia.) These competencies encompass a wide range of areas and might include the abilities to assist with ADLs and help maintain intrinsic capacity, enable older people to make decisions and live autonomously, and the ability to work as part of a multidisciplinary team.

Once core competencies and other training objectives have been determined, accreditation can be used to help ensure that these are integrated into the basic or preservice curricula for professional care workers. The capacity of educational institutions may need to be developed to make it possible for care workers to receive this type of training.

For existing care workers, engaging in continuing education and receiving ongoing supervision are important aspects of training. At the managerial level, auditing and feedback can be used to verify that continuing learning is happening and that caregivers' knowledge is being updated to meet changing needs. Some countries may elect to formally licence care workers, which would provide another mechanism for ensuring the continual improvement of skills.

In addition to training, care guidelines must be developed and made more widely available. Multidisciplinary guidelines have been developed in several countries, spanning areas such as nutrition, continence, alternatives to restraints, dealing with challenging behaviours and preventing elder abuse. Research shows that systematic implementation is feasible (69–71).

Finally, it will be essential to ensure that these guidelines and protocols are being followed. One mechanism to achieve this may be through the licencing or accreditation of care providers and facilities. Many middle-income

Box 5.6. Person-centred care for people living with dementia

Person-centred care values older people as individuals with unique experiences, needs and preferences (*66*). They are seen in the context of their daily lives and are helped to maintain relationships with their friends, family and community. In place of ageist attitudes, their dignity and autonomy are respected and embraced in a culture of shared decision-making.

People with dementia are often deprived of this approach to care and instead may be treated as non-persons, particularly in the advanced stages of dementia when their symptoms become most prominent.

Research indicates that providing training in person-centred care and offering ongoing support to caregivers can change their attitudes and actions towards people with dementia. Studies also have reported that caregivers who engage in person-centred interventions have lower job stress and increased personal and professional satisfaction.

Through training, caregivers can learn that people with dementia continue to experience a full range of emotions, even during advanced stages of cognitive decline, and that they continue to communicate through their behaviours, even when they have difficulty speaking. Although people with dementia may eventually lose their capacity to make truly informed choices about complex matters, most can make reliable decisions about their preferences. Even if their capacity for understanding language is severely impaired, the nonverbal behaviour that accompanies being asked about their preferences or opinions will do much to convey to people with dementia that they matter (*67*).

In all interactions, caregivers can assess whether they are practising person-centred care by asking themselves the following questions (*68*):

- Does my behaviour and the manner in which I am communicating show that I respect and value this person?
- Am I treating this person as a unique individual with a history and a range of strengths and needs?
- Am I making a serious attempt to see my actions from the perspective of the person I am trying to help? How might this person interpret what I am doing?
- Does my behaviour and interactions help this person feel socially confident and supported?

countries have experienced a proliferation of private agencies, which offer training to care workers and then arrange placements with families. In many countries, these private agencies are almost entirely unregulated. Similarly, in low-income countries, residential facilities are generally unregulated and the quality of care is generally poor. Accrediting these facilities is crucial for providing a higher quality of care.

Supporting unpaid caregivers

Various forms of support can be developed for unpaid caregivers. Support may include providing education, training and respite care, as well as offering flexible working arrangements and cash payments.

Most informal caregivers need education and training, typically about the older person's health condition and its consequences, its expected progression, and ways to help the person manage at home. Caregivers also need information on how to use a person-centred perspective when providing care for older people and on how to work within a multidisciplinary team.

Evidence indicates that providing caregivers with basic information about the older person's health condition and teaching them how to deal with challenging behaviours, such as those seen in cases of dementia, alleviates their stress (*72, 73*). In addition, caregivers might be taught a range of practical skills, such as how to safely transfer a person from a chair to their bed or how to help with bathing. Information about community-based resources available to the older person or to the caregiver might also be provided. Education and training can occur one-on-one, in a classroom, via the Internet (Box 5.5) or as part of a support group for caregivers. Extensive evi-

Box 5.7.   Respite care for people with dementia and their caregivers

Respite care mostly occurs in older people's homes, but it can also be provided at day centres or residential facilities. Within these group settings, people with dementia are able to interact in a safe environment with others who share similar problems.

In high-income countries such as the United States, day centres and the provision of short-term respite care in residential facilities were developed several decades ago to aid people with dementia and their informal caregivers. Facilities that offer one or more days of respite each week or respite for up to several weeks enable family members who act as caregivers to take a break while the person with dementia stays in a supervised and safe environment. This contributes to the ultimate aims of supporting ageing in place for people with dementia, ensuring that they receive high-quality care, and reducing the likelihood of health problems in family caregivers.

During the past decade, lower-income countries have increasingly focused on developing day centres. For example, Alzheimer's Pakistan has established its first day centre for people who have dementia with technical collaboration from Alzheimer's Australia in Western Australia (77). The centre is designed for people with all stages of dementia who need care and supervision during the day. It allows families to have a regular break from their caregiving responsibilities and enables them to continue their employment. Care workers provide education, support groups and counselling for families. They also offer a broad package of services for people with dementia, including door-to-door transportation to and from the centre; activities such as painting, cooking, gardening, reading the newspaper, and daily exercise; and help with personal care. Lunch and tea are provided. Also included are medical and psychological services, as well as the provision of prescribed medication. The centre and its related services are paid for by Alzheimer's Pakistan and provided free of charge to clients, although people who can afford to pay are encouraged to share the costs. Nonetheless, the centre's financial structure is fragile because Alzheimer's Pakistan relies completely on private donations and other external fundraising.

Day-care centres for people with dementia have also been developed in Singapore. The local Alzheimer's Disease Association has established four centres throughout the city, with an emphasis on locating them near publicly-funded housing. The centres provide care to people with dementia and other conditions, for example people who are recovering from strokes, 5 days a week (Monday to Friday) and also on certain Saturdays. Transport is available for those who need it. Activities include occupational therapy, encompassing physical, cognitive and social domains; art therapy; and planned outings. One centre also serves as a day rehabilitation centre, and has a physiotherapist on the staff. Individualized care plans and a well-being profiling tool are used to provide person-centred services and monitor clients' outcomes. Support groups are offered for caregivers, and those who require counselling or additional respite care are referred to designated social workers. The centres are funded by the Ministry of Health through subsidies given to people with dementia who qualify through means testing (78).

dence from high-income countries shows that these types of interventions have a beneficial impact on informal caregivers (73–76).

Respite care is another form of support. It allows primary informal caregivers to have short periods away from their responsibilities. The main goal of respite care is to help reduce stress among informal caregivers while still meeting the daily needs of those who need care. Volunteers or professionals sometimes provide respite care at the older person's home. In other situations, the older person is admitted temporarily

to a residential facility. Adult day care is another form of respite care in which older people spend part of their day engaged in social programmes (Box 5.7 provides an example of respite care being provided for older people with dementia). Although several studies have tried to establish the impact of respite care on the burden and well-being of caregivers, the findings have been mixed (79–81): outcomes seem to depend on the quality of care provided and how well the service meets the needs of family caregivers (82). Research is needed to determine how respite-care programmes can be designed to be most helpful. Where respite services are available, it is important to ensure that family caregivers are aware of them and that they are provided in a culturally sensitive way (*83*).

Promoting integrated care through case management and broader collaboration

Case management is a key tool for ensuring that older people's care is person-centred and integrated across the health care and social sectors (*84, 85*). Major functions include case-finding, proactive care planning and monitoring, and ensuring the ongoing involvement of a case manager. Research has shown that case management has a beneficial impact on an older person's psychological health and well-being (*86, 87*), and on the satisfaction and well-being of caregivers (*87, 88*). It also has the potential to delay nursing-home placement, and to reduce admission rates and shorten lengths of stay in nursing homes (*89–91*). Cost savings have been found in the medium-term (*91*).

Some case-management programmes target not only older people but also their caregivers. In the Netherlands, for example, case managers have an important role in providing education and support to older people and their informal caregivers (*92, 93*).

Throughout the care continuum, case-management planning must enable older people to make their own choices, thereby supporting their autonomy. This holds true for all older people, even for those with significant declines in capacity (*94*). For example, although people with severe dementia might not be able to decide whether they need surgery, they may still have the capacity to choose what to eat or what to wear. Adhering to this principle can be challenging. Yet a *Healthy Ageing* approach demands that people who provide long-term care should help older

Box 5.8. What is palliative care?

Palliative care aims to improve the quality of life of people experiencing a significant decline in their intrinsic capacity and who have a limited life prognosis; it also aims to help patients and their families by preventing or relieving physical, psychosocial or spiritual suffering. This concept has been evolving: previously, palliative care focused mainly on people with terminal cancer and on institutional and specialist care. During the past decade, however, its scope has expanded considerably to include a wider range of health conditions, care settings and caregivers' groups. Now, it also addresses the well-being of families.

WHO estimates that around 40 million people need palliative care every year (*98*). Approximately 80% live in low- and middle-income countries, and some 67% are aged 60 years or older. Yet health systems in most countries address this need inadequately: an estimated 42% of countries have no palliative care services whatsoever, and services in a further 30% reach only a small percentage of the population in need (*99*). Training in palliative care is often limited or non-existent; and a lack of access to opioid analgesics and other medications used in palliative care affects 80% of the world's population (*99*). Other barriers include a lack of awareness of the need for palliative care and misconceptions about the nature of palliative care.

Palliative care uses an interdisciplinary approach to address the holistic needs of recipients and their families (*100*). Ideally, this begins in primary-care settings when the prognosis becomes clear. Those involved in planning for palliative care aim to ensure that older people make informed and autonomous decisions that are consistent with their values and preferences. Care is then delivered across a range of settings, with an emphasis on community-based care; and it is offered by a range of caregivers, including trained community caregivers or volunteers. These principles of palliative care can be applied in all health-care and long-term care settings, and are embedded within the approaches outlined in this chapter.

people make the choices they are capable of (*94*), and caregivers must continually assess "when advocacy is justified, and unjustified patronizing starts" (*95*).

In addition to case management, advance care planning is an important part of caring for people who have a significant decline in their intrinsic capacity. It refers to formal discussions that aim to assist people in establishing personal decisions about their future treatment and palliative care (*96, 97*) (Box 5.8). The main aim of advance care planning is to uphold older people's autonomy and personal decision-making, after they cannot speak for themselves, by clarifying their wishes, needs and preferences before they reach a point where they are unable to do so. Skilled facilitators who engage key decision-makers and include older people and their

---

Box 5.9.   An integrated home-health and social-care system for older people in Turkey

In Turkey, several institutions provide services and support to older people living at home. These services are provided free of charge and funded through a mix of expenditures from the general budget, taxes, municipal budgets and premiums paid by employers and employees. The Ministry of Health provides health care at home, which is offered by multidisciplinary teams of professionals; the Ministry of Family and Social Policies provides social support, assistance and care across a range of settings, including in older people's homes; and municipalities provide social support and other services, such as home health care; psychological support; home repairs and maintenance; help with housework, personal care and cooking; and social activities (*102–104*).

In 2015, the Ministries of Health, Family and Social Policies and the Interior, and the Union of Municipalities of Turkey instituted a new protocol that called for electronic data sharing among the various institutions and organizations providing home care (*105, 106*). The system will be piloted initially in nine provinces, followed by countrywide implementation. The government will use data-sharing software to help ensure that older people receive home health care, social support and any other public services that they need. Data integration will also enable the delivery of a holistic coordinated approach, thereby improving efficiency and reducing the duplication of services.

When an older person or a family applies for a specific service, their information will be entered in the database. If the initial care team thinks that someone would benefit from another service, they will notify the relevant institution via the database. In this way, older people's needs will be met quickly.

This protocol is a good example of how a country can enhance the delivery of comprehensive and integrated long-term care, which includes health care and social care and support. Turkey's holistic, collaborative and multidisciplinary approach offers the following advantages.

- It improves access to services and the availability of professional care for older people.
- It is people-centred, coordinated and flexible, and adapted to each person's circumstances and needs.
- It respects the rights and dignity of older people, enabling them to participate in decisions about their needs and allowing them to receive many of the services in their own home.
- It supports families who care for their older relatives, and it helps improve the social participation of older people.
- It increases the quality of life for, and well-being of, older people.
- It protects older people and improves their safety.
- It makes the best use of facilities, people and other resources through data sharing, which enables the coordination of care.

Although this is a new system in Turkey and it has not yet been evaluated, the protocol demonstrates some general points.

- Even in a developing country with a fragmented system of long-term care, a comprehensive care and support system can be provided free of charge.
- Multisectoral approaches are key to providing long-term care, and the pilot demonstrates how governments can provide the stewardship necessary for collaboration between institutions and organizations.
- The government's most important responsibilities within the system are to create the mechanism for coordination, determine who needs health care, social care and support, and to work with partners to help provide the required services.

caregivers can improve the effectiveness of advance care plans (*101*).

Although care-management strategies and the principles that underpin them will help ensure that long-term care becomes more person-centred and integrated, health care and social care and support also need to be aligned and integrated at the administrative level. This calls for a more unified approach. One option might be for a single government agency, for example a ministry of health or of social services, to have the lead responsibility for the entire system of long-term care not just part of it. However, these formal governance structures are not the only way to facilitate integration (Box 5.9).

Ensuring collaboration between informal and professional caregivers is another aspect of integration. Evidence indicates that the effective transfer of information among different caregivers improves the integration and coordination of care (*88*). Therefore, establishing shared information systems may be a critical strategy for building truly integrated services.

Importantly, family care and professional care are not mutually exclusive. Informal caregivers may be empowered by professional caregivers, and their work may be complemented by the work of professional caregivers; equally, professional care workers may be guided by family members and their care may be supplemented by family caregivers.

Ensuring sustainable and equitable financing

The costs of responding to age-related care-dependency are already high and set to increase substantially. And as described previously in this chapter, when governments do not finance services, someone else must pay. Because the burden of poor health in older age falls disproportionately on disadvantaged people, this burden of care is likely to fall disproportionately on the poor, as well as on women. Therefore, identifying equitable ways of sharing the burden of caregiving is critical. This will generally require either risk-pooling or targeting resources specifically to those most in need.

This does not mean, however, that governments must necessarily assume all expenses for long-term care. To a large degree this is a political issue, reflecting wider social choices about how the overall cost of care should be distributed. But even where the role of government is largely limited to stewardship, this is not without cost: effective governance requires strong and adequately resourced coordination and oversight.

As with health financing (*107*), the financing of long-term care must consider three main targets: how to generate sufficient financial resources; how to ensure that care is both accessible and affordable, even for the poorest in society; and how to use resources in a cost-effective and equitable manner.

If there is a strong social consensus that long-term care is an important public good and a high social priority, then governments can generate resources for long-term care by diverting general tax resources from areas that are less of a priority. Alternatively or additionally, governments may decide to establish compulsory saving schemes or insurance for long-term care. Several OECD countries have adopted universal insurance schemes to successfully generate financial resources; they include Germany, Japan, Luxembourg, the Netherlands and the Republic of Korea (*14*) (Box 5.10). For example, within 4 years of the inception of an insurance scheme for long-term care in the Republic of Korea, it was providing care to 5.5% of the population aged 65 and older, with an overrepresentation of poor older people, women and those living alone, thus indicating that the scheme was reaching vulnerable groups (*110*). Among those using the service, 89% reported that they were satisfied with the quality of care, and 93% of families reported a reduction in their burden of care (*111*).

However, in Latin America and sub-Saharan Africa, the experiences with contributory insur-

Box 5.10. Financing health care and long-term care for ageing populations: the Netherlands

In the Netherlands, older people receive health care and long-term care through different municipal schemes that cover their health-care needs, inpatient long-term care and social care and support. In addition, the country's welfare system provides income support to those who lack other means (*108*). In an effort to address rising costs and changing needs, the Netherlands introduced far-reaching reforms to these various schemes in 2015 (*109*).

The health-insurance system (known as Zorgverzekeringswet), which covers basic health-care needs for the entire population, is being implemented by private (mainly not-for-profit) health-care insurers. It will extend coverage to include personal and nursing care. Health insurers are responsible for providing most intensive home-care needs, such as help getting out of bed, showering and getting dressed, as well as providing community nursing.

On top of this health insurance, people have the option of enrolling in voluntary health insurance, which covers services that are not included in the public schemes. Voluntary insurance covers dental care for adults and physiotherapy. Around 85% of the population is enrolled in these voluntary plans, including a relatively high proportion of older people.

The accompanying scheme for long-term care has undergone drastic reforms. Previously, it was a compulsory scheme that covered long-term care for older people, people with mental disorders and people with disability. The new scheme (known as Wet Langdurige Zorg) will cover only the most intensive forms of residential long-term care (and fewer people will be eligible for residential care). Outpatient personal and nursing care have been transferred to the health insurance system, as described above.

Social support, including certain home-care services and respite care, has been devolved to municipalities under a tax-funded appropriation (and is known as Wet Maatschappelijke Ondersteuning). This must be used to ensure that people can live in their own homes for as long as possible and receive the assistance that they need to do so. With these reforms, local authorities are being given a predominant role in providing community-based long-term care.

Older people may draw a personal budget from all three schemes but only for their long-term care needs. The personal budget enables individuals to buy and organize their own care according to their preferences. As budget holders, older people are free to hire their family members or anyone else to provide care.

The main lessons from the experience of the Netherlands are as follows.

1. Providing broad coverage for health care and long-term care has many benefits and contributes to social solidarity.
2. Several different schemes might be necessary to cover all the needs of older people. In these circumstances, it is crucial to ensure there is collaboration among the various schemes and that an integrated and holistic approach is used.
3. It is important to respect the wishes of the older people who want to live at home for as long as possible.

ance schemes for pensions and health services have been mixed (*112*). Schemes have often generated large financial deficits and required substantial bailouts from general revenue. One reason is that there have been high levels of evasion, possibly reflecting low levels of trust in public insurance systems. If it is difficult to persuade people to contribute to an insurance fund that offers tangible benefits, such as retirement pensions, it may be even harder to encourage them to make

lifetime contributions towards potential long-term care that many may never need.

In very poor countries, limited public resources and competing priorities make it unlikely that substantial government funds will be devoted to long-term care in the foreseeable future. However, opportunities likely exist to raise awareness of financial commitments to long-term care among development partners and nongovernmental organizations. Even in the least-resourced settings, governments can convene potential partners, make their case and galvanize financial support.

Regardless of how revenue is collected, broad-based risk-pooling helps spread the financial costs of long-term care across the whole of society. This helps protect poor and marginalized people, and reduces the risk of financial catastrophe for older people and their families.

Ensuring that interventions are cost effective helps ensure that resources are spent judiciously. For example, enabling older people to remain at home both enhances their quality of life and can be more affordable than residential care, although this is not necessarily the case (113).

Beyond this, initiatives such as older people's associations (Box 5.4), which draw on the human and social capital inherent in older populations to meet the needs of older people, might offer sustainable and low-cost care options in the near-term. Although currently largely limited to low- and middle-income countries, these mechanisms for drawing on what is often an overlooked resource may also be useful in more developed settings.

Financing a universal system of long-term care may appear daunting in low- and middle-income countries. Yet for several reasons these settings have cost advantages over high-income countries. First, population ageing is less advanced and so the demand for long-term care is lower. Second, most forms of long-term care do not require expensive equipment or specialist technology: the primary and essential input is human labour, and the costs for this are considerably lower in less-developed economies. Third, these countries have opportunities to learn from the past mistakes of high-income countries: namely, they can emphasize the use of more cost-effective services that support family caregivers. In Chile, for example, it has been estimated that the cost of a universal home-based social-care system would be around 0.45% of GDP, which

is roughly equivalent to 10% of the total health budget (114).

Changing mindsets about long-term care: a political and social challenge

The problems and injustices of current systems of long-term care often do not receive the attention they should. In part, this is because many of those who are directly affected lack political voice or organized representation. Care-dependent older people, migrant care workers and family caregivers confined to their homes face many barriers to participating in political debates. Most national governments lack a focal influential agency that can highlight and champion these issues. In many cases, the division of roles and responsibilities among national and local government departments is unclear and confusing. This hinders the coordination of an integrated system of health care and social care and support, and obscures lines of government accountability. Where policy debate occurs, it is often focused on fiscal concerns. Less attention is paid to the important benefits provided by an effective system of long-term care (Box 5.11).

Media representations of long-term care issues are often ageist, narrow and ill-informed (115). Increasing society's awareness of the inaccuracy and destructive potential of common ageist stereotypes is one way to confront these negative attitudes (116). When physical and cognitive impairment, depression and pain are viewed as inevitable aspects of ageing, older people are unlikely to be taken seriously and will become marginalized, in particular in societies where independence and self-sufficiency are highly valued (117). The widespread fear of dying and personal discomfort in talking about dying, including among health-care workers, further perpetuate this problem (118).

The media, however, can offer solutions to the problem it repeatedly reinforces by challenging ageist attitudes and supporting informed debate

Box 5.11. Key benefits of taking action on long-term care

1. Enables dignity in older age: the rights of older people are respected.
2. Reduces hospitalizations and associated costs: the use of long-term care shortens the length of hospital stays, reduces readmission rates and supports older people in returning home. All of these reduce the associated health-care costs. For older people over the age of around 70 years in countries with accessible long-term care services, health-care costs decrease with age.
3. Reduces poverty: long-term care that is based on ensuring equitable access to and utilization of care services provides a safety net for older people and protects them – and their families – from poverty in late life. It also helps share the risk of catastrophic health-care costs, reduces burdens on families and promotes social cohesion.
4. Improves the quality of care and quality of life: a well-designed system of long-term care that offers different options for care supports families in sustaining quality care at home, relieves the burden on caregivers and improves the quality of life of older people and their caregivers.
5. Improves dementia care: home-based coaching and support enable family members who act as caregivers to manage challenging behaviours at home and reduces crises and caregivers' distress.
6. Improves end-of-life care: long-term care that is consistent with the principles of palliative care enables older people to be free from pain and distress at the end of life. If provided in home-care or residential-care settings, it helps to avoid unnecessary, expensive and stressful admissions to hospitals for end-of-life care.
7. Enhances employment: if managed proactively, the demand for professional care workers creates jobs and enhances access to long-term care services. As such, it is a win-win solution for governments and the public. Also, lifting some of the burden from caregivers may free them to enter (or re-enter) the workforce.
8. Supports innovation and commerce: many innovative technologies are being developed to address the needs of older people who have significant losses in capacity. These products help fill a gap for older people and in turn become marketable to others with similar needs.

about long-term care. A study from the United States, for example, showed that geographical differences in media coverage of long-term care were significantly associated with policy reforms that prioritized community-based care (*119*).

Conclusion

This chapter has made the case that long-term care needs to evolve in fundamental ways. In many low- and middle-income countries, formal long-term care services are essentially non-existent. The task of supporting care-dependent older people typically falls to female relatives, who are mostly untrained and unpaid for this work. In some high-income countries, comprehensive public services are available, but sustainability is of great concern as populations age. In all settings, the nature and quality of care often fall short. The need to opti-

mize trajectories of intrinsic capacity and support autonomy and dignity may be overlooked entirely.

Promoting new ways of thinking about long-term care – including shifting to a central objective of optimizing functional ability – is an important first step. Beyond this, action is needed on several fronts.

First, all countries need a fully integrated system of long-term care. For most countries, this implies the development of a national plan. Governments can convene stakeholders to discuss and decide what needs to be done and who will be responsible for what. At a minimum, the plan should outline the services to be provided, who will provide them, how these services will be financed, how universal access will be facilitated, how quality will be ensured, and how the system will be coordinated to ensure the provision of integrated and comprehensive long-term care.

Box 5.12. National Dementia Strategy, Scotland

Scotland's National Dementia Strategy: 2013–2016 has the following key outcomes (*120*).

1. More people with dementia will be living at home longer and with good life quality.
2. Communities will be accessible and supportive to people with dementia, which will contribute to improved awareness of dementia and reduced stigma.
3. People should be assured of timely and accurate diagnosis.
4. There will be better post-diagnosis support for people with dementia and their families.
5. More people with dementia and their families and caregivers will be involved as equal partners in care.
6. There will be better respect for and promotion of the rights of people with dementia in all settings, together with improved compliance with the legal requirements with regard to treatment.
7. People with dementia will be treated with dignity and respect in hospitals and other institutional care settings.

The strategy contributes to Scotland's 2020 vision for health and care (*121*): that is, all people, including those with dementia, will be enabled to live well and longer at home or in home-like settings. An integrated health care and social care system is the key strategy for realizing this vision; supported self-management and community-based health care are features of this integrated approach.

Both strategies are underpinned by Scotland's Charter of Rights for People with Dementia and their Carers (*122*), which sets out the existing human and other legal rights of people with dementia and their caregivers. At the centre of this human rights-based approach is the right of people with dementia and their caregivers to be treated as equal citizens within their communities, to be supported to live as well as possible and to be enabled to remain connected to their communities and family and social support networks.

Alzheimer Scotland has been instrumental in moving this agenda forward. For example, its Five Pillars Model of Post Diagnostic Support is the basis for the Scottish government's commitment to provide every person diagnosed with dementia with a guaranteed minimum of 1 year of post-diagnosis support (*120*). This model enables individuals and their families to develop robust personal plans designed to support each person with dementia to live well and independently for as long as possible. More broadly, Alzheimer Scotland has spearheaded awareness-raising campaigns and initiatives on dementia-friendly communities and becoming a friend to people with dementia to help develop a better understanding of dementia and combat negative societal perceptions across the country. It also has developed national standards of care for people with dementia (*123*) and a training framework that outlines the knowledge, skills and behaviours expected of all health care and social-care workers. More than 500 dementia champions, supported by dementia nurse consultants, are working within the National Health Service as change agents to promote best practices to improve the experience, care and treatment of, and outcomes for, people with dementia and their families; their work aims to reduce the use of psychoactive medications and promote non-drug therapies.

Scotland's National Dementia Strategy: 2013–2016 demonstrates several points discussed in this report.

1. A national strategy or plan is important for organizing stakeholders and agreeing priority areas for action.
2. Improvement efforts should span a wide range of services and settings – not only social services but also acute health care provided in hospitals and in the community – including all organizations or settings that older people are likely to visit.
3. A human rights-based approach is a key overarching strategy for improving long-term care.

The second priority is to find ways to create and sustain a workforce prepared to provide long-term care. This can be accomplished by adequately preparing paid care workers for their roles, paying them a fair wage and creating reasonable working conditions. Giving care workers meaningful authority to make decisions and meaningful career pathways are other ways to improve recruitment and retention. Crucially, family caregivers must be supported; this can be accomplished by providing education, training, respite care, legislation to support flexible working arrangements or leaves of absence, and cash payments for services rendered.

Third, actions must be taken to promote the rights of older people and their caregivers. It is unacceptable to treat care-dependent older people in a depersonalized, degrading or abusive manner. Instead, long-term care must be designed to facilitate older people's dignity, autonomy and personal wishes, while keeping them connected to their community and social networks. Similarly, the mainly female care workforce must be treated equitably and justly.

Countries have considerable scope for diversity, innovation and flexibility in deciding how to take action in these areas (Box 5.12). Further suggestions for action are provided in Chapter 6. In all countries, a wide range of stakeholders will likely be involved in the process. But only governments can establish and steward long-term care systems as a whole.

References

1. Leveille SG, Penninx BW, Melzer D, Izmirlian G, Guralnik JM. Sex differences in the prevalence of mobility disability in old age: the dynamics of incidence, recovery, and mortality. J Gerontol B Psychol Sci Soc Sci. 2000 Jan;55(1):S41–50. doi: http://dx.doi.org/10.1093/geronb/55.1.S41 PMID: 10728129

2. Rodrigues MA, Facchini LA, Thumé E, Maia F. Gender and incidence of functional disability in the elderly: a systematic review. Cad Saude Publica. 2009;25 (Suppl. 3):S464–76. doi: http://dx.doi.org/10.1590/S0102-311X2009001500011 PMID: 20027393

3. Current and future caregiver needs for people with disabling conditions. Geneva: World Health Organization; 2002 (Longterm care series).

4. Prince M, Prina M, Guerchet M. World Alzheimer report 2013. Journey of caring: an analysis of long-term care for dementia. London: Alzheimer's Disease International; 2013 (https://www.alz.co.uk/research/WorldAlzheimerReport2013.pdf, accessed 17 June 2015).

5. Low LF, Fletcher J. Models of home care services for persons with dementia: a narrative review. Int Psychogeriatr. 2015 Feb 12. doi: http://dx.doi.org/10.1017/S1041610215000137 PMID: 25672570

6. Szanton SL, Wolff JL, Leff B, Roberts L, Thorpe RJ, Tanner EK, et al. Preliminary data from community aging in place, advancing better living for elders, a patient-directed, team-based intervention to improve physical function and decrease nursing home utilization: the first 100 individuals to complete a Centers for Medicare and Medicaid Services Innovation Project. J Am Geriatr Soc. 2015 Feb;63(2):371–4. doi: http://dx.doi.org/10.1111/jgs.13245 PMID: 25644085

7. Pot AM. Improving nursing home care for dementia: is the environment the answer? Aging Ment Health. 2013;17(7):785–7. doi: http://dx.doi.org/10.1080/13607863.2013.828679 PMID: 23971862

8. De Bruin SR, Oosting SJ, Tobi H, Blauw YH, Schols JM, De Groot CP. Day care at green care farms: a novel way to stimulate dietary intake of community-dwelling older people with dementia? J Nutr Health Aging. 2010 May;14(5):352–7. doi: http://dx.doi.org/10.1007/s12603-010-0079-9 PMID: 20424801

9. Nakanishi M, Nakashima T, Sawamura K. Quality of life of residents with dementia in a group-living situation: an approach to creating small, homelike environments in traditional nursing homes in Japan. Nihon Koshu Eisei Zasshi. 2012 Jan;59(1):3–10. PMID: 22568106

10. Verbeek H, Zwakhalen SM, van Rossum E, Kempen GI, Hamers JP. Small-scale, homelike facilities in dementia care: a process evaluation into the experiences of family caregivers and nursing staff. Int J Nurs Stud. 2012 Jan;49(1):21–9. doi: http://dx.doi.org/10.1016/j.ijnurstu.2011.07.008 PMID: 21820656

11. Willemse BM, Depla MF, Smit D, Pot AM. The relationship between small-scale nursing home care for people with dementia and staff's perceived job characteristics. Int Psychogeriatr. 2014 May;26(5):805–16. doi: http://dx.doi.org/10.1017/S1041610214000015 PMID: 24507445

12. Smit D, Willemse B, de Lange J, Pot AM. Wellbeing-enhancing occupation and organizational and environmental contributors in long-term dementia care facilities: an explorative study. Int Psychogeriatr. 2014 Jan;26(1):69–80. PMID: 24053758

13. te Boekhorst S, Depla MF, de Lange J, Pot AM, Eefsting JA. The effects of group living homes on older people with dementia: a comparison with traditional nursing home care. Int J Geriatr Psychiatry. 2009 Sep;24(9):970–8. doi: http://dx.doi.org/10.1002/gps.2205 PMID: 19452499

14. Colombo F, Llena-Nozal A, Mercier J, Tjadens F. Help wanted? Providing and paying for long-term care. Paris: OECD Publishing; 2011.

15. Health at a glance 2013: OECD indicators. Paris: OECD Publishing; 2013.

16. Erol R, Brooker D, Peel E. Women and dementia: a global research review. London: Alzheimer's Disease International; 2015 (http://www.alz.co.uk/sites/default/files/pdfs/Women-and-Dementia.pdf, accessed 17 June 2015).

17. Mayston R, Guerra M, Huang Y, Sosa AL, Uwakwe R, Acosta I, et al. Exploring the economic and social effects of care dependence in later life: protocol for the 10/66 research group INDEP study. Springerplus. 2014;3(1):379. doi: http://dx.doi.org/10.1186/2193-1801-3-379 PMID: 25105086

18. Redondo N, Lloyd-Sherlock P. Institutional care for older people in developing countries: repressing rights or promoting autonomy? The case of Buenos Aires, Argentina. Norwich, England: University of East Anglia, School of International Development; 2009 (Working paper 13; https://www.uea.ac.uk/documents/6347571/6504346/WP13.pdf/40c878ad-25f5-4967-b338-fca4246103d9, accessed 17 June 2015).

19. Herd R, Hu Y, Koen V. Providing greater old age security in China. Paris: OECD Publishing; 2010 (Economics Department working paper No. 750; http://www.oecd.org/officialdocuments/publicdisplaydocumentpdf/?doclanguage=en&cote=eco/wkp(2010)6, accessed 17 June 2015).

20. Wong YC, Leung J. Long-term care in China: issues and prospects. J Gerontol Soc Work. 2012;55(7):570–86. doi: http://dx.doi.org/10.1080/01634372.2011.650319 PMID: 22963116

21. Nienhaus A, Westermann C, Kuhnert S. Burn-out bei Beschäftigten in der stationären Altenpflege und in der Geriatrie. [Burnout among elderly care staff: a review of its prevalence]. Bundesgesundheitsblatt Gesundheitsforschung Gesundheitsschutz. 2012 Feb;55(2):211–22. (in German).doi: http://dx.doi.org/10.1007/s00103-011-1407-x PMID: 22290165

22. Vernooij-Dasssen MJ, Faber MJ, Olde Rikkert MG, Koopmans RT, van Achterberg T, Braat DD, et al. Dementia care and labour market: the role of job satisfaction. Aging Ment Health. 2009 May;13(3):383–90. doi: http://dx.doi.org/10.1080/13607860902861043 PMID: 19484602

23. Baumbusch J, Dahlke S, Phinney A. Nursing students' knowledge and beliefs about care of older adults in a shifting context of nursing education. J Adv Nurs. 2012 Nov;68(11):2550–8. doi: http://dx.doi.org/10.1111/j.1365-2648.2012.05958.x PMID: 22364192

24. The long-term care workforce: can the crisis be fixed? Problems, causes and options. Washington (DC): Institute for the Future of Aging Services; 2007 (http://www.leadingage.org/uploadedFiles/Content/About/Center_for_Applied_Research/Center_for_Applied_Research_Initiatives/LTC_Workforce_Commission_Report.pdf, accessed 17 June 2015).

25. The 2012 Ageing Report: economic and budgetary projections for the 27 EU Member States (2010–2060). Brussels: European Union; 2012. doi: http://dx.doi.org/10.2765/19991

26. Wimo A., Prince M. World Alzheimer report 2010: the global economic impact of dementia. London: Alzheimer's Disease International; 2010 (https://www.alz.co.uk/research/files/WorldAlzheimerReport2010.pdf, accessed 17 June 2015).

27. Leichsenring K, Billings J, Nies H, editors. Long-term care in Europe: improving policy and practice. London: Palgrave Macmillan; 2013 (http://www.palgraveconnect.com/pc/doifinder/10.1057/9781137032348.0001, accessed 17 June 2015).

28. Scheil-Adlung X, Bonan J. Can the European elderly afford the financial burden of health and long-term care: assessing impacts and policy implications. Geneva: International Labour Organization; 2012 (ESS paper No. 31; https://www.ilo.org/gimi/gess/RessourcePDF.do?ressource.ressourceId=30228, accessed 17 June 2015).

29. World social protection report 2014/15: building economic recovery, inclusive development and social justice. Geneva: International Labour Organization; 2014. (http://www.ilo.org/global/research/global-reports/world-social-security-report/2014/lang--en/index.htm, accessed 17 June 2015).

30. Ogawa T. Ageing in Japan: an issue of social contract in welfare transfer or generational conflict? In: Lloyd-Sherlock P, editor. Living longer: ageing, development and social protection. London: Zed Books; 2004 (http://zedbooks.co.uk/node/21198, accessed 17 June 2015).

31. Mitchell O, Pigott J, Shimizutani S. Developments in long-term care insurance in Japan. Sydney: University of New South Wales, Australian School of Business; 2008 (UNSW Australian School of Business Research Paper No. 2008 ECON 01; http://dx.doi.org/10.2139/ssrn.1115186, accessed 17 June 2015).

32. Simizutani S, Inakura N. Japan's public long-term care insurance and the financial condition of insurers: evidence from municipality-level data. Government Auditing Review. 2007;14:27–40.

33. Hayashi M. Japan's long-term care policy for older people: the emergence of innovative "mobilisation" initiatives following the 2005 reforms. J Aging Stud. 2015 Apr;33:11–21. doi: http://dx.doi.org/10.1016/j.jaging.2015.02.004 PMID: 25841725

34. Adressing dementia: the OECD response. Paris: OECD Publishing; 2015.

35. Willemse BM, Downs M, Arnold L, Smit D, de Lange J, Pot AM. Staff-resident interactions in long-term care for people with dementia: the role of meeting psychological needs in achieving residents' well-being. Aging Ment Health. 2015;19(5):444–52. PMID:25117793 PMID: 25117793

36. Cohen-Mansfield J, Bester A. Flexibility as a management principle in dementia care: the Adards example. Gerontologist. 2006 Aug;46(4):540–4. doi: http://dx.doi.org/10.1093/geront/46.4.540 PMID: 16921008

37. Hancock GA, Woods B, Challis D, Orrell M. The needs of older people with dementia in residential care. Int J Geriatr Psychiatry. 2006 Jan;21(1):43–9. doi: http://dx.doi.org/10.1002/gps.1421 PMID: 16323258

38. Meyer G, Köpke S, Haastert B, Mühlhauser I. Restraint use among nursing home residents: cross-sectional study and prospective cohort study. J Clin Nurs. 2009 Apr;18(7):981–90. doi: http://dx.doi.org/10.1111/j.1365-2702.2008.02460.x PMID: 19284433

39. Pellfolk T, Sandman PO, Gustafson Y, Karlsson S, Lövheim H. Physical restraint use in institutional care of old people in Sweden in 2000 and 2007. Int Psychogeriatr. 2012 Jul;24(7):1144–52. doi: http://dx.doi.org/10.1017/S104161021200018X PMID: 22414562

40. de Veer AJ, Francke AL, Buijse R, Friele RD. The use of physical restraints in home care in the Netherlands. J Am Geriatr Soc. 2009 Oct;57(10):1881–6. doi: http://dx.doi.org/10.1111/j.1532-5415.2009.02440.x PMID: 19682126

41. Feng Z, Hirdes JP, Smith TF, Finne-Soveri H, Chi I, Du Pasquier JN, et al. Use of physical restraints and antipsychotic medications in nursing homes: a cross-national study. Int J Geriatr Psychiatry. 2009 Oct;24(10):1110–8. doi: http://dx.doi.org/10.1002/gps.2232 PMID: 19280680

42. Hamers JP. Review: nurses predominantly have negative feelings towards the use of physical restraints in geriatric care, though some still perceive a need in clinical practice. Evid Based Nurs. 2015 Apr;18(2):64. doi: http://dx.doi.org/10.1136/eb-2014-101827 PMID: 24997212

43. Kurata S, Ojima T. Knowledge, perceptions, and experiences of family caregivers and home care providers of physical restraint use with home-dwelling elders: a cross-sectional study in Japan. BMC Geriatr. 2014;14(1):39. doi: http://dx.doi.org/10.1186/1471-2318-14-39 PMID: 24674081

44. Johannesen M, LoGiudice D. Elder abuse: a systematic review of risk factors in community-dwelling elders. Age Ageing. 2013 May;42(3):292–8. doi: http://dx.doi.org/10.1093/ageing/afs195 PMID: 23343837

45. Dias A, Dewey ME, D'Souza J, Dhume R, Motghare DD, Shaji KS, et al. The effectiveness of a home care program for supporting caregivers of persons with dementia in developing countries: a randomised controlled trial from Goa, India. PLOS ONE. 2008;3(6):e2333. doi: http://dx.doi.org/10.1371/journal.pone.0002333 PMID: 18523642

46. Guerra M, Ferri CP, Fonseca M, Banerjee S, Prince M. Helping carers to care: the 10/66 dementia research group's randomized control trial of a caregiver intervention in Peru. Rev Bras Psiquiatr. 2011 Mar;33(1):47–54. doi: http://dx.doi.org/10.1590/S1516-44462010005000017 PMID: 20602013

47. Gavrilova SI, Ferri CP, Mikhaylova N, Sokolova O, Banerjee S, Prince M. Helping carers to care–the 10/66 dementia research group's randomized control trial of a caregiver intervention in Russia. Int J Geriatr Psychiatry. 2009 Apr;24(4):347–54. doi: http://dx.doi.org/10.1002/gps.2126 PMID: 18814197

48. Morley JE. Aging in place. J Am Med Dir Assoc. 2012 Jul;13(6):489–92. doi: http://dx.doi.org/10.1016/j.jamda.2012.04.011 PMID: 22682696

49. Schulz R, Wahl HW, Matthews JT, De Vito Dabbs A, Beach SR, Czaja SJ. Advancing the aging and technology agenda in gerontology. Gerontologist. 2014;pii: gnu071. doi: http://dx.doi.org/10.1093/geront/gnu071 PMID: 25165042

50. Pot AM, Willemse BM, Horjus S. A pilot study on the use of tracking technology: feasibility, acceptability, and benefits for people in early stages of dementia and their informal caregivers. Aging Ment Health. 2012;16(1):127–34. doi: http://dx.doi.org/10.1080/13607863.2011.596810 PMID: 21780960

51. Zwijsen SA, Niemeijer AR, Hertogh CM. Ethics of using assistive technology in the care for community-dwelling elderly people: an overview of the literature. Aging Ment Health. 2011 May;15(4):419–27. doi: http://dx.doi.org/10.1080/13607863.2010.543662 PMID: 21500008

52. Baek SH, Sung E, Lee SH. The current coordinates of the Korean care regime. J Comp Soc Welf. 2011;27(2):143–54. doi: http://dx.doi.org/10.1080/17486831.2011.567019

53. Community-based social care in East and Southeast Asia. Chiang Mai, Thailand: HelpAge International, East Asia and Pacific Regional Office; 2015 (http://ageingasia.org/eaprdc0019/, accessed 17 June 2015).

54. Hussein S, Manthorpe J. An international review of the long-term care workforce: policies and shortages. J Aging Soc Policy. 2005;17(4):75–94. doi: http://dx.doi.org/10.1300/J031v17n04_05 PMID: 16380370

55. Westermann C, Kozak A, Harling M, Nienhaus A. Burnout intervention studies for inpatient elderly care nursing staff: systematic literature review. Int J Nurs Stud. 2014 Jan;51(1):63–71. doi: http://dx.doi.org/10.1016/j.ijnurstu.2012.12.001 PMID: 23273537

56. Rodrigues R, Huber M, Lamura G, editors. Facts and figures on healthy ageing and long-term care: Europe and North America. Vienna: European Centre for Social Welfare Policy and Research; 2012 (http://www.euro.centre.org/data/LTC_Final.pdf, accessed 17 June 2015).

57. Thompson B, Tudiver F, Manson J. Sons as sole caregivers for their elderly parents. How do they cope? Can Fam Physician. 2000 Feb;46:360–5.%20http://www.ncbi.nlm.nih.gov/pmc/articles/PMC1987702/pdf/canfamphys00002-122.pdf PMID: 10690492

58. Bettio F, Simonazzi A, Villa P. Change in care regimes and female migration: the 'care drain' in the Mediterranean. J Eur Soc Policy. 2006;16(3):271–85. doi: http://dx.doi.org/10.1177/0958928706065598

59. The WHO global code of practice on the international recruitment of health personnel. Geneva: World Health Organization; 2010 (World Health Assembly Resolution WHA63.16; http://www.who.int/hrh/migration/code/code_en.pdf?ua=1, accessed 17 June 2015).

60. Morita A, Takano T, Nakamura K, Kizuki M, Seino K. Contribution of interaction with family, friends and neighbours, and sense of neighbourhood attachment to survival in senior citizens: 5-year follow-up study. Soc Sci Med. 2010 Feb;70(4):543–9. doi: http://dx.doi.org/10.1016/j.socscimed.2009.10.057 PMID: 19944506

61. Older people's associations. In: HelpAge International [website]. London: HelpAge International; 2015 (http://www.helpage.org/tags/older+people's+associations/, accessed 27 July 2015).

62. Boots LM, de Vugt ME, van Knippenberg RJ, Kempen GI, Verhey FR. A systematic review of Internet-based supportive interventions for caregivers of patients with dementia. Int J Geriatr Psychiatry. 2014 Apr;29(4):331–44. doi: http://dx.doi.org/10.1002/gps.4016 PMID: 23963684

63. Pot AM. Mastery over dementia: an internet intervention for family caregivers of people with dementia. Alzheimers Dement. 20010:6(4)(Suppl.):S90. doi: http://dx.doi.org/10.1002/gps.4016 PMID: 23963684

64. Blom MM, Zarit SH, Groot Zwaaftink RB, Cuijpers P, Pot AM. Effectiveness of an Internet intervention for family caregivers of people with dementia: results of a randomized controlled trial. PLOS ONE. 2015;10(2):e0116622. doi: http://dx.doi.org/10.1371/journal.pone.0116622 PMID: 25679228

65. Pot AM, Blom MM, Willemse BM. Acceptability of a guided self-help Internet intervention for family caregivers: mastery over dementia. Int Psychogeriatr. 2015;4:1–12. doi: http://dx.doi.org/10.1017/S1041610215000034 PMID: 25648589

66. Kitwood T. Dementia reconsidered: the person comes first. Buckingham: Open University Press; 1997 (http://www.mheducation.co.uk/9780335198559-emea-dementia-reconsidered, accessed 17 June 2015).

67. Greenblat C. Love, loss and laughter: seeing Alzheimer's differently. Guildford (CT): Lyons Press; 2012 (http://www.lyonspress.com/book/9780762779079, accessed 17 June 2015).

68. Brooker D. Person-centred dementia care: making services better, second edition. London: Jessica Kingsley Publishers; 2015 (http://www.jkp.com/uk/person-centred-dementia-care.html, accessed 17 June 2015).

69. Zwijsen, SA, Smalbrugge M, Eefsting JA, Twisk JW, Gerritsen DL, Pot AM, et al. Coming to grips with challenging behavior: a cluster randomized controlled trial on the effects of a multidisciplinary care program for challenging behavior in dementia. J Am Med Dir Assoc. 2014;15(7):531. doi: http://dx.doi.org/10.1001/jama.2012.4517 PMID: 22618925

70. Köpke S, Mühlhauser I, Gerlach A, Haut A, Haastert B, Möhler R, et al. Effect of a guideline-based multicomponent intervention on use of physical restraints in nursing homes: a randomized controlled trial. JAMA. 2012 May 23;307(20):2177–84. doi: http://dx.doi.org/10.1001/jama.2012.4517 PMID: 22618925

71. Flores-Castillo A. Cuidado y subjetividad: una mirada a la atención domiciliaria. [Care and subjectivity. a look at care at home.] Santiago (Chile): Naciones Unidas; 2012 (CEPAL – Serie Mujer y desarrollo No. 112; http://archivo.cepal.org/pdfs/2012/S1200015.pdf, accessed 17 June 2015) (in Spanish).

72. Chien LY, Chu H, Guo JL, Liao YM, Chang LI, Chen CH, et al. Caregiver support groups in patients with dementia: a meta-analysis. Int J Geriatr Psychiatry. 2011 Oct;26(10):1089–98. doi: http://dx.doi.org/10.1002/gps.2660 PMID: 21308785

73. Brodaty H, Arasaratnam C. Meta-analysis of nonpharmacological interventions for neuropsychiatric symptoms of dementia. Am J Psychiatry. 2012 Sep;169(9):946–53. doi: http://dx.doi.org/10.1176/appi.ajp.2012.11101529 PMID: 22952073

74. Van't Leven N, Prick AE, Groenewoud JG, Roelofs PD, de Lange J, Pot AM. Dyadic interventions for community-dwelling people with dementia and their family caregivers: a systematic review. Int Psychogeriatr. 2013 Oct;25(10):1581–603. doi: http://dx.doi.org/10.1017/S1041610213000860 PMID: 23883489

75. Kroes M, Garcia-Stewart S, Allen F, Eyssen M, Paulus D. Dementia: which non-pharmacological interventions? Brussels: Belgian Health Care Knowledge Centre; 2011 (KCE reports 160C; https://kce.fgov.be/sites/default/files/page_documents/kce_160c_dementia_0.pdf, accessed 17 June 2015).

76. Dementia: a public health priority. Geneva: World Health Organization; 2012 (http://whqlibdoc.who.int/publications/2012/9789241564458_eng.pdf, accessed 17 June 2015).

77. Day care centre.In: Alzheimer's Pakistan [website]. Lahore: Alzheimer's Pakistan; 2014 (http://alz.org.pk/day-care-centre/, accessed 2 June 2015).

78. Dementia day care: New Horizon Centres. In: Alzheimer's Disease Association [website]. Singapore: Alzheimer's Disease Association; 2010 (http://www.alz.org.sg/support-services/dementia-day-care-new-horizon-centres, accessed 2 June 2015).

79. Maayan N, Soares-Weiser K, Lee H. Respite care for people with dementia and their carers. Cochrane Database Syst Rev. 2014;(1):CD004396.http://www.ncbi.nlm.nih.gov/entrez/query.fcgi?cmd=Retrieve&db=PubMed&list_uids=24435941&dopt=Abstract PMID: 24435941

80. Shaw C, McNamara R, Abrams K, Cannings-John R, Hood K, Longo M, et al. Systematic review of respite care in the frail elderly. Health Technol Assess. 2009 Apr;13(20):1–224. doi: http://dx.doi.org/10.3310/hta13200 PMID: 19393135

81. Mason A, Weatherly H, Spilsbury K, Arksey H, Golder S, Adamson J, et al. A systematic review of the effectiveness and cost-effectiveness of different models of community-based respite care for frail older people and their carers. Health Technol Assess. 2007 Apr;11(15):1–157. doi: http://dx.doi.org/10.3310/hta11150 PMID: 17459263

82. Tretteteig S, Vatne S, Rokstad AM. The influence of day care centres for people with dementia on family caregivers: an integrative review of the literature. Aging Ment Health. 27 Mar 2015. doi: http://dx.doi.org/10.1080/13607863.2015.1023765 PMID: 25815563

83. Huang HL, Shyu YI, Chang MY, Weng LC, Lee I. Willingness to use respite care among family caregivers in Northern Taiwan. J Clin Nurs. 2009 Jan;18(2):191–8. doi: http://dx.doi.org/10.1111/j.1365-2702.2008.02538.x PMID: 19120749

84. Beland F, Hollander MJ. Modelos integrados de asistencia para ancianos frágiles: perspectiva internacional. [Integrated models of care delivery for the frail elderly: international perspectives]. Gac Sanit. 2011;25(Suppl. 2):138–46. (in Spanish). doi: http://dx.doi.org/10.1111/j.1365-2702.2008.02538.x PMID: 19120749

85. Eklund K, Wilhelmson K. Outcomes of coordinated and integrated interventions targeting frail elderly people: a systematic review of randomised controlled trials. Health Soc Care Community. 2009 Sep;17(5):447–58. doi: http://dx.doi.org/10.1111/j.1365-2524.2009.00844.x PMID: 19245421

86. You EC, Dunt D, Doyle C, Hsueh A. Effects of case management in community aged care on client and carer outcomes: a systematic review of randomized trials and comparative observational studies. BMC Health Serv Res. 2012;12(1):395. doi: http://dx.doi.org/10.1186/1472-6963-12-395 PMID: 23151143

87. Somme D, Carrier S, Trouve H, Gagnon D, Dupont O, Couturier Y, et al. Niveau de preuve de la gestion de cas dans la maladie d'Alzheimer: revue de literature. [Level of evidence for case management in Alzheimer's disease: a literature review.] Psychol Neuropsychiatr Vieil. 2009 Dec;7(Spec. No. 1):29–39. (in French). PMID: 20061231

88. Eklund K, Wilhelmson K. Outcomes of coordinated and integrated interventions targeting frail elderly people: a systematic review of randomised controlled trials. Health Soc Care Community. 2009 Sep;17(5):447–58. doi: http://dx.doi.org/10.1111/j.1365-2524.2009.00844.x PMID: 19245421

89. You EC, Dunt DR, Doyle C. Case managed community aged care: what is the evidence for effects on service use and costs? J Aging Health. 2013 Oct;25(7):1204–42. doi: http://dx.doi.org/10.1177/0898264313499931 PMID: 23958520

90. Pimouguet C, Lavaud T, Dartigues JF, Helmer C. Dementia case management effectiveness on health care costs and resource utilization: a systematic review of randomized controlled trials. J Nutr Health Aging. 2010 Oct;14(8):669–76. doi: http://dx.doi.org/10.1007/s12603-010-0314-4 PMID: 20922344

91. Reilly S, Miranda-Castillo C, Malouf R, Hoe J, Toot S, Challis D, et al. Case management approaches to home support for people with dementia. Cochrane Database Syst Rev. 2015;(1):CD008345.http://www.ncbi.nlm.nih.gov/entrez/query.fcgi?cmd=Retrieve&db=PubMed&list_uids=25560977&dopt=Abstract PMID: 25560977

92. Peeters JM, Francke AL, Pot AM. Organisatie en invulling van casemanagement dementie in Nederland. [Organization and content of case-management for people with dementia in the Netherlands.] Utrecht: Nivel/Trimbos-instituut; 2011 (in Dutch).

93. Verkade PJ, van Meijel B, Brink C, van Os-Medendorp H, Koekkoek B, Francke AL. Delphi research exploring essential components and preconditions for case management in people with dementia. BMC Geriatr. 2010;10(1):54. doi: http://dx.doi.org/10.1186/1471-2318-10-54 PMID: 20696035

94. Peisah C, Sorinmade OA, Mitchell L, Hertogh CM. Decisional capacity: toward an inclusionary approach. Int Psychogeriatr. 2013 Oct;25(10):1571–9. doi: http://dx.doi.org/10.1017/S1041610213001014 PMID: 23809025

95. Diesfeldt H, Teunissen S. Wislbekwaamheid. [Capacity.] In: Pot AM, Kuin Y, Vink MT, editors. Handboek Ouderenpsychologie. [Handbook of geropsychology]. Utrecht: De Tijdstroom; 2007 (https://www.tijdstroom.nl/boek/handboek-ouderenpsychologie#.VYmmSPlVhHw, accessed 17 June 2015) (in Dutch).

96. Hayhoe B, Howe A. Advance care planning under the Mental Capacity Act 2005 in primary care. Br J Gen Pract. 2011 Aug;61(589):e537–41. doi: http://dx.doi.org/10.3399/bjgp11X588592 PMID: 21801576

97. Advance care planning. London: Royal College of Physicians; 2009 (National Guideline No. 12; https://www.rcplondon.ac.uk/sites/default/files/documents/acp_web_final_21.01.09.pdf, accessed 17 June 2015).

98. Strengthening of palliative care as a component of integrated treatment throughout the life course: report by the Secretariat. Geneva: World Health Organization; 2013. (http://apps.who.int/gb/ebwha/pdf_files/EB134/B134_28-en.pdf, accessed 17 June 2015).

99. Humphreys G. Push for palliative care stokes debate. Bull World Health Organ. 2013 Dec 1;91(12):902–3. doi: http://dx.doi.org/10.2471/BLT.13.021213 PMID: 24347727

100. Amblàs-Novellas J, Espaulella J, Rexach L, Fontecha B, Inzitari M, Blay C, et al. Frailty, severity, progression and shared decision-making: a pragmatic framework for the challenge of clinical complexity at the end of life. Eur Geriatr Med. 2015 Apr;6(2):189–94. doi: http://dx.doi.org/10.1016/j.eurger.2015.01.002

101. Lorenz KA, Lynn J, Dy SM, Shugarman LR, Wilkinson A, Mularski RA, et al. Evidence for improving palliative care at the end of life: a systematic review. Ann Intern Med. 2008 Jan 15;148(2):147–59. doi: http://dx.doi.org/10.7326/0003-4819-148-2-200801150-00010 PMID: 18195339

102. Evde Bakim Hizmetleri Sunumu Hakkinda Yönetmelik. [The regulation of home care services.] In: Mevzuat Geliştirme ve Yayin Genel Müdürlüğü [website]. Ankara: Mevzuat Geliştirme ve Yayin Genel Müdürlüğü [Ministry of Health, Turkey.]; 2005 (http://www.mevzuat.gov.tr/Metin.Aspx?MevzuatKod=7.5.7542&MevzuatIliski=0&sourceXmlSearch=evde%20bak%C4%B1m, accessed July 3 2015) (in Turkish).

103. [Ankara Metropolitan Municipality.] Yaşlı Hizmetleri ve Şefkat Evleri. [Services for the elderly and care homes.] In: Ankara Büyükşehir Belediyesi [website]. Ankara: Ankara Büyükşehir Belediyesi; 2013 (in Turkish) (http://www.ankara.bel.tr/sosyal-hizmetler/yasli-hizmetleri, accessed 2 July 2015).

104. [Ministry of Family and Social Policies, Mardin province, Turkey.] Engelli Evde Bakım Hizmetleri Nelerdir? [What are home care services for the disabled?] In: T.C. Aile ve Sosyal Politikalar Bakanlığı Mardin İl Müdürlüğü [website]. Mardin: T.C. Aile Ve Sosyal Politikalar Bakanlığı Mardin İl Müdürlüğü; 2012 (in Turkish) (http://www.mardin-aile.gov.tr/engelli-evde-bakim-hizmetleri-1.html, accessed 2 July 2015).

105. [Ministry of Family and Social Policies, Turkey.] Evde Sağlık ve Sosyal Destek Hizmetlerinde İşbirliği Protokolü İmzalandı. [Cooperation protocol signed for home health and social support services.] In: T.C. Aile ve Sosyal Politikalar Bakanlığı [website]. Ankara: T.C. Aile ve Sosyal Politikalar Bakanlığı; 2014 (in Turkish) (http://www.aile.gov.tr/haberler/evde-saglik-ve-sosyal-destek-hizmetlerinde-isbirligi-protokolu-i%CC%87mzalandi, accessed 2 July 2015).

106. [Ministry of Health, Turkey.] Evde Sağlık ve Sosyal Destek Hizmetlerinin İşbirliği İçerisinde Yürütülmesine Dair Protokol İmzalandı. [Implementation protocol for home health and social support services.] In: T.C. Sağlık Bakanlığı [website]. Ankara: T.C. Sağlık Bakanlığı; 2015 (in Turkish) (http://www.saglik.gov.tr/TR/belge/1-39760/evde-saglik-ve-sosyal-destek-hizmetlerinin-isbirligi-ic-.html, accessed 2 July 2015).

107. The world health report 2000. Health systems: improving performance. Geneva: World Health Organization; 2000 (http://www.who.int/whr/2000/en/, accessed 17 June 2015).

108. van Ewijk C, van der Horst A, Besseling P. The future of health care. The Hague: CPB Netherlands Bureau for Economic Policy Analysis; 2013 (CPB Policy Brief 2013/03; http://www.cpb.nl/en/publication/the-future-of-health-care, accessed 17 June 2015).

109. Verbeek-Oudijk D, Woittiez I, Eggink E, Putman L. Who cares in Europe? A comparison of long-term care for the over-50s in sixteen European countries. The Hague: The Netherlands Institute for Social Research; 2014. (http://www.scp.nl/english/Publications/Publications_by_year/Publications_2014/Who_cares_in_Europe, accessed 17 June 2015).

110. Kim H, Kwon S, Yoon NH, Hyun KR. Utilization of long-term care services under the public long-term care insurance program in Korea: implications of a subsidy policy. Health Policy. 2013 Jul;111(2):166–74. doi: http://dx.doi.org/10.1016/j.healthpol.2013.04.009 PMID: 23706386

111. Lee HS, Wolf DA. An evaluation of recent old-age policy innovations in South Korea. Res Aging. 2014 Nov;36(6):707–30. doi: http://dx.doi.org/10.1177/0164027513519112 PMID: 25651545

112. Lloyd-Sherlock P. When social health insurance goes wrong: lessons from Argentina and Mexico. Soc Policy Adm. 2006;40(4):353–68. doi: http://dx.doi.org/10.1111/j.1467-9515.2006.00494.x

113. Kuo YC, Lan CF, Chen LK, Lan VM. Dementia care costs and the patient's quality of life (QoL) in Taiwan: home versus institutional care services. Arch Gerontol Geriatr. 2010 Sep-Oct;51(2):159–63. doi: http://dx.doi.org/10.1016/j.archger.2009.10.001 PMID: 20042244

114. Matus-López M, Pedraza CC. Costo de un sistema de atención de adultos mayores dependientes en Chile, 2012–2020. [Cost of a health care system for dependent older adults in Chile, 2012–2020.] Rev Panam Salud Publica. 2014 Jul;36(1):31–6. PMID:25211675 (in Spanish). PMID: 25211675

115. Mebane F. Want to understand how Americans viewed long-term care in 1998? Start with media coverage. Gerontologist. 2001 Feb;41(1):24–33. doi: http://dx.doi.org/10.1093/geront/41.1.24 PMID: 11220811

116. Butler RN. Psychiatry and the elderly: an overview. Am J Psychiatry. 1975 Sep;132(9):893–900. doi: http://dx.doi.org/10.1176/ajp.132.9.893 PMID: 1098483

117. Allen JO. Ageism as a risk factor for chronic disease. Gerontologist. 2015 23 Jan; pii: gnu158. doi: http://dx.doi.org/10.1093/geront/gnu158 PMID: 25618315

118. Leclerc BS, Lessard S, Bechennec C, Le Gal E, Benoit S, Bellerose L. Attitudes toward death, dying, end-of-life palliative care, and interdisciplinary practice in long term care workers. J Am Med Dir Assoc. 2014 Mar;15(3):207–13. doi: http://dx.doi.org/10.1016/j.jamda.2013.11.017 PMID: 24461725

119. Miller EA, Nadash P, Goldstein R. The role of the media in agenda setting: the case of long-term care rebalancing. Home Health Care Serv Q. 2015;34(1):30–45. doi: http://dx.doi.org/10.1080/01621424.2014.995259 PMID: 25517684

120. Scotland's National Dementia Strategy: 2013–2016. In: Scottish Government [website]. Edinburgh: Scottish Government; 2013 (http://www.gov.scot/Resource/0042/00423472.pdf, accessed 13 July 2015).

121. 2020 Vision. In: Scottish Government [website]. Edinburgh: Scottish Government; 2015 (http://www.gov.scot/Topics/Health/Policy/2020-Vision, accessed 13 July 2015).

122. Charter of Rights for People with Dementia and their Carers in Scotland. In: Alzheimer Scotland [website]. Edinburgh: Alzheimer Scotland, Action on Dementia; 2015 (http://www.dementiarights.org/charter-of-rights/, accessed 13 July 2015).

123. Standards of care for dementia in Scotland: action to support the change programme. In: Scottish Government [website]. Edinburgh: Scottish Government; 2011 (http://www.gov.scot/Resource/Doc/350188/0117212.pdf, accessed 13 July 2015).

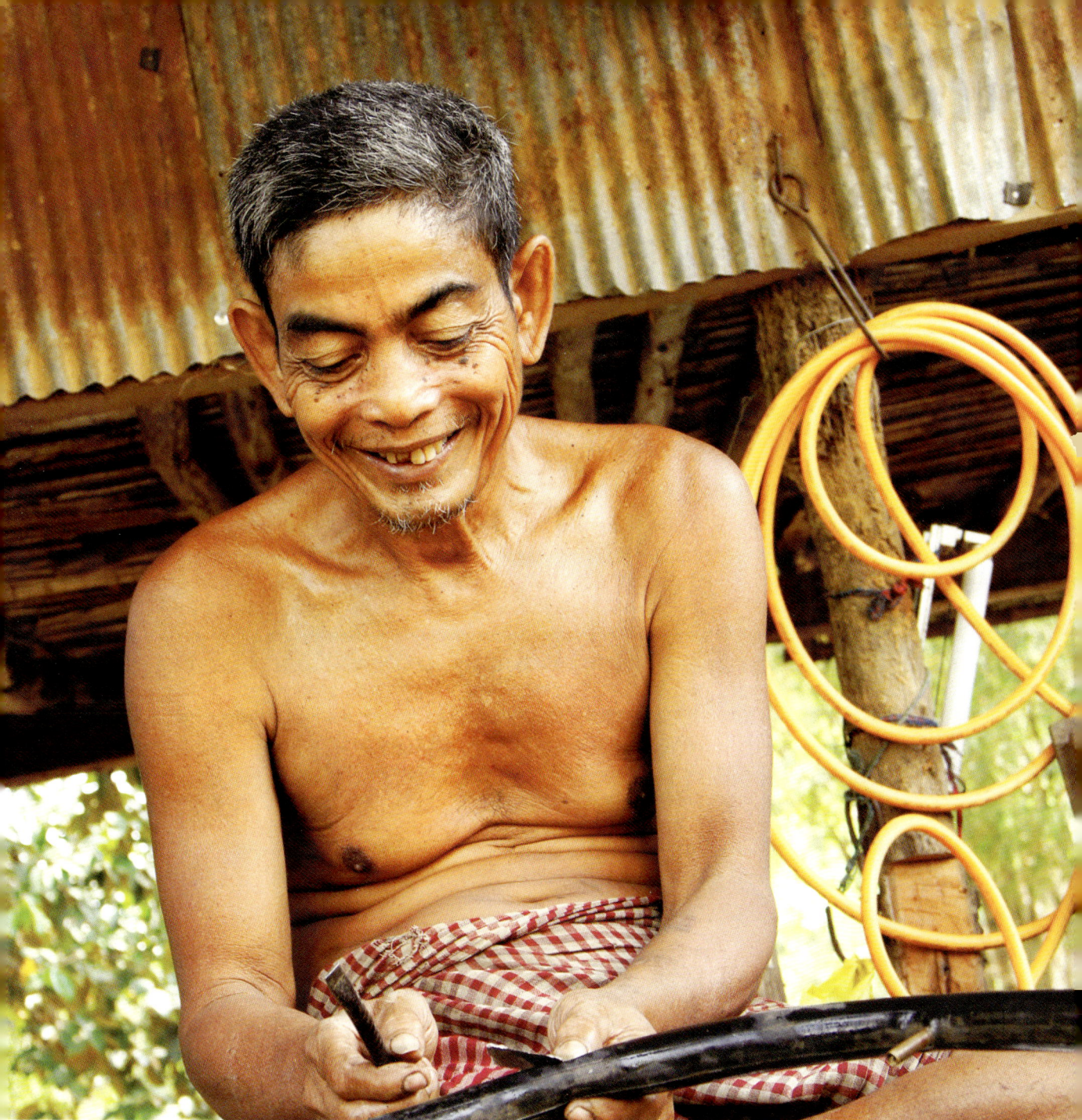

Chapter 6
Towards an age-friendly world

Yeun, 59, Cambodia

Yeun cares for two grandchildren and lives alone.

"I was born in this village and have lived here all my life. I have never been to the capital Phnom Penh - only to nearby Battambang City. The community organiser from HelpAge asked me if I wanted to start a new business.

When I said yes, the older people's association arranged for me to undergo an apprenticeship with someone who knew how to fix bicycles. Once I was ready, the older people's association gave me a grant of US$220 (880,000 Cambodian riels) to buy tools and an air pump- everything I needed to start fixing bicycles.

I used to repair shoes, but I did not make enough money. At that time, people used to wear a lot of second-hand shoes, but not so much now. I like my bicycle repair business much more as I can make two or three times as much money now. Using the profits from this business, I was able to buy more tools and replace some of the old ones. I was able to put a tin roof on my house to keep the rain out. Also, because I live on the side of the river, my house can easily be flooded, but using the earnings from my business I was able to raise my house higher. Now, I even lend money to my children.

In the village, people bring me all kinds of vehicles - almost anything with wheels. I get at least two to three customers a day. The most difficult thing about repairing a puncture is removing the tyres. It took me a while to master that skill, but now I am an expert.

I think older people should never give up and always keep hope. Even if you are disabled as I am, you can live with your efforts, you can live with your skills. With a little help I was able to set up this business; I think others can do the same."

6

Towards an age-friendly world

Introduction

Chapter 4 and Chapter 5 outlined the importance of health care and long-term care and what can be done to strengthen these systems. This chapter outlines the crucial role of further aspects of an older person's environments and how other sectors can contribute to harnessing the opportunities and addressing the challenges of population ageing.

The process of *Healthy Ageing* argues that all sectors share a common goal: to build and maintain functional ability. Therefore, this chapter is structured around five key domains of functional ability that are essential for older people to:

- meet their basic needs;
- learn, grow and make decisions;
- be mobile;
- build and maintain relationships;
- contribute.

These abilities are essential to enable older people to do the things that they value. Together they enable older people to age safely in a place that is right for them, to continue to develop personally, to be included and to contribute to their communities while retaining their autonomy and health.

Although the five abilities are treated separately in the text, they are strongly interconnected. For example, participating in work may be essential for meeting basic needs. Meeting basic needs is a prerequisite for learning and growth. Opportunities to learn and grow are also opportunities to develop relationships.

Three important considerations permeate these discussions. First, what older adults can do physically or mentally – their intrinsic capacity – is only part of their potential. What they are actually able to do (their functional ability) will depend on the fit between them and their environments. Second, a paradigm shift is needed in the way that society understands ageing. Pervasive ageist stereotypes of older people as uniformly frail, burdensome and dependent are not supported by evidence (Chapter 1) and limit society's ability to appreciate and release the potential human and social resources inherent in older populations. Yet these negative attitudes influence decision-making, choices about public policy and public attitudes and behaviours (*1*). Third, the effect of environments will influence one older person differently from the next depending on factors such as gender, ethnicity or level of education. This may result in unequal access to material or psychological support, or limit behavioural options and, thus, affect an older person's ability to experience *Healthy Ageing* (2). Without considering these inequitable relationships, policies in all sectors risk widening the gaps demonstrated in Chapter 1 and Chapter 3.

This chapter also builds on WHO's approach, used during the past decade, to develop age-friendly cities and communities. Much of this work is built around key municipal-level services: transportation, housing and urban development, information and communication, and health and community services. This chapter complements this approach by framing age- friendly actions towards meeting the goal of enhancing functional ability and by extending these concepts in a way that is relevant for all sectors and that can encourage them to work together. The discussion is therefore relevant for any level of government or any sector, public or private.

The actions we discuss take many forms but enhance functional ability in two fundamental ways.

1. By building and maintaining intrinsic capacity, by reducing risks (such as high levels of air pollution), encouraging healthy behaviours (such as physical activity) or removing barriers to them (for example, high crime rates or dangerous traffic), or by providing services that foster capacity (such as health care).

2. By enabling greater functional ability – in other words, by filling the gap between what people can do given their level of capacity and what they could do in an enabling environment (for example, by providing appropriate assistive technologies, providing accessible public transport or developing safer neighbourhoods). In doing these things, it is important to acknowledge that although population-level interventions

may improve environments for many older people, many will not be able to benefit fully without individually tailored support.

The purpose of this chapter is to provide an overview of the five abilities and explore the evidence about what works to foster them. It is intended to help decision-makers reflect on current practices and to provide support for possible ways to move forward. The lessons learnt and shared by members of the WHO Global Network of Age-friendly Cities and Communities (Box 6.1) are reflected in many of the examples.

Ability to meet basic needs

Perhaps the most fundamental of abilities is the ability of older people to manage and meet their immediate and future needs to ensure an adequate standard of living as defined in United Nations Article 25 of *The universal declaration of human rights* (7).This ability includes older people being able to afford an adequate diet, clothing, suitable housing, and health-care and long-term care services. It also extends to having support to minimize the impact of economic shocks that may come with illness, disability, losing a spouse or the means of livelihood (7).

The inability of older people to meet their basic needs can be both a cause and an effect of reduced capacity (8–11). But their environments, too, play a crucial part. "Poor social policies, unfair economic arrangements [where the already well-off and healthy become even richer and the poor who are already more likely to be ill become even poorer] and bad politics" (12) make meeting basic needs in older age much harder and, hence, decrease what older people can and could do.

The most important basic needs identified by older people, beyond health care and long-term care, are personal and financial security, and adequate housing (13, 14). This section explores briefly what we know about these three important areas, their implications for *Healthy Ageing* and the potential for action.

Box 6.1.   Age-friendly cities and communities

An age-friendly city or community is a good place to grow old. Age-friendly cities and communities foster healthy and active ageing and, thus, enable well-being throughout life. They help people to remain independent for as long as possible, and provide care and protection when they are needed, respecting older people's autonomy and dignity.

The WHO Global Network of Age-friendly Cities and Communities was established in 2010 to support municipalities that wished to transform these ambitions into reality, involving older people in the process and maximizing their opportunities at the local level. The network seeks to do this by:

- **inspiring** change and showing what can be done and how it can be done;
- **connecting** cities and communities worldwide to facilitate the exchange of information and experience;
- **supporting** cities and communities to find solutions by providing innovative and evidence-based technical guidance.

The network builds on previous work by WHO, and by 2015 included more than 250 cities and communities in 28 countries. Network members commit to:

- engage with older people and other stakeholders across sectors;
- assess the age-friendliness of their cities and identify priorities for action;
- use the assessment findings to engage in evidence-based planning and policy-making across a range of fields to adapt their "structures and services to be accessible to and inclusive of older people with varying needs and capacities" (3).

Age-friendly interventions are responsive to local needs. For example in New York City, the Department of Transportation's **Safe Streets for Seniors** programme has developed measures to improve the safety of older pedestrians in particular areas of the city where older people had been involved in accidents that resulted in severe injuries or fatality. Between 2009 and 2014, more than 600 dangerous intersections were redesigned and pedestrian fatalities among older people decreased by 21% (4).

Initiatives in other cities, have focused on enhancing mobility by making transportation affordable for and accessible to older people, including in rural areas. For example, in Winnipeg, Canada, **Handi-transit** provides transportation for older people who are not well served by public transport or who can no longer drive (5).

To address the challenges of social isolation and loneliness, many communities have developed telephone hotlines as well as befriending schemes in which volunteers visit older people. Another way of tackling social isolation and loneliness is through schemes that offer activities of interest to older people. An example is the **Men's Sheds** in Australia and Ireland that target men at risk of social isolation, offering activities of interest to them, such as wood turning, repairing vintage vehicles, compiling heritage memorabilia and classes on information technology (6). Further examples of local interventions are shared on the network's portal (http://agefriendlyworld.org/en/about-us/).

Financial security, housing, personal security

Lack of financial security in older age is a major obstacle to *Healthy Ageing* and to reducing health inequity (12). The prevalence of poverty among older people compared with that in the general population varies significantly across the world. In Europe, one in every five older persons has an income below the poverty line, with people older than 80 years being the most severely affected.

Individual European countries, however, show differences. In the majority of countries in the European Union, older people are at higher risk of poverty than the general population, but older people appear relatively well protected from poverty in some of these countries, including the Czech Republic, France, Hungary, Luxembourg, the Netherlands and Poland (15). This suggests that local policies make a significant difference. In high-income countries in general, an individual's level of financial security tends to change little across the life course – that is, those that were affluent in early life remain affluent in later years, and those who were poor remain poor (*15, 16*). In countries in sub-Saharan Africa households comprising only older people generally have less financial security than households comprising a mix of ages (*17*). In Latin America, poverty rates among older people tend to be lower than among the general population (*18*).

Specific groups are at greater risk of not being able to meet their basic need for financial security. Across all contexts, women are more likely than men to be poor, and less likely to have gained pension rights during their working life. For example, older women in OECD countries are 33% more likely to be poor than men of the same age (*15, 19*). In sub-Saharan Africa, older people living with grandchildren (known as skip-generation households) are at increased risk of poverty (*17*). In OECD countries older people living alone, who most often are widowed older women, are at increased risk of poverty, with rates exceeding 40% in many countries, including Australia, Ireland, Japan, Mexico, the Republic of Korea and the United States (*15*).

Around the world, older people with low incomes find it particularly problematic to meet their basic need for adequate housing (Box 6.2). For poor older people, housing is often the biggest household expenditure and the main determinant of how much food is available and whether the heat will be turned on when it is cold (*21, 22*). Ensuring that older people live in housing that is an appropriate and manageable size for their household, and that is affordable to heat, is associated with improved health, and may promote improved social relationships within and beyond the household (*23*). When older people have a fixed income they are particularly affected by the level at which rents are set and the costs of utilities, maintenance or the modifications that are necessary to accommodate a loss of capacity. Making improvements to housing that result in an increase in rent that is beyond older people's

---

Box 6.2. The right to adequate housing

The right to adequate housing requires more than just four walls and a roof (Article 11.1 of the *International covenant on economic, social and cultural rights*) (*20*). It includes the right to have a safe and secure house and community in which to live in peace and dignity. The right to adequate housing encompasses a range of concepts relevant to older people (*21*), such as:

- guaranteeing legal protection of tenure against forced evictions, harassment and other threats;
- being sufficiently affordable such that the costs do not threaten or compromise the occupants' enjoyment of other basic needs;
- ensuring access to safe drinking water, adequate sanitation, energy for cooking, heating, lighting, food storage and refuse disposal;
- ensuring habitability – that is, guaranteeing physical safety, providing adequate space, protecting against threats to health and against structural hazards, and not being located in polluted or dangerous areas;
- ensuring accessibility and usability, for example, by taking into consideration declines in capacity;
- facilitating access to transportation, shopping, employment opportunities, health-care services and other social facilities;
- respecting the expression of cultural identity.

---

ability to pay can cause significant distress and negatively impact their health (*24*).

Poorer people are also more likely to live in deprived neighbourhoods where there is less access to safe environments that might allow them to be physically active; where there are fewer resources, such as hospitals, that might help them cope with adverse events; and where there is less access to healthy food that might allow them to eat a nutritious diet (*25*). The characteristics of neighbourhoods and communities can also have an impact on crime and stress levels, and result in older people restricting their movements. When combined, these impacts from personal and neighbourhood poverty have been shown to increase the risk of symptoms of depression (*26*). Those with the least financial security or poorest intrinsic capacity are often least able to meet their need for adequate housing. For example, higher rates of disability occur among those who are poorest and who are the least able to pay for adequate housing or improve their housing situation (27, 28). Therefore, their disadvantages accumulate (29).

Personal security is another crucial issue for older people. It, too, is more threatened in deprived neighbourhoods but is nonetheless relevant to all, and its absence has significant consequences for health, well-being and survival (30). Abuse and crime can cause injury, pain, stress and depression. When older people, particularly women, are victims of violent crime, the consequences are often more severe than for other age groups: older women are more likely to have a higher need for medical care, to be admitted into a nursing home and to die as a result of an assault (31). Victims of elder abuse have twice the risk of death compared to those not reporting abuse (32). The fear of crime, and actually having been the victim of a crime, a disaster or abuse can increase the risk of social isolation and feelings of vulnerability, and seriously undermine both older people's ability to participate in their families and communities and community efforts to improve their health (33, 34).

However, because older people do not form a homogeneous group, their experiences and the health implications of crime, fear and abuse are not uniform. Factors such as age, sex, level of physical or mental capacity, socioeconomic status, ethnic or religious background, and being part of a sexual minority, are all important influences on risk and how it is experienced. In general, those who are more likely to experience threats to personal security include older people with poor physical and mental health, who are care-dependent, who are socially isolated and who are poor.

Disasters can make it more difficult for all older people to meet their basic needs for food, water, sanitation, shelter and health-care services. Older people who are less resilient and who experienced difficulty meeting their basic

needs prior to a disaster may be inadequately prepared to mitigate the effects of a disaster (for example, by hurricane-proofing their house) or to cope afterwards. Disasters may also create or exacerbate threats to their personal security, for example, when older people are forced by a disaster to live in temporary shelters (35).

What works in improving financial security

Having no significant money worries is important throughout the life course, but this is increasingly so in older age when the ability to generate income often declines. Evidence suggests that having up to a certain amount of money makes people happier and reduces mental health problems, such as depression and anxiety (36, 37). Money can also increase choices related to other abilities, such as decisions about relationships, learning options and work.

Financial security in older age can be accumulated from a wide variety of sources: pensions, social insurance benefits, earnings, assets and intergenerational transfers. Research has shown that in high-income countries, higher-income households are more likely to draw from diverse sources, while poorer households have greater reliance on income from social security (27). In low-income countries, access to social insurance benefits and other social safety nets is particularly limited.

For older adults who have not been able to accumulate sufficient income through contributory pensions, savings, intergenerational transfers or other sources, social-protection support can enable them to meet their basic needs. Social protection is a fundamental human right and can be critical for older people, allowing them to manage financial risks and protecting them from poverty (7, 20). A range of approaches is needed to ensure social protection, which can include a social pension, means-tested benefits, and protection from the costs of health care and social care. However, reliance on these approaches should not stigmatize older adults. The discussion that follows focuses on the strategies being used in diverse contexts to provide support to poor older adults, and reflects both universal and targeted approaches. This section should be read in conjunction with the section on the Ability to contribute which looks at, among other things, how to support older people to remain in the workforce in ways that do not undermine *Healthy Ageing*.

Social pensions (that is, noncontributory cash transfers to older people) can raise the social status of older people within households, enable older people to continue to have a role in household decision-making, and improve access to services (*12, 38, 39*). They can also contribute to gender equity because women tend to live longer but often have less access to contributory pensions. Especially in low-income countries, social pension systems can also improve the well-being of other household members, including children: the extra money that comes into the household can, for example, help children enrol in school and can be used to improve their nutrition (*40*). Thus, a social pension given to an older person can help to break an intergenerational cycle of poverty. A range of countries have established social pension schemes that can be used to provide care for vulnerable older people. For example, in Chile poor women and men receive a social pension if they are not provided for by the formal pension systems that provide benefits only after years of employment and contributions. Older women tend to be poorer than older men, so they benefit proportionately more from the programme, especially in rural areas (*18*). Thus, this is an example of a policy on ageing that is effective in combating the inequities highlighted elsewhere in this report.

Both funding and financing instruments can be strengthened to address these vulnerabilities (*41*). Namibia provides a universal pension to people aged older than 60, and it is not means-tested. Approximatley 88% of eligible persons receive the pension, and it is the main source of income for 14% of rural households and 7% of households in urban areas. In addition to being an important means of reducing poverty, it often indirectly benefits the children who live in skip-generation households because their parents are away working or have died of AIDS (*18*). For example, a study conducted in South Africa found that girls living with grandmothers who received a social pension had improvements in their height and weight for their age (*42*). Nepal, despite conflict and its aftermath, has also maintained and developed social pensions for older people (*43*). The Republic of Korea introduced a basic old-age pension in 2008, which is a means-tested noncontributory social pension, as one mechanism for providing social protection. This pension has improved older people's ability to meet their basic needs, such as for heating and nutritious food, particularly among the oldest age group (*44*). In Kazakhastan, pensions have also been shown to have an important role in reducing poverty among older people (*45*).

However, addressing the financial needs of poor older people requires more than offering pensions (Box 6.3). Different forms of direct and indirect support are needed; these may include:

- making available in the community programmes for retraining that are adapted to the needs of older workers and can enable them to work for longer;
- changing employers' attitudes about the value and contributions of older workers;
- providing social assistance within the home and community for the poorest and the oldest people (categories that frequently overlap) and for those without family support. Women are often a large part of this group (*47*). For example, in Jordan, targeted cash transfers (that is, direct payments of money to eligible people) favour poor women and households headed by older people, but this benefit is delivered within a context of family and community networks and the significant additional social support

provided by religious organizations and nongovernmental organizations (*18*);

- providing essential health care at a nationally defined minimum level that meets the criteria of availability, accessibility, acceptability and quality (Chapter 4) (*48*);
- developing policies that provide unemployment insurance and health insurance, including coverage for catastrophic health expenditures (*48*);
- connecting informal workers with different forms of social security and pension coverage (*49*). In India, for instance, the national pension scheme has been extended to include informal workers (*50*);
- providing assistance to families that care for older family members (Chapter 5).

Box 6.3.   Promoting accountability to older people and uptake of pensions in Bangladesh

In Bangladesh, the Resource Integration Centre, a nongovernmental organization, has worked with older people in 80 villages to form associations. The associations elected members to monitor older people's entitlements, such as the old-age allowance, widow's allowance and access to health services. They found that significantly fewer people were receiving entitlements than were eligible: less than 1 in 10 in one area. The older people's associations meet regularly with local governments to help people claim pension entitlements; as a result, pension uptake has increased fivefold, and banks have improved their procedures for serving older people (*46*).

What works in ensuring adequate housing

Older people want housing that enables them to be safe and comfortable regardless of their age, income or level of capacity. For some this may mean the desire to age in place – that is, to remain in their homes and communities as they get older (*28, 51–54*). For others, ageing in place

may not be desirable. For example, their housing may no longer suit them if their neighbourhood has experienced decline or gentrification and if the community networks and services that they relied on have been eroded. For others, their housing may be so inadequate that it is detrimental to them, which may be particularly common in resource-poor settings. In these settings, limited basic amenities, multiple safety risks and overcrowded intergenerational households may restrict both comfort and security (*55*) (Source: I Aboderin, [African Population and Health Research Center] Older men and women's experience of older age in three sub-saharan cities [unpublished data], 27 July 2015).

Policies need to enhance the fit between the needs and preferences of older people and their housing, and will require mechanisms to address the inevitable changes that occur both in people and places over time (*56*). Benefits of increased fit can include improvements in mental health, reductions in injuries, the ability to maintain attachments to both home and community, and increased autonomy and independence (*54*).

A discussion on general housing policies and programmes, and what works in providing adequate housing and safe and secure neighbourhoods is important but beyond the scope of this report. The focus here is on what could be done to ensure that policies consider population ageing and specifically focus on poor older people and those who have lost capacity. The actions to be taken will involve many different organizations, governance arrangements, funding instruments, types of accommodation and providers. Any action that is chosen will depend on the context.

Facilitate older people's choices

Older people in every income group and across all contexts should have access to a range of options for adequate and affordable housing. These may include market-driven housing for those who can afford it, social housing, assisted-living facilities, continuing-care communities (which provide residential options that are responsive to different levels of capacity, such as independent living, assisted living or care homes) and shared-living arrangements, including hostels and care homes.

The United Nations' *Convention on the rights of persons with disabilities and optional protocol* recognizes the equal right of all persons with disabilities to live in their community, to choose where and with whom they want to live, and to not be obliged to reside in a particular living arrangement (*57*). Article 19 of the convention also includes provisions for a range of in-home, residential and other community services to support living and inclusion in the community, and these may provide cost-effective options for enabling older people to age in place. For example, telecare (that is, the remote provision of services) has been shown to increase older people's ability to stay in their homes, even people who have dementia. In Bradford, England, a pilot project that provided telecare to older adults found that 26% of those in the telecare programme were able to stay in their own home, thus avoiding an unwanted admission to a care home (*58*). A further 13% of those in the programme avoided hospital admission, and there was a 29% reduction in the number of hours needed for home care. This was a pilot project, but if expanded to full capacity it is estimated that the programme would save significant resources (*58*).

Develop policies that support housing modifications and access to assistive technologies

The accessibility of housing and the usability of modifications and assistive devices is of particular importance for older adults because they are likely to spend more time in their homes or immediate neighbourhood when compared with younger people, and may have less intrinsic capacity with which to navigate barriers such as uneven floors or roads with potholes (*59*). Declines in intrinsic capacity are the most common reasons why older people become unable to cope in their existing residence and need to move (*60*). Many older people live in housing that was built

a long time ago and has features that may be hazardous – such as rugs, narrow doors, inaccessible bathrooms or poor light – and act as barriers to independence as people age and lose capacity (*52, 61*). When people experience a significant loss of capacity, previously minor household barriers may become major obstacles to managing their daily needs. This may mean that older people are unable to return home after being hospitalized or that they need to transition to more supportive housing (*62*).

Home modifications (that is, conversions or adaptations made to the permanent physical features of people's homes to reduce the demands from the physical environment) can have a multitude of benefits: it may make tasks easier; reduce risks to health, such as falls (Box 6.4); provide better security; help maintain independence over time; and have positive impacts on social relationships and networks, thus facilitating continued engagement with society (*24, 61, 72*). Home modifications have been found to be cost effective (Box 6.5). They generally target one or more of the following three issues:

- physical accessibility – for example, by removing obstacles (such as stairs to the entrance) and providing mobility and safety aides (such as grab bars in showers and near toilets);
- comfort – for example, by improving energy efficiency, such as installing insulation and draught proofing (*25*);
- safety – for example, by reducing airborne dust, or introducing and maintaining mechanisms to reduce injury, such as installing nonslip flooring in bathrooms.

Older people can plan ahead and integrate the changes needed to ensure accessibility – for example, by adding handrails when they renovate the bathroom – or they can introduce changes as their capacity declines. Because older people's capacity can decline rapidly, it is necessary to ensure that assessments are timely and changes are made promptly so that older people

Box 6.4.   Reducing falls through environmental intervention

The immediate environment plays an important part in protecting older people against falls. A systematic review of multifaceted population-level interventions assessed in studies conducted in Australia, Denmark, Norway and Sweden showed reductions of between 6% and 75% in fall-related injuries (*63*).

In addition to treating health conditions and controlling medications, a range of environmental interventions have been shown to be helpful in reducing risks for community-dwelling older adults (*64*). These include providing:

- education to individual older people to enhance their knowledge and reduce their fear of falling (*63, 65, 66*);
- home visits by health professionals to high-risk individuals (*65, 67, 68*). Joint assessments conducted by certified health providers and an older person can be more comprehensive and result in better follow-up action than either self-assessment alone or an assessment made only by a health practitioner (*69*);
- information about reducing hazards in the home (*65, 68*);
- training for municipal service providers, health-care workers and new housing planners about how to remove hazards in the home and public spaces (*70*);
- opportunities for physical activity (*65*), such as community walking programmes (*67*) or Tai chi classes (*66*) (Box 6.12);
- improvements in the physical environment of the neighbourhood, for example improving lighting in public places and making roads and walkways more accessible and safer (*67*);
- community education about falls prevention and management using brochures, posters, and television and radio (*68, 70, 71*), and by engaging with local media, community agencies and services (*65, 67, 71*).

can maximize their trajectories of functioning and age in place (*72*). Because the home can be an important base from which to foster connectedness, older people must have control over any decisions about proposed modifications (*61*).

The following are examples of policies or programmes being implemented to assist older people in making home modifications. Programmes should ensure that information about the services available to help with modifications is offered in formats that are accessible and easy to understand.

- Loans, grants or direct transfers (subsidies): these are made directly to older people or to landlords whose older residents meet defined criteria, such as income level, and landlords must agree not to increase an older person's rent as a result of the adaptations (*74, 75*). These have been used in many countries in Europe, North America and the Caribbean and can specifically target older people who are poor but own their house, and landlords with low-income tenants. For example, in Germany the Pflegeversicherung (national care insurance based on the social code book XI) subsidizes home modifications for all who require long-term care at home including older people and others. Individuals can apply for up to €4000 to fund housing modifications. If an individual's capacity declines and needs change, individuals can reapply for support up to the same amount. The demand for home-modification subsidies has increased nearly fourfold, from €39 million in 1998 to €143 million in 2013, and now represents 0.62% of overall expenses under the Pflegeversicherung (*Source*: B Hernig [Verband der Ersatzkassen] personal communication with Matthias Braubach, May 13, 2015).
- Schemes to maintain housing in good condition: cleaning and repair services are offered by schemes in Australia (*76*), the Bahamas and Barbados (*77*), and the United Kingdom (*78*) to support frail or vulnerable older people who may have concerns about having strangers in their homes or managing the financial side of the repairs.

Box 6.5. Money well spent: the effectiveness and value of making housing modifications

A study in 2000 examined the effectiveness of using public funding to make housing modifications for older people and others with reduced capacity in England and Wales (73). The study interviewed people who had major adaptations made to their homes, and used information from postal questionnaires returned by those who had minor adaptations, administrative records, and the views of visiting professionals. The main measure of effectiveness was the degree to which the problems experienced by the respondent before adaptation were overcome by the adaptation without causing new problems. The study found that:

- minor adaptations (such as adding handrails, ramps, over-bath showers, and entry systems) produced a range of lasting, positive consequences for virtually all recipients – 62% of respondents suggested that they felt safer from the risk of accident, and 77% perceived a positive effect on their health;

- major adaptations (such as bathroom conversions, extensions, or the addition of a lift) in most cases had transformed people's lives. Before the adaptations, people used words such as "prisoner", "degraded", and "afraid" to describe their situations; following the adaptations, they spoke of themselves as "independent", "useful", and "confident";

- where major adaptations failed, it was typically because of weaknesses in the original specification. For example, extensions were too small or too cold to use, or failed to provide proper bathing facilities;

- the evidence from respondents suggested that successful adaptations keep people out of hospital, reduce the strain on carers and promote social inclusion;

- the benefits were most pronounced when careful consultations with users took place, where the needs of the whole family had been considered, and where the integrity of the home had been respected.

Adaptations appear to be a highly effective use of public resources, thus justifying the investment.

Efforts to improve the accessibility of housing may need to be accompanied by the provision of assistive technologies (79), such as canes, walkers, shower chairs, bath boards, nonslip bath mats, adapted toilet seats; or for people with cognitive impairment, calendars that use symbols. For devices to be appropriate, suitable and of high quality they must meet the needs and preferences of older persons, be suitable to their environments, and adequate follow-up must ensure they are used safely and efficiently (80).

Other technologies can also help increase an older person's safety and security in the home. For example, sensors and cameras can monitor the home and analyse data to determine whether, for example, an older person has fallen, set off a smoke alarm or wandered away. One systematic review of smart-home technology found that older people were open to having these technologies in their homes if there were tangible benefits and if their privacy concerns were addressed (79).

Research has shown that providing a comprehensive package of housing adaptations and assistive technologies for older people would be cost-effective because of the resultant reductions in the need for formal care (81).

Develop policies that expand options for adequate housing for older adults

Older people around the world vary enormously in their needs, preferences, living arrangements and financial situations. Policies aimed at ensuring that they have adequate housing therefore need to offer a range of solutions (51). Because housing for older people with low incomes poses a particular challenge to *Healthy Ageing*, this section looks specifically at affordable and social housing. Strategies to make housing affordable require that either the ability of older people to pay for adequate housing is improved or that social housing is provided. These strategies are likely to require collaboration among governments, social services and the private sector.

Different countries have approached affordability in varied ways, but consideration has been given to both supply and demand. Strategies that enhance demand include increasing the money available to older people to rent or buy adequate housing. Uruguay, for example, provides housing benefits that are based on a person's income and that can be used to pay part or all of the rent (*77*). Other countries in the region also provide direct subsidies for home improvements. Governments can also influence the cost of rent or its impact on older people. Countries such as the United States have provided subsidized housing vouchers to help renters age in place. For older homeowners with low incomes, property tax relief programmes are an option (*27*). In South Africa, subsidies are available for recipients of an old-age grant that enables them to build or buy a house. Other strategies to increase older people's disposable income include using an unencumbered house as an asset that can be traded for cash or against which a loan can be raised (*82*).

Implementing a policy that supports older people in moving into more suitable housing may be an option. For example, the Netherlands provides a specific housing allowance to assist older people in moving to more adequate housing (*25*). In Nicaragua a law provides older people, or households with an older person, with preferential access to social housing projects (*77*).

Ensuring there is an adequate supply of appropriate and affordable housing – which may include market-based housing, low-cost housing or housing in assisted-living rental villages – is increasingly difficult, especially in many regions where the stock of social housing has been reduced (*83*). However, there are a range of financing options, such as loans, subsidies and incentives, that can be used to increase the availability of affordable and social housing (*27, 53, 84*).

Policies and programmes can also be put in place to improve the existing stock of housing or neighbourhoods so that they meet the conditions for adequate housing. Across the life course, improving housing in disadvantaged areas may provide a population-based strategy for improving health and reducing health inequalities.

Efforts that go beyond housing to improve distressed areas may be more cost effective than strategies that move people from lower socioeconomic backgrounds to better-off areas (*25*).

It is cheaper to build new housing that is accessible and energy efficient than it is to retrofit housing. In many countries, laws and standards on disability and accessibility stipulate the need to provide access to all people. Even if the renewal rates for housing stock are low and a focus on building new housing is not feasible in the short term, it is important to ensure that state-supported housing adheres to universal design principles, is energy efficient and is capable of harnessing innovations in housing design that can support people as they age. Building codes that require accessible features can also be used to ensure that developers of market-rate houses build more age-friendly homes and arrange for age-friendly renovations. Architects, builders and town planners must be sensitized to the importance of ensuring accessibility. This is particularly relevant for large-scale urban renewal projects and during reconstruction after a disaster.

What works in meeting the need for personal security

Older people need to be and to feel safe (that is, able to avoid injury) and secure (that is, able to avoid harm) in their homes and in their communities. Injuries, elder abuse, crime and disasters all undermine older people's personal security. This section describes three issues that challenge an older person's personal security: crime (for example, robbery, assault and homicide); elder abuse (for example, physical, sexual, psychological, emotional, financial and material abuse, and abandonment and neglect); and disasters. Safety related to road traffic injuries and falls is addressed in the sections on the Ability to be mobile and What works in ensuring adequate housing.

Although the evidence is limited about what works to safeguard the personal security of older adults, the following discussion draws on evidence that suggests that certain strategies benefit older people and also have a limited risk of unanticipated negative effects.

Crime

Although older people are more likely to have fears about crime than younger members of a community, they may be less likely to be actual victims of crime and related violence (*85*). However, the lower prevalence of crime observed against older people may not reflect an age-related decline in risk so much as an increase in fear-driven behaviours that reduce exposure (for example, older people may spend more time at home) (*30*). The fear of crime is heightened by greater inequalities, negative intergenerational attitudes and relationships, and a media culture that sensationalizes crimes (*86*).

Increasing older people's personal safety and the security of their property requires taking action at home and within the broader community. Measures such as fitting locks or alarms should be accompanied by efforts to maintain the home so that it does not appear neglected or easy to enter. For example, the Security and Advice For the Elderly project, in Nottinghamshire, England, found a 93% decrease in residential burglaries among low-income older people who had been provided with stronger locks and who took other precautionary measures (*87*). Decisions taken about town planning and land use may also enhance older people's personal safety if measures include designing safe well-lit and accessible structures and landscapes. To increase older people's safety it is important to ensure that local authorities provide safer spaces and identify and respond to security problems (Box 6.6).

It is important to reduce older people's fear of crime while encouraging them to maintain vigilance in the face of real risks. Older people who are active and involved in their communities and who are made to feel involved are less likely to fear crime. Isolated individuals are more likely to lose confidence and trust, and they can be specifically targeted when facilitating com-

> ### Box 6.6. Older people getting to know their local police officer: New Delhi, India
>
> Sangam Vihar in South Delhi, India, is one of the largest unauthorized settlements in India and has no government services, including water, electricity and sewage. A community survey revealed that older adults were especially concerned about safety, and that they had very little contact with local law enforcement.
>
> With local political support, a programme to facilitate contact between older adults and community police officers was implemented in six wards in Sangam Vihar; it included around 1800 older adults. With the support of two local police stations, older adults met their local police officers, and were given cards with the phone numbers of all street-patrol police officers. To encourage older adults to use the phone numbers when necessary, they practised by calling their local police officer. The police stations created a register of the participating older adults so that they would be recognized if they called. In addition, the police officers identified older adults living alone, and periodically visited their homes. A small follow-up study conducted 4 months after implementation indicated that more than 50% of older adults still had their contact card. Although this programme shows promise, further research is needed to understand the impact on personal security.
>
> *Source*: B Grewel, L Warth, personal communication, June 2015.

munity involvement with the aim of reducing fear. For example, in Queensland, Australia, the Department of Health and Ageing produced an information kit on crime and safety, and trained community organizations to use the kit to dispel myths and fears about the extent of crimes perpetrated against older people (*87*). Another strategy includes engaging the media to minimize sensationalist reporting of crimes against older people and to promote positive images of older people participating in their communities (*86*).

Strategies to prevent crime and reduce fear may best be implemented at the level of local government and as part of a community safety strategy (*87*). Programmes that draw on the abilities of all stakeholders – such as the government, private sector, nongovernmental organizations, older people's associations and the police – may be most effective (*87*).

Elder abuse

At least 1 in 10 older people living in the community appear likely to experience elder abuse, with women being most vulnerable (Chapter 3) (*88*). This is likely to be an underestimation as only one in 24 cases of elder abuse is reported (*89*). The prevalence in care settings and among people with dementia is likely to be much higher.

The public-health response to elder abuse is limited by the almost complete absence of reliable evidence on the effectiveness of prevention programmes. The strategies below draw on considerable evidence from case studies and from clinical evidence, and require engagement with local media, community agencies and services:

- multidisciplinary teams – professionals from various disciplines pool their expertise and assist in resolving cases of elder abuse;
- helplines – these can provide information to anonymous callers and referrals for actual and potential victims;
- bank use – this can be monitored to detect suspicious patterns and may help to identify older people at risk of financial abuse (Box 6.7);
- support for caregivers of older people at risk of abuse – in the form of training,

---

Box 6.7.   Fighting elder financial abuse in California

The financial abuse of older people (also called senior fraud) spans a broad spectrum of conduct. Unusual transactions are the most obvious indicator, such as a client who usually withdraws US$ 2000 and then suddenly withdraws US$ 30 000. Other more subtle forms of financial abuse may be more difficult to identify. These include phone or Internet scams that target older people, an older person being forced to sign a deed or will, an older person's property or possessions being used without permission, or even someone making a promise of providing lifelong care in exchange for money and then not following through on the promise.

In the United States, the financial abuse of older people is considered to be one of the fastest growing crimes, with older adults losing an estimated US$ 2.9 billion annually, and only 1 in 6 cases being reported (*74*). According to a large study on the financial abuse of older people in the United States, the most common perpetrators are not outsiders, but family members (58%), most often the adult children of the older person (25%). Other common perpetrators include friends and neighbours (17%) and paid home-care workers (15%). Financial abuse was found to disproportionately affect older African American adults and those living below the poverty line. Older adults who struggle to live independently were also found to be at higher risk of being exploited. When older people need assistance with shopping and meal preparation, potential perpetrators may gain access to their finances (*90*). In California, the government, elder-care organizations, and business and private citizens have successfully implemented a series of coordinated measures to counteract the financial abuse of older people.

- A new state law was passed mandating that banks report the suspected financial abuse of older people in the same way that teachers are mandated to report suspicions of child abuse.
- A civil-society organization produced a guide for non-professionals who help manage the finances of older adults to provide standards of practice and tips on how to protect older people's funds from financial exploitation.
- A major older people's organization sponsored a series of events to raise awareness about the financial abuse of older people as a key factor affecting their health and well-being.
- A new national Consumer Financial Protection Bureau was opened with an Office for the Financial Protection of Older Americans, which supports state-level efforts and helps to protect all older Americans.

The California experience has demonstrated that a multisectoral approach involving a variety of actors at different levels is essential to address the complex challenge of the financial abuse of older people.

information and respite care that can help reduce caregivers' stress and enable them to manage their responsibilities better;

- emergency shelter – provided for victims of elder abuse.

Further research is urgently required on the magnitude of abuse and the risk factors as well as what works in prevention and care.

Disasters

The number of disasters is increasing worldwide and places older people at particular risk, both of reductions in capacity and ability (Chapter 3). Disasters undermine older people's capacity and chance of survival as a result of disaster-related injuries, poor basic surgical care, emergency-induced mental health and psychological problems, the breakdown in services for preventing and managing chronic conditions and for providing social support. In addition, older people who experience disasters may be more susceptible to communicable diseases and to a worsening of their existing conditions. For example, adults aged 60–79 years were four times more likely to die (rising to 11 times more likely for those aged older than 80) than younger adults during recent cholera outbreaks in Haiti and Zimbabwe and were twice as likely to experience severe dehydration (*91*).

Disasters can also seriously limit the full range of older people's abilities even in comparison with younger individuals experiencing the same circumstances; this is because older people may lose essential assistive devices, such as spectacles, hearing aids and mobility devices; or they may be left behind or given inadequate support when a community is forced to evacuate or when the capacity of care settings is reduced (*92*). The vulnerability of older people with limitations in capacity becomes even more acute during emergencies when they are separated from their families and their usual sources of informal care and support (*93*).

Although older people vary significantly in their health status as well as their ability to cope during disasters, they are also an important and often untapped resource. In general, the knowledge older people have of their culture and community, their experience with past disasters, as well as their positions of respect within their families and communities, can be drawn upon during emergencies and disasters (*33*). Indeed, in Sri Lanka a study of persons affected by the Indian Ocean tsunami in 2004, found that older people were more frustrated by the lack of work than by their perceived vulnerabilities: "Many older people expressed a strong desire to go back to work, especially because the tsunami had pushed their family deeper into poverty" (*94*). Providing sustained psychosocial support to older people was also important to aid recovery (*95*).

To respond to this diversity among older people, all sectors need to include, assist and support them to harness their potential contributions where possible and to support them when assistance and protection are required. This will require a range of specific activities, such as those outlined in Table 6.1, but will also require a range of changes to systems to ensure that the long-term needs of the community are met.

A priority for action is to ensure that issues related to older people are included in policies for emergency risk management, funding appeals and budgets, legislation and programmes. Where there are policies on ageing, they should also cover emergency risk management (*92*). Older people should be involved in the development of policies, legislation and programmes, and in monitoring implementation. This may require capacity building of older people and their organizations (Box 6.8).

Mechanisms for ensuring intersectoral coordination that include older people in decision-making can facilitate their involvement before, during and after disasters. It may be particularly useful to consider developing coordination mechanisms between health care and long-term

Table 6.1.   Specific actions that can improve older people's access to a range of basic services during disasters (35, 92)

Area	Examples of possible actions
Health services	Enable older people living in the community and in institutions to access primary health-care services, and prevent secondary conditions and comorbidities, as well as benefit from services needed to manage capacity loss, such as rehabilitation, including the provision of assistive devices.
Nutrition and food security	Ensure that older people have access to appropriate food and nutritional support (for example, access to supplementary feeding sites for those who have difficulty standing).
Shelter, facilities and site planning	Include accessibility considerations when planning sites and developing facilities and shelters to ensure the safety and dignity of older people and the ease of use.
Water and sanitation	Specifically consider people with disability to enable safe and appropriate access to water and sanitation for all people (for example, consider providing adapted water containers or ensuring that help is available from the community). This can be important for older people who have difficulty accessing water pumps or toilets, or carrying water supplies for cooking.
Protection	Raise awareness about elder abuse and follow the actions listed in the section on Elder abuse. Ensure that caregivers and older people are reunited.
Emergency preparedness (including early warnings)	Raise awareness and provide guidance on emergency preparedness to older people, their caregivers and the broader community. Preparedness may include, for example, understanding safe evacuation routes or having a buffer stock of drugs for chronic diseases or spare batteries for hearing aids. Include older people in analyses of potential hazards, as well as in response and recovery planning measures.
Recovery and rehabilitation	Facilitate poor older people's access to livelihood programmes and include access considerations when built environments are reconstructed.

care systems. For example, nursing homes may be useful sites for sheltering community-dwelling individuals who require care during and immediately following a disaster (96).

Identifying and recruiting older people, and staff and volunteers, who understand ageing and the local culture, and providing orientation and training for aid workers on *Healthy Ageing* can help strengthen human resources. For example, during the 2006 conflict in Lebanon, older people were regarded as a valuable source of social support for families and communities because of their knowledge and experience that "allow[ed] them to make contributions across areas of care, coping strategies, counselling and rehabilitation" (97). Involving older people in making decisions about their community can also help them to overcome any sense of separation and associated psychological trauma (Box 6.8).

It is important to ensure that information reaches older people before, during and after disasters, and information about older people

Box 6.8.   Older people supporting their own recovery and that of their communities: Mozambique

After flooding in Mozambique in 2000, councils representing older people were organized in each village, and older people were included in the planning and implementation of all community activities aimed at recovery, including the distribution of animals, agricultural seeds and tools, and credit for income-generating activities. Older people also worked with community groups to identify others in their age group who were vulnerable, carry out home visits to identify problems, and provide access to food, blankets and clothing. In this way older people supported their own recovery, the recovery of their peers and of their communities (33).

should inform any responses. When communicating to older people it is important to consider those with low literacy and sensory loss, and ensure that information and communication can reach them about early warnings, risks, impacts, responses (including specific support available for older adults), recovery efforts and their legal rights. Gathering data that are disaggregated by age and capacity level and consulting older people during participatory assessments and during monitoring and evaluation activities can ensure that better responses are made. Providing community education about disaster risk-management through brochures, posters, television and radio can be used to increase the visibility of older people and highlight both their needs and capacities (*33*).

It will also be important to consider the different needs of individuals and subgroups; applying a human rights-based approach to all actions can help to identify, monitor, prevent and respond to threats during and after disasters, such as an increased risk of elder abuse.

Abilities to learn, grow and make decisions

The abilities to learn, grow and make decisions include efforts to continue to learn and apply knowledge, engage in problem solving, continue personal development, and be able to make choices. Continuing to learn enables older people to have the knowledge and skills to manage their health, to keep abreast of developments in information and technology, to participate (for example, by working or volunteering), to adjust to ageing (for example, to retirement, widowhood or becoming a caregiver), to maintain their identity and to keep interested in life (*98*). Continued personal growth – mental, physical, social and emotional – is important for enabling older people to do what they value, and the ability to make decisions is key to older people's sense of control (*99*).

Age is associated with positive and negative changes in capacity (or the perceptions of it), which influence these abilities. Research has shown that with age a number of cognitive pro-

cesses deteriorate, including the speed of processing (the slowing of which can be minimized with use), working memory, executive functions, attention and inhibition. In contrast, automatic, intuitive cognitive processes remain stable or even improve. Likewise, social and emotional growth typically increase with age because of the self-knowledge, skills in self-regulation and stable social relationships that older people have developed over the years (*100*).

Investing in these abilities can have positive impacts on all aspects of life: health, recreation, relationships, and civic and work life. Older people who continue to learn report heightened self-confidence and self-actualization, and learning keeps older people more involved in community activities, reduces their dependency on family and government-funded social services, and enhances their health and well-being (*101*, *102*). It does this by building the knowledge, experience and skills of older people both within and outside the workforce, extending social networks and by promoting shared norms and tolerance of others (*101–103*). There is also good evidence that ensuring that learning remains a lifelong pursuit helps to combat stereotypes and ageism (*102*), can help increase levels of trust between generations and provide a sense of common identity and respect for differences while ensuring that the talents of every individual are put to best use (*104*). Beyond learning, being able to control their lives is also central to older people's well-being (*99*). The abilities to learn, grow and make decisions are strongly associated with older people's autonomy, dignity, integrity, freedom and independence (*105*, *106*).

What works in fostering the abilities to learn, grow and make decisions

Hence, learning and personal growth are important areas for investment by both governments and individuals, alongside learning for paid employment (section on the Ability to contribute). Thus, policy-makers need to consider how resources are distributed across the life course and not only to younger populations, which is currently the case (*104, 107*). For example, in the United Kingdom only 1% of the 2009 education budget was spent on the oldest one third of the population (*104*). The diversity of learning opportunities needs to be adapted to the diversity of adult learners and to recognize their strengths. As such, the ability to learn is equally relevant across the spectrum of older people and just as important, for example, to older people who are illiterate yet wish to maximize their health as it is to older people who can't independently decide what they would like to wear or eat because of the effects of a health condition, or those who finally have time to undertake study for an academic degree.

There are however a number of barriers that need to be addressed to facilitate older people's involvement in lifelong learning. These barriers include (*108*):

- their own attitudes – older people may have negative attitudes about returning to learning because they see themselves as too old, lack confidence or motivation, fear competition with younger adults or in some cases fear that their limited educational background may be exposed;
- physical and material barriers – these may include the costs of educational opportunities, a lack of time, a lack of information about what is available, the location where educational services are available and problems with the availability and accessibility of transportation;
- structural barriers – these may include a lack of opportunities for pursuing their interests, instruction that is delivered in ways that are not acceptable to older people, and problems with inaccessible and unfamiliar locations.

Strategies for addressing these barriers are numerous and outlined below.

Challenge negative attitudes and stereotypes

Stereotypes of older people as forgetful and less able to learn and decide remain prevalent across diverse stakeholders (*100*), whether they be older people themselves, family members, friends, health care and other care providers, teachers or instructors (*106*). However, these are generally social constructs and not consistent with the capacity of older people. For example, a study in the United States on memory performance that compared older adults aged 60–75 years with younger adults aged 17–24 years showed there were no real differences when participants were encouraged to learn compared with when they were encouraged to remember (*109*). In another study, priming older adults with a positive account of memory enabled them to identify effective memory strategies, thus significantly reducing the gap between older and younger participants in a memory task (*110*). Older people also have more to remember, and their experiences can lead to better judgement in making some decisions.

It will be important to challenge stereotypes through communication campaigns that increase knowledge about and understanding of the process of ageing, in the media and among the general public, policy-makers, teachers and service providers (Chapter 7, Box 7.3).

Improve literacy in older adults

Literacy levels, including levels of health literacy, are lower among older age groups than other sections of the population (*24, 102, 111*). Levels of health literacy relate to the capacity to obtain, interpret and understand basic health information and services, and to have the competence to use such information and services to enhance health (*24*). Older people with low levels of health literacy are more likely to report not receiving vaccinations or cancer screening, and health literacy is a more meaningful predictive factor than educational level for older people's use of preventive services (*24*).

Basic literacy and health literacy provide important foundations for learning and decision-making. Literacy can be improved by formal individual programmes, but innovative population-based approaches may also help. For example, in India, where illiteracy is high among older people, particularly among older women living in rural areas, regular television screenings of Bollywood movies with same-language subtitles have been shown to have a positive impact on reading skills in adults as well as children (*112*).

Health programmes focusing on health literacy have been shown to improve eating habits and increase physical activity (*24*), encourage better management of chronic and degenerative diseases (*111*), and enhance a person's ability to cope when negative health events occur. Health literacy can be improved by working with older adults to enhance their self- management skills, improve their links to clinical care, and by providing ongoing social support (Chapter 4 and Chapter 5).

If the health information given to patients reflects real-life situations and is tailored to sociocultural contexts, it is more likely to have an impact on people with lower socioeconomic status (*113*). Educational leaflets written in simple language aimed at those with low levels of literacy can help older adults better discuss their problems with health practitioners, and they have been shown to increase the uptake of preventive health interventions, such as pneumococcal vaccination (*114*).

However, outreach to older people is often needed. This may be achieved by identifying and nurturing the networks that support older people or by specifically targeting older people (*113, 115*). In Ireland, for example, the Adult Education Guidance Initiative specifically targets older people who are already taking part in literacy programmes and provides them with additional guidance on personal development, stress management and interview techniques (*102*).

Invest in accessible opportunities for lifelong learning and growth

Lifelong learning comprises learning across all phases of life and includes the spectrum of formal, non-formal and informal learning (*107*). Hence, it is a process that can occur at any time or place and addresses both an individual's needs and those of the community.

Learning opportunities, which historically have focused on the first two decades of life, need to be made more inclusive to enable older people to develop new skills and knowledge and to maintain a sense of self, identity and meaning. Expanding learning opportunities will require that public policies fully engage with the implications of population ageing, and acknowledge that for some people ageing can mean an extension of their working life and for others a phase in which they spend up to one third of their lives in retirement.

To address the material and structural barriers to learning, media and approaches will also need to be adapted to older learners, and making reasonable accommodation can ensure that older people with disability can effectively participate in learning opportunities (*57*). A variety of media can be used to design courses and foster learning, including providing open universities (that is, universities with no entry requirements) for older people, developing older people's groups and having them act as partners in health promotion activities, and using massive open online courses (known as MOOCs), which have the potential to reach people across countries and socioeconomic divides.

Working within groups and with peers, and being able to share experiences, are important parts of learning for adults. Self-management skills can be improved by using peer-to-peer support and longer-term group involvement (lasting 3 years or longer); for example, these have been shown to help people who have lost their sight, and also to reduce falls (*116*). In Britain, peer mentors for ageing south Asians have used their language skills and community knowledge, to encourage their peers to take up and sustain physical activity programmes (P Ong, unpublished paper on Older people as a resource for their own health, 2015).

Older adults tend to be committed learners who are less focused on assessments (117). However, taking on a new learning challenge requires an older person to be motivated, to have information about opportunities, and to have a supportive environment. Making the physical locations for learning attractive and accessible will facilitate broader participation. To address declines in capacity, for example in hearing and vision, information should be available in alternative formats (such as, large print, or electronic books) that adhere to clear print guidelines; additionally, using microphones in classes, ensuring that only one person speaks at a time, and using accessible websites can all facilitate learning. Training approaches and materials should be developed to enable participants irrespective of their capacity to learn. A range of bottom-up and top-down legislative and policy mechanisms that are already used in many countries may also apply to learning for older adults, such as consumer protection policies, and nondiscrimination legislation that applies to public buildings, educational settings or ICT (80).

Lastly, the perspective of time associated with a person's age may also affect goals for learning and personal development. Perhaps because of this perspective, learning may be more desirable if it is relevant to an older person's life and can be used in the present rather than accessed in the future. Older adults particularly value experiential learning if it enables them to build on the past experiences that they value.

Facilitate choice and control

The process of *Healthy Ageing* demands that older people take or share in making decisions that affect their lives, including how to spend their time, what treatments they have, what they learn and where they live (99). However, choices about health care and where and how to live can be complex, and this complexity can influence the desire of older people to maintain responsibility for decision-making. Ensuring that information is easy to understand and relevant will be critical to overcoming concerns about decision-making and enabling older people to make the right choices for themselves (Box 6.9). It is also essential that caregivers or family members do not provide or withhold information to control older people rather than enabling them to make decisions (119).

Significant losses in capacity, particularly mental capacity, can present operational and ethical challenges to the right to self-determination for older people. When individuals do not have the capacity to exercise choice independently, then support for decision-making may be required (57, 120). The use of supported decision-making strategies emphasizes that an individual does not lose legal capacity but may need support to take decisions (57). Supported decision-making is not substituted decision-making. The person or persons providing support must attempt to take decisions that are deeply in the character of the older person and that take account of their past and present values and preferences. It is important to build mechanisms within families and communities to support decision-making and to establish safeguards regarding duties of care, the process of designating support persons and mechanisms to adjudicate disputes (80).

Less severe declines in capacity can also make it more difficult for an older person to make their own decisions, shape their environments and create opportunities. Although family and friends, appropriate housing and safe communities can make a difference, there are a number of policy strategies that can be considered, including developing older people's organizations, using innovative financing mechanisms, such as personal budgets, or providing support to plan ahead in the case of illness or disability.

Older people's organizations have been established in many countries and can facilitate older people's participation in community deci-

Box 6.9. Health promotion for older people: not business as usual

Ageing often requires the need to make significant lifestyle changes, such as taking new medications, following a different diet or changing an exercise regimen. Older people may also have unique motives for making these lifestyle changes. For example, they may not wish to be a burden to their family and this may provide an additional incentive for maintaining their physical capacity. They may also want to live to see their grandchildren grow up so that they can influence the next generation. Unlike younger adults – who may not see the impact of their negative behaviours until the future– older adults may see immediate and potentially life-threatening effects (*100*).

Ensuring that health messages reach older people in ways that they can accept is essential for changing attitudes and behaviours. The implications for health-promotion messages are as follows (*118*).

- Use communication processes that rely on heuristics and intuition. These processes may be more effective than those that rely on large amounts of information processing and thinking.
- Make messages more relevant to older people. Targeting messages (for example, about the importance of physical activity in later years) can make the message appear more relevant and appealing.
- Trial positive messaging for older adults. Many older adults are motivated to avoid processing negative information. Emphasizing gains to promote preventive behaviours, (such as eating a healthy diet) and the use of testing (such as screening for cancer), may be more effective in older adults.
- Tailor messages to specific older people. Matching information to an individual's characteristics can influence how older people think and feel about a health issue; this can be more effective especially if the message addresses how by modifying behaviour an older person may become more emotionally satisfied.
- Manage emotional distress. Emotional distress can be both a catalyst for and a saboteur of change; hence, it needs to be managed successfully to encourage behavioural change and maintenance of that change.
- Consider an older person's social support. As people age, their social networks decrease in size and the networks may be more effective at promoting stability than change. Social support can facilitate or endanger behavioural change – for example by providing emotional support and helping to manage emotional distress – or by discouraging change – for example if one person in a couple wants to stop smoking and the other does not.

Further research that examines the role of different factors in the older person and the environment, to motivate older adults to make and sustain positive behavioural changes, offers much promise.

sion-making (*121, 122*), help older people access resources, and ensure that they are actively engaged in public policy debates and the development of their communities (*123*) (Box 6.10). For example, the advocacy of older people's associations in Serbia resulted in the development of age-friendly systems of health care and social care, while older citizen's monitoring programmes in Bangladesh and Ghana increased older people's awareness about the policy environment and placed older adults at the forefront of decision-making and monitoring in their community (*121, 126, 127*).

Personal health budgets (that is, cash payments given to individuals, usually by the government, to pay for services) can also give older people greater choice and control over the way in which their needs are met (*128*). The United Kingdom's national personal budget survey in 2013 found that personal budgets may benefit older people in many ways, including improving their physical health, feeling independent, adequately supported, respected and safe both inside and outside their home. They can also enable choice and the maintenance of relationships (*128*).

Older people can also be enabled to influence decisions about their lives that may arise when they have lost the capacity necessary to make informed choices. Advance care planning, including advance directives and living wills, allows older adults to discuss and document their wishes for decisions about future treatment and end-of-life care should they lose their capacity to make those decisions (*129, 130*).

Box 6.10. Intergenerational clubs: improving the lives of older people in Viet Nam

Viet Nam's National Action Plan on Ageing (2012–2020) aims to improve the care and support provided to older people. Intergenerational self-help clubs are a promising intervention. The model for these clubs was refined through a series of pilot programmes led by HelpAge International between 2005 and 2012. The clubs help develop and build the capacity of local civil society organizations to:

- engage in community development processes;
- represent community members' interests in dialogue with local and national governments;
- address the community's needs, ranging from health care to access information and services to improving older people's abilities to build and maintain relationships and to actively participate in community life.

Yen Thang village in Thanh Hoa province, Viet Nam, established an intergenerational club in March 2014 to encourage disadvantaged community groups to take a leading role in local development. The club has had a positive impact on older people, who have been encouraged to take regular physical exercise, conduct self-care activities and have health check-ups. Club members reported that over a period of 9 months they had increased their knowledge about noncommunicable diseases and self-care; they had improved their awareness of and access to information about their rights and entitlements; and that they took regular physical exercise and had regular health check-ups (*124*). A total of 45 of 49 members of the club obtained health insurance as a result of their membership. Furthermore, club members reported having greater confidence in participating in or leading activities to help themselves or their communities (*124*).

This club is one of nearly 700 that exist across 13 provinces in Viet Nam. National targets that are part of the plan require that, by 2015, 15% of the country's communes establish these clubs or similar community-based models that provide both care and support to older people, with the proportion to increase to 50% by 2020 (*125*).

Evidence suggests that advance care planning can facilitate the delivery of long-term care that is aligned with a patient's wishes and improve a patient's satisfaction with care. Factors that contribute to success in advance care planning include an older person having health literacy, preparing plans before any cognitive decline has developed, allowing an older person sufficient time with their health care providers to ensure that the provider understands the person's wishes, having good documentation, and reviewing plans regularly with health providers to update the plans as required (*131*). For example, in a randomized controlled trial in Australia that compared advance care planning with usual care, 86% of older people had their end-of-life wishes respected compared with only 30% in the control group (*132*). In the United States, another randomized controlled trial that included 139 patients newly admitted to a nursing home found that only two patients in the group that had developed an advance care plan received treatment that was not in accordance with their wishes compared with 17 patients in the control group (*133*). Even though these are small studies, the results are encouraging.

Ability to be mobile

The ability to be mobile is important for *Healthy Ageing*. It refers to movement in all its forms, whether powered by the body (with or without an assistive device) or a vehicle. Mobility includes getting up from a chair or moving from a bed to a chair, walking for leisure, exercising, completing daily tasks, driving a car and using public transport (*134*). Mobility is necessary for doing things around the house; accessing shops, services and facilities in the community (such as parks); and participating in social and cultural activities.

The changes in physical and mental capacities that are common in older age can limit mobility. However, capacity can be built, and the power of environments to extend what a person can do is perhaps most easily illustrated by the ability to be mobile. For example, using a walker or wheelchair can enable older people to move around in and outside their home; providing public transportation that is accessible both physically and financially can enable older people to get where they need to go; and ensuring that buildings have ramps, handrails, elevators and appropriate signage can make it easier for older people to use them regardless of capacity loss. If these adaptations or supports are not available, then declines in mobility can result in further decrements in health, such as increasing the risk of falls (64) and depression (135); these decrements can have negative consequences for older people's autonomy, social engagement, civic participation and well-being, thus affecting all other domains of functional ability (136–140).

The losses associated with declines in mobility extend beyond the individual. When older people are not able to move around, their social networks are also affected and the community may lose valuable contributions, as well as need additional resources to support older people in their daily lives (141). Facilitating the ability of older people to be able to get around when and how they choose, and at an affordable cost, are important provisions of the United Nations *Convention on the rights of persons with disabilities and optional protocol* (57). Public health has a crucial part to play in maximizing the mobility of older people.

What works to maintain mobility in older age

Mobility is influenced not only by an older person's intrinsic capacity and the environments they inhabit but also by the choices they make. Decisions about mobility are, in turn, shaped by the built environment, the attitudes of the older person and of others, and having both a motivation and the means to be mobile (such as by using assistive devices or transportation) (142, 143). If older people perceive there are barriers

to being mobile – for example, a lack of respect from drivers or conductors on public transportation – and believe that the risk of injury is heightened by physical activity, then they may restrict their movements. Overprotective caregivers who do not allow older people to move around very much, either for fear that they might fall or because they want to spare the older person the effort, can also reduce older people's movements (137, 144).

Strengthen what older people can do: their capacity to move

Physical and cognitive capacities are both important for getting around, whether by walking or by driving or by using other means of transportation, and there is good evidence about what works to help maintain capacity.

Physical activity is crucial. The loss of muscle mass, decreased flexibility, and problems with balance and coordination can all make getting around more difficult. WHO provides recommendations on engaging in physical activity to maintain health that consider different starting points and levels of capacity (145). Box 6.11 summarizes the evidence about what works to help maintain physical capacity, taking into consideration interventions made at the level of the individual and the environment.

Rehabilitation may be helpful in restoring and maintaining capacity in older adults who have declines in mobility associated with conditions such as a stroke, a cardiac event or injury (157). Such services may include medical rehabilitation and therapy, such as training, exercises, education and counselling. When introducing rehabilitation services in contexts where they have not been available, the focus should be on prioritizing cost-effective approaches and delivering them in locations that are as close as possible to where people live (80).

A key determinant of declines in mobility in automobile-dependent societies is ceasing to drive in older age. Physical and cognitive capacities – both perceived and actual – impact on

Box 6.11. **Maintaining mobility through physical activity**

Older people's participation in physical activity is increasingly linked to the environment in which they live (146–148). Individual, social, and physical-environmental factors have been found to be equally important influences on the amount that older people walk (149). Environmental characteristics associated with increasing the physical activity of older people include providing safe spaces for walking (such as footpaths and parks); ensuring easy access to local facilities, goods and services; seeing other older people exercising in the same neighbourhood; and regularly participating in exercise with friends and family (149–152).

Older people can maintain mobility by making simple changes in their lives (24, 153).

They should try to stay as active as possible. Engaging in moderate-intensity exercise effectively increases strength, aerobic capacity, flexibility and balance for walking and standing among older adults. Even short walks can help maintain physical and cognitive functions. Aerobic exercise and exercises used to strengthen muscles and to improve balance are all important; however, resistance training is particularly important if capacity is declining.

- Older adults should meet the recommended physical activity guidelines for their age and any health conditions. (For additional information, see http://www.who.int/dietphysicalactivity/factsheet_recommendations/en/.)
- Older people should engage in physical-activity programmes that target visual attention, limb flexibility, coordination, the speed of movement and executive functions because these can also improve driving performance and driving safety (154, 155).
- In the event of losing the use of their lower extremities, older adults should be trained to use adaptive equipment, such as hand controls.

Policy-makers can create environments that promote physical activity (153, 156) by:

- addressing barriers to activity and promoting changes that facilitate safe walking for recreation, transport and physical exercise;
- creating community events to promote physical activity and raise awareness of the benefits;
- providing exercise programmes to address cardiorespiratory fitness, muscle strength and balance, and resistance training programmes, particularly for the oldest old people and people recovering from acute health events. When these programmes combine prescribed exercise and adherence interventions they may be more effective;
- promoting counselling interventions in clinical settings;
- promoting positive attitudes towards physically active ageing and older people's participation in physical activity.

decisions about mobility (142). Including mobility as part of disease-prevention and health-promotion activities is important for ensuring coordinated action (150).

Building cognitive capacity shows particular promise for extending safe mobility among older adults who drive (158, 159). Other options for prolonging the ability to drive include physical interventions, such as increasing physical activity (154); providing driver education training; and occupational therapy interventions, such as improving transfers into the driver's seat or improving the position of seating. Knowledge about safe driving and driving performance can be improved by raising awareness about

common problems encountered by older drivers, especially when this is accompanied by on-road driver education (160). Training to maintain or enhance the cognitive speed of processing has also been shown to enhance the performance of everyday abilities, including driving (159). Counselling may also be helpful in developing a gradual transition plan for safer driving, such as driving only during daylight hours or at times when there is less traffic and only on well-known routes (160).

In identifying when older people may no longer have the ability to drive safely, it is important to judge each situation on its merits, and consider a range of options. Restrictions or screening based on chronological age should be adopted only with caution, given the wide range of capacity experienced by older people and the importance of mobility to them. It is worth noting that the rate of involvement in motor vehicle accidents in the United States shows little increase before the age of 75 years at which time these adults are still less likely than younger adults to be involved in a traffic crash, and most of the increased deaths observed in older people from car crashes arise from their increased physical vulnerability (161).

Provide assistive technologies to aid mobility

The availability of appropriate mobility devices has a significant influence on older people's mobility (162, 163); devices include walking canes, walkers, white canes for those who have lost vision, and wheelchairs. When assistive devices are available, affordable and appropriate to older people's needs and their environments, their mobility, independence and participation can be greatly enhanced. Guidance on how to increase and improve the provision of assistive devices is outlined in WHO's position paper on mobility devices (164) and the *World report on disability* (165).

Reduce barriers in the built environment

Physical activity and patterns of mobility among older people are influenced by land-use patterns, aesthetics, the accessibility and connectivity of urban design, as well as the perceived level of safety (163). The effect of these factors differs across communities and studies, and the effects of specific variables, such as housing and population density, are not clear or consistent (156). However, adhering to the principles of universal design can help (Box 6.12). Other potential ways to facilitate mobility include ensuring that:

- neighbourhoods are free from signs of decay, such as litter and graffiti;
- environments are pedestrian-friendly by using features such as high-visibility

crossings, raised medians or pedestrian refuge islands; by reducing speed limits and installing traffic-calming measures; by keeping footpaths and kerbs well maintained (including using kerb cuts); by ensuring that overpasses and underpasses are accessible; by ensuring that signals at street crossings allow adequate time for crossing; and by providing auditory aids at crossings (Box 6.1 and Box 6.13) (170–172);

- aesthetically-pleasing features are included in streets and parks, such as trees, gardens or vegetation;
- neighbourhoods are designed to allow easy access from homes to a large number of destinations, such as shops, health services, community centres, and religious organizations;
- there are a large number of intersections, thus enabling more options for crossing roads, and adequate facilities for older people, such as places to rest and public toilets.

Improve the availability and accessibility of transportation

Improvements to transportation may include developing national and local transport policies that promote access to public transportation, affordable private transport or transport provided by family, friends and neighbours (Box 6.1). Operational differences are likely to exist between rural and urban settings, but generally improvements can be made in terms of:

- improving the physical accessibility of vehicles, stations, stops and their staging areas;
- increasing the relevance and convenience of public transport by making changes to routes or timetables, or both;
- improving financial accessibility by offering free or reduced-price fares;
- ensuring that information about the system is accessible (for example, schedules) (80);
- providing priority seating for people with reduced capacity;

Box 6.12. Universal design: making it work in Ireland, Norway and Singapore

Universal design is a process that increases usability, safety, health and social participation through the design and operation of environments, products and systems to be usable by all people, to the greatest extent possible, without the need for adaptation or specialized design (*57, 166, 167*).

Making universal design work requires a high level of political commitment, resources and capacity development, as illustrated by the following examples from Norway, Singapore and Ireland.

Norway is working towards the ambitious goal of achieving universal design by 2025 (*168*). High-level commitment, and shared responsibilities for planning, implementation and monitoring across different sectors and levels of government are key strategies being used to ensure success. Three government bodies share the responsibility for delivering on this goal: the Ministry of Children, Equality and Inclusion (specifically the National Resource Centre for Participation and Accessibility); the Ministry of Climate and Environment; and the Ministry of Local Government and Modernisation. During the past two decades, increasingly inclusive legislation has been passed, culminating in 2008 when Norway made inaccessibility a form of discrimination by introducing the Anti-Discrimination and Accessibility Act. In 2010 the act was extended to include the concept of universal design, and an action plan was developed that targeted the built environment, public transportation, the accessibility of information and technology, and the refurbishing of municipal housing.

Funding is needed to transform policy into practice, in particular where the retrofitting of existing structures is required to ensure access. The Singapore government's Accessibility Fund (financed with 40 million Singapore dollars) supports public departments and private businesses by lowering the financial burden of modifying existing structures to make them accessible to older adults and people with disability (*169*). For example, the fund covers the costs of constructing or refurbishing elevators in older buildings or providing bathroom facilities that are accessible to people using wheelchairs. Businesses in buildings built before 1990 complete a simple application form to become eligible for support from the fund. The fund is also being used by the government to ensure accessibility across all public spaces and essential facilities by 2016.

Sensitization and training of product designers, service providers and urban planners is important for enhancing the accessibility of products, services and the built environment. Ireland's Centre for Excellence in Universal Design supports professional development by integrating universal design principles into curricula to sensitize a range of professionals to universal design, including architects, urban planners and designers (*2*). Efforts to raise awareness also include an annual competition for college students to find the best innovation or invention using the principles of universal design, and funding and publicizing relevant research.

Around the world, other institutions have also taken on the task of expanding the use and awareness of universal design principles, including an ongoing 5-year collaboration between the Center for Universal Design at North Carolina State University in the United States and the Beijing Institute of Technology to translate materials about universal design, share curricula and facilitate exchanges among faculty and students.

- educating transport operators to consider that some passengers may require help or more time to get on or off public transport.

Furthermore, improving older people's mobility requires considering accessibility throughout the entire travel chain. Subsidized on-call transportation services or taxi vouchers may fill some gaps in the coverage of public transportation or meet the needs of those who have a more significant loss of capacity (*3*).

Create opportunities for older people to participate

Being employed and taking part in civic activities, as well as in leisure and entertainment activities, can motivate older people to stay mobile and socially connected. Being involved in activities outside the home encourages older people to walk

Box 6.13. Making sure older people get where they want to go: Sri Lanka

The level of accessibility of public buildings is important in ensuring that older people can gain access to services and for social participation. The Wellawaya Age- and Disabled-Friendly City project in Sri Lanka is helping to ensure accessibility by providing ramps, tactile paving and accessible toilet facilities to improve access not only to community centres for older people, which are popular meeting places for peers to socialize, but also to places of worship, such as the mosque of Wellawaya and two Buddhist temples, and to public services, such as the police station, the bus station and community medical centres.

more and exercise, and can contribute to improved intrinsic capacity (Box 6.1 and Box 6.14). Participation can be facilitated by ensuring that a variety of events are available, affordable and physically accessible as well as catering to the diverse interests of older people (3).

Abilities to build and maintain relationships

Maintaining relationships is often identified by older people as central to their well-being, and as people age, they may give increasing priority to this ability (178). A broad range of relationships are important to older people, including their relationships with children and other family members, intimate relationships, and informal social relationships with friends, neighbours, colleagues and acquaintances, as well as more formal relationships with community-service providers.

This ability is also strongly interconnected with, and can have an impact on, all other abilities (179–185). For example, the quantity and quality of interpersonal relationships, and the levels of trust within, and feeling of belonging to, a network of people with shared interests can influence the enjoyment of other abilities, such as being mobile and contributing to the community (186).

Box 6.15 summarizes some of the mechanisms and pathways by which social networks may affect older people's health and well-being (187).

Social relations are an important component of *Healthy Ageing* because when they are positive they can yield resources, such as trust and social support. Relationships with family are differentially important to those with friends and neighbours. Family relationships are typified by both solidarity and ambivalence (188). Older people benefit directly from positive interactions with social networks and indirectly by residing in a community with a high degree of social cohesion and participation (186, 189, 190). Strong social networks can enhance older people's longevity and quality of life, protect against functional decline and promote resilience (179–185). Notwithstanding the benefits of relationships, older people may find some of them burdensome. For example, providing long-term care for a spouse may affect the mental health of caregivers and their ability to take advantage of other opportunities, such as learning (191). Raising their grandchildren can place additional financial, emotional and physical strains on grandparents (192).

The abilities to build and maintain relationships and social networks are closely related to a range of competencies, including the abilities to form new relationships and to behave in ways that are socially appropriate. It is also closely related to levels of intrinsic capacity. When faced with declining capacity, older people may find it harder to maintain social networks, which consequently often shrink (179–185).

Loneliness – that is dissatisfaction with the quantity and quality of social relations and social isolation (193) – that is lack of social contact are likely to indicate the absence of strong social networks. These are associated with decreases in health status and quality of life, although loneliness and social isolation are distinct characteristics and may have independent impacts on health (194). Estimates of the prevalence of social isolation among com-

Box 6.14. Older people helping children read and learn: the United States of America

Experience Corps is a volunteer programme in the United States that places older volunteers in public elementary schools, giving them meaningful roles that are designed to help schools meet the needs of their students as well as increasing the social, physical, and cognitive activities of the volunteers. The programme is designed to have an impact in areas such as improving:

- children's interest in reading and discovering books;
- children's literacy;
- children's ability to solve problems;
- children's ability to play nonviolently;
- school attendance.

Teams of 7–10 volunteers are assigned to each school, thus ensuring that sufficient volunteers are available to have an effect across all grades within the school. Volunteers commit to spending at least 15 hours each week at the school for the duration of the school year; they receive training and a stipend to reimburse the costs of travel and meals. Volunteers receive 30 hours of skills training that encourages mental flexibility, coordination, visual–spatial learning and problem-solving. The volunteers meet regularly to plan, solve problems and socialize. Physical activity is stimulated by virtue of participating in the programme, and includes commuting to the school and moving around the school, for example, by going up and down the stairs.

This programme has demonstrated positive effects on the health of older people. A number of randomized trials have evaluated the impact of participating in Experience Corps. Benefits for participants compared with controls have shown:

- an increase in physical strength and capacity (*173, 174*);
- increased cognitive activity;
- maintenance of walking speed;
- improvements in social networks – that is, volunteers had people that they could turn to for help (*174*);
- fewer depressive symptoms (*173*).

Volunteers are attracted to Experience Corps by the chance to make a meaningful contribution to society and assist children in achieving academic success. Satisfaction levels among volunteers are as high as 98%, and 80% of those surveyed returned during the following school year (*175*). Traditional health-promotion programmes that focus explicitly on physical activity tend to have significantly lower retention rates.

Initiated in 1996 in five cities in the United States, the programme has expanded to 17 cities and inspired similar initiatives internationally. For example, in Japan a programme called REPRINTS places teams of 6–8 older volunteers in kindergartens and elementary schools to read to young children. A follow-up assessment found that those who volunteered most intensively had a significantly higher frequency of contact with their own grandchildren and other children in their neighbourhoods, as well as better self-rated health compared with those who did not volunteer or only did so minimally (*176*).

Volunteering opportunities, if well-designed, can be a win-win for older people and their communities. Programmes like Experience Corps and Reprints, need not be costly to put in place, and they have the potential to yield positive returns in terms of health gains and social benefits for the older and younger generations alike (*145, 177*).

munity-dwelling older people range from 7 to 17%, depending on the definitions and outcome measures used; approximately 40% of older people report feeling lonely (*195*). The causal links are difficult to determine but loneliness, social isolation, behavioural risk factors, and poor health weave an interdependent web that can have a significant impact on an older person's risk of functional limitations, disability and death (*186, 190, 196*).

Older people's access to resources through social networks

Older people can obtain different types of support through their social networks. There are four primary types of support (*179*):

- instrumental support to help with the activities of everyday life, such as shopping, getting to appointments, household chores and paying bills;
- appraisal support, for help with decision-making, getting appropriate feedback or problem solving;
- informational support, which includes advice or information about particular needs;
- emotional support, which includes love and friendship, understanding, caring and recognition.

Networks can also exert social influence. The values, norms and attitudes prevalent in a person's network may influence individuals in ways that either promote or damage health; for example, excessive alcohol consumption may be accepted or encouraged within a social group or friends may discourage older people from leaving the house for fear of falling.

By offering opportunities for social engagement, social networks define and reinforce meaningful roles within the family, community and beyond, which in turn provide a sense of value, belonging and attachment.

Networks further facilitate access to income and material goods. This access may include cash loans to pay for medical treatment, help in paying for long-term care or by providing access to accommodation, food or income.

Social networks are embedded within larger social and cultural contexts that determine their structure and function. In communities with limited social protection and access to health care, social networks may have a comparatively stronger role in providing access to essential resources and services.

What works to build and maintain relationships

Identify and tackle loneliness and social isolation

Evidence supports the use of interventions to address loneliness and social isolation, although these cannot focus on simply one aspect of the complex web connecting these distinct characteristics without considering the contributing role and impact on other characteristics. Given the prevalence of loneliness and social isolation, it may be important to identify people at risk, such as those who have recently retired or become bereaved. Identifying individuals, through health-care or social-care services, is more straightforward than answering the question of how to assist older people who are lonely and or socially isolated. Research in this area is limited but some principles of effective interventions have emerged from the research (*195, 197–199*).

- Group interventions (for example, providing social support, community-based exercise programmes or skills development) tend to be more effective than individual interventions, perhaps because they provide opportunities for social engagement and developing new social ties (Box 6.1).
- Both in-person and technology-assisted interventions (for example, using the phone or Internet) can be effective (Box 6.16).

The Telephone Rings at 5: Portugal

The Telephone Rings at 5 offers a reliable source of companionship and mental stimulation to older adults in Setúbal, Portugal, who have difficulty leaving their homes. The programme, which is free and requires only that participants have a telephone, connects four older adults each day with a volunteer moderator from the community. Topics discussed vary depending on the day and the expertise of the volunteer, and include current events, culture, health and sport. In addition, the programme offers what are known as guided tours, in which pictures of a local area of interest are mailed to participants in advance and the moderator leads the group through a virtual visit and discussion (*200*). This programme ran as a successful pilot from 2011 to 2013, and others like it continue to provide service through Senior Centers Without Walls in communities such as Manitoba, Canada (*201*), and Oakland, California (*202*).

- It is important to identify and nurture the types of networks that support older people, for example in managing their own care (*113, 115*).
- Participatory interventions are more effective than nonparticipatory interventions, and interventions with a theoretical foundation tend to be more effective than those without.

- Access to appropriate assistive devices helps (*164, 203*).
- Facilitating access to and confidence and competence in using ICT has also been shown to be effective (*204*).

Box 6.17. Reviving the principles of give and take between the generations: Germany

Multigenerational centres in Germany are reviving the principles of give and take between the generations that were common in extended families in the past. They provide young and old with a public space in the neighbourhood in which all generations can meet, build and maintain relationships, and benefit from their different competencies, experiences and interests.

Since 2006, more than 450 multigenerational centres have been established and subsidized by the German government, creating an infrastructure for social cohesion in cities and communities across the country. The services and activities offered include informal care for older adults who are care-dependent, education, help with accessing domestic services and opportunities for volunteering.

At the heart of each multigenerational centre is the "Offener Treff", a public living room, in which generations can connect in a relaxed atmosphere. For many it provides a first informal contact with the services on offer as well as volunteering opportunities. Intergenerational activities that facilitate connections and mutual support are emphasized. These are particularly valuable for children and youth who have limited opportunities for meeting and sharing with older generations, for example when grandparents live far away. In multigenerational centres older people may teach adolescents traditional crafting techniques or recipes, and the younger people might, in turn, tutor older people in the use of computers or smartphones.

About 15 000 volunteers participate in the programme and are central to the success of the centres. Volunteers help with 60% of the activities that are offered, and 20% are run exclusively by volunteers. These activities include, for example, preparing meals, reading stories to children and mentoring youth in their occupational choices. For many, the centres are the first point of contact with volunteering opportunities and they often open doors to reconnection with the labour market. This dynamic is actively supported by the training, counselling and networking opportunities available to volunteers.

The multigenerational centres further act as points for the coordination of information and services in the community. Each is oriented towards the needs of the local community. For example, a counselling service for people living with dementia was established in the Groß-Zimmern multigenerational centre to inform families providing care at home about support services. Others centres provide childcare or care services for older people, for example offering flexible services that complement general day-care services and make it easier for parents to continue to work and to care for their relatives. The centres foster connections and cooperation with local businesses, service providers, cultural and educational institutions, and the media. In the centre in the city of Bielefeld, young retirees offer a volunteer service to their older peers, undertaking small repairs, such as changing light bulbs, which complement services offered by local business.

Multigenerational centres provide support across all stages of the life course, and for older people in particular they provide supportive services and information that can facilitate active participation in community life and provide opportunities for engaging meaningfully in the community, but they also support activities of daily living that can enable older people to stay longer in their homes and communities. By fostering relationships between the generations, these centres also contribute to overcoming negative stereotypes and ageist attitudes in the community (*206*).

Create opportunities for meaningful social roles and reciprocal relationships

Reciprocal relationships are important for an older person's sense of self-worth and as a motivator for continued social engagement (*205*). Box 6.14 and Box 6.17 describe successful programmes that encourage reciprocal relationships. Time banks, through which people trade their time and services for other services, have also been shown to foster reciprocal relationships and build social capital in communities (*207*). Creating opportunities for social interaction by introducing dedicated facilities, special events, classes and gathering places can also enhance social connections (Box 6.1 and Box 6.17).

Consider the impact of public buildings, transport, housing and medical facilities on social networks

Older people's need for social support tends to increase with declines in capacities (cognitive, mental, social and physical) and when environments, such as social venues and transport, are not accessible. Barriers need to be identified and

Box 6.18. A city for seniors: Switzerland

Cité Seniors in Geneva, Switzerland, is an information and meeting centre for older adults, offering a space to socialize, learn and access information about a wide variety of topics. *Cité Seniors* provides events year-round, including seminars, debates, cultural outings and a variety of training courses. More than 25 courses and hands-on workshops are available about topics such as computer skills, creative arts and overall well-being. A new programme is available each semester, and an on-site registration day provides the opportunity to learn about activities and to sign-up for events. *Cité Seniors* also provides meeting space for Geneva's platform of older people's associations – *la Plateforme des associations d'aînés de Genève* – which has a membership of more than 35 000 people. The facility is used by around 25 000 people each year and welcomes all generations. *Cité Seniors* forms part of a wider infrastructure of neighbourhood-based senior meeting centres (*212*).

eliminated, and policies used to create supportive environments. Transport policies that include accessible public transport and the development of nonmotorized transport (for example, cyclopousse in Lyons, France) (*208*), the use of universal design principles in the built environment and the development of walkable neighbourhoods, and the availability of assistive devices (see the section on the Ability to be mobile) can all contribute to fostering social networks (*156, 199, 209–211*). Neighbourhoods that facilitate social interaction and mutual support can be achieved both through implementing appropriate urban design and developing social services, such as senior centres (Box 6.18).

Improve access to information and communications technologies

Communicating by telephone or Internet is important for maintaining relationships (*213–215*). A range of interventions has been shown to strengthen older people's access to these resources, including the use of appropriate assistive devices to compensate for sensory impairments that might have a negative impact on communication and relationships, increasing the coverage and affordability of ICT services and improving the availability of accessible information, especially by advertising events and facilities that provide opportunities for social interaction.

Ability to contribute

This ability covers a myriad of contributions that older people make to their families and communities, such as assisting friends and neighbours, mentoring peers and younger people, and caring for family members and the wider community. The ability to contribute is closely associated with engagement in social and cultural activities, which are discussed in terms of other abilities in the sections about the Abilities to build and maintain relationships and the Abilities to learn, grow and make decisions.

Volunteering and working are two important ways that adults use to find fulfilment in older age and are used in this section to illustrate the ability to contribute. The term "work" is used in its broadest sense, and includes unpaid work in the home or in a family enterprise, paid work for another person or organization in the formal or informal economy, and self-employment (165). Volunteering is unremunerated work that older people choose to do for people outside their household and for the wider community (216).

Although the evidence is limited, research from high-income countries suggests that working and volunteering in later life can have positive health outcomes (217). For example, age-related changes in physical, mental and cognitive capacities can be reduced by the physical and intellectual activities associated with work (127). A longitudinal study in Japan of older men who worked, found that engaging in paid work for less than 35 hours per week contributed to older people maintaining their physical and mental health (218). Older people in high- and middle-income countries may value work more once they have retired, and many older people desire to return to work after retirement, particularly if the work is not physically demanding and they can reduce the number of hours that they work (219, 220).

Thus, facilitating different types of work for older people may have significant benefits if capacity allows and if the conditions are met for decent work (221). However, these are big ifs. As described in Chapter 1, there is also evidence that, for example, most older people in the United Kingdom experience some form of disability well before the current retirement age, and the risk of disability before retirement age is far greater for people living in disadvantaged areas. Moreover, not only are disadvantaged older people more likely to experience a lower level of intrinsic capacity, they are less likely to have the skills or levels of education that provide the flexibility and opportunity for work that is health-promoting. Work environments in low- and middle-income countries are likely to be too hazardous and exhausting to have positive effects.

Health and volunteering have a reciprocal relationship. Older adults who are in better health are more likely to volunteer, and people are healthier and happier because they volunteer (222, 223). Researchers have argued that the altruistic nature of volunteering contributes to its beneficial health effects (224, 225). Because volunteering is socially valued, publicly recognized and provides more choice than working or caregiving, it may have even stronger positive impacts than other forms of social contribution (226, 227). Studies among older adults have demonstrated that volunteering enhances self-rated physical health (228–230), reduces hypertension (231), increases physical strength and gait speed (232, 233), and reduces depressive symptoms (234–236). The positive effects of volunteering on physical and mental health have also been seen in those older than 80 years (229). A longitudinal study of Americans aged 60 years and older found that the greater the time spent in productive activities, the greater the gains in well-being (237). Volunteering benefits older people in a variety of other ways: they report gaining a sense of control, feeling appreciated, having a purpose, and having an opportunity to learn and to give something back (238).

Although the emphasis of policies in many countries is on extending older people's abilities to contribute, this requires other abilities to be enhanced as prerequisites. It also requires a range of policies and practices that facilitate older people's ability to work and volunteer in ways that promote *Healthy Ageing*.

What works in facilitating the ability to contribute

Older adults' decisions to work are influenced by their interests, financial need, health, the nature of the work being offered and the implications for their pensions.

Making policies work requires approaches that create opportunities for older adults who can and want to contribute, and that support employers willing to recruit, train and retain workers and volunteers. Policies should also tackle inequities: for example, in general, women have less accumulated financial resources and across their lifespan are likely to spend more time providing care to elders and children than their male counterparts.

The following policy options may not be generalizable to older people who have always taken part in the informal labour market.

Challenge ageism and create inclusive environments that embrace age diversity

Employers often have negative attitudes towards older workers (239). Age discrimination persists even though older workers are not necessarily less healthy, educated, skilful or productive than their younger counterparts (240, 241). Older women face particular challenges in employment because of their sex and age.

Strategies to combat ageism can include introducing laws that make age discrimination illegal, increasing opportunities for intergenerational teams, and introducing campaigns to challenge the myths and inaccurate stereotypes that hinder older people's ability to participate (242). A number of studies have focused on exposing young people to older adults in order to combat negative stereotypes. Extended contact has been found to decrease negative attitudes and to moderate perceptions (243). Exposure to positive examples of older workers can improve implicit beliefs about older adults (244). An intervention that provided information about the myths and realities of ageing, which was followed by a discussion about ageism aimed at changing attitudes, was found to successfully change younger people's perceptions about ageing (245).

Numerous high- and middle-income countries have implemented anti-discrimination laws to combat ageism. For example, for countries within the European Union, the Employment Equality Framework Directive 2000/78/EC aims to combat discrimination in the workplace that is based on disability, sexual orientation, religion and age, and all European Union member states are required to implement this in their national laws (246). The United States, which has one of the highest rates of labour participation among people older than 65 years, has some of the strongest anti-discrimination laws and enforcement; for example, the 1967 Age Discrimination in Employment Act prohibits employment discrimination against people aged 40 years and older. Other countries, such as the Netherlands, have gone so far as to proactively screen vacancy announcements to prevent age discrimination (247).

Abolish mandatory retirement ages

Age is not a reliable indicator when judging workers' potential productivity or employability. The OECD has recommended the eventual elimination of all mandatory retirement policies in order to benefit workers, employers and economies (247). Many countries, including those that have taken actions to increase workforce participation among older people, still have mandatory retirement ages or support industries with mandatory retirement ages. Organizations of the United Nations also have mandatory retirement ages. Policies enforcing mandatory retirement ages do not help create jobs for youth, as was initially envisaged, but they reduce older workers' ability to contribute and reduce an organization's opportunities to benefit from the capabilities of older workers.

Reform pension systems that incentivize early retirement or penalize a return to work

The availability and design of pension systems can either increase or decrease participation in the labour force. In low-income countries, many adults need paid work (also in the sense of agrarian or subsistence work) throughout their lives because there is no social safety net and they cannot afford to retire (248). In contrast, wealthier countries that have expanded the coverage and generosity of their pension system enable older workers to withdraw from the labour force at earlier ages (249). Policies requiring mandatory retirement reduce the opportunities for and motivation of older people to continue working. For example, in Japan if all other factors are held constant, mandatory retirement has been found to reduce by 20% the probability of men aged 60–69 years remaining in the workforce (86). Participation in the labour force is likely to be reduced if older people are eligible for a pension but the system restricts earnings while drawing a pension (86). Pension systems that do not incentivize early retirement or do not penalize retirees who return to work can be particularly influential on older adults' willingness to work. In Sweden, for example, individuals can stop receiving all or part of their pension and continue to work at any age, without constraints on their earned income (250).

Support gradual retirement options and flexible work arrangements

One of the desired options that people approaching traditional retirement ages have identified is the flexibility of part-time work. Phased-retirement schemes remain to be evaluated but have the potential to allow companies to retain experienced employees (251, 252). Policies that provide the option of partial retirement – that is, a gradual move from work to retirement – and remove financial barriers can allow individuals to move in and out of work. Pathways towards gradual retirement may include older people changing the industry in which they work, moving to self-employment or reducing the number of hours that they work. Japan, Norway and Sweden, for example, have been particularly successful at implementing formal partial-retirement schemes and training programmes to help older workers improve their skills and remain longer in the labour force (242, 253).

Older employees may want flexible working arrangements for a number of reasons. For example, they may need or wish to take on caregiving responsibilities for their parents, partners or grandchildren. Flexible work arrangements may include allowing people to work part-time or to have flexibility in their working hours, or to work from home or outside an office. They may also include flexible pay practices; for example, as older employees change their responsibilities, their pay may change consistent with their contribution to the workplace. Particularly progressive employment programmes consider the work–life balance as well as caregiving responsibilities (86), and help societies achieve a better fit between the desires of older people for work and what employers offer. The experiences in Finland and other European countries suggest that improving the fit between the preferences and abilities of older workers and their jobs requires not only the active intervention of policy-makers but also of human resource managers (254).

Consider incentives that encourage employers to retain, train, hire, protect and reward older workers

Many countries with labour shortages, high rates of long-term unemployment and overstretched pension systems, offer incentives to employers to hire older workers. The incentives differ from country to country but typically involve exempting employers from certain taxes, offering bonuses, or providing access to government contracts. Wage subsidies that are used as an alternative to private or public job-training programmes for older workers have been proposed as a cost-effective option but they require evaluation (*255*). Some countries offer incentives for hiring specific populations of older workers, including women, those with lower incomes and those who have been incarcerated. Some countries have employment-protection acts that specifically incentivize employers to hire unemployed women who are older than 50 years and unemployed men who are older than 55 (*248*); these countries include Austria, Bulgaria, France, Greece, Hungary, Lithuania and Slovakia. France, which has one of the lowest job-mobility rates for older workers in the OECD, provides financial aid and access to government contracts for employers who hire unemployed people who are older than 50. Singapore implemented an incentive programme that did not constrain wage levels, and companies benefited from state incentives but older workers were paid below market-level wages.

Help older adults plan for the second half of life and invest in lifelong learning

Increased life expectancy has great significance for both the length of people's working lives and how they may choose to reinvent themselves over that time. Offering appropriate and accessible advice about careers throughout the life course can help people to make informed decisions about life transitions, including engaging in lifelong learning and work.

Although each generation of older adults becomes better educated than the preceding generation, a critical ingredient in helping workers remain employable and employed is lifelong learning, particularly for older workers and most particularly for those in less-skilled jobs (*247*). Employers need to invest in older employees to ensure that they remain engaged, that their knowledge is up to date and that they can remain flexible and responsive to work requirements. In addition to providing education and training, consideration can be given also to providing mentoring, buddy programmes and job rotation. Although different approaches have been under-

taken in a number of countries, it is still not clear which work in policy and practice (*49, 247, 256*).

Invest in health and functioning

Across all countries, poor health is the most frequent reason why people are forced to retire, followed by layoffs and the inability to find a new job (*257*). Ensuring that the workforce is healthy is a precondition for enabling older adults to work longer and an essential consideration for any proposed changes in retirement age or access to pensions. Absenteeism for health-related reasons occurs less often in older workers, but when it occurs the duration is often longer. Investing in activities that promote *Healthy Ageing*, including making attitudinal and behavioural changes, will be crucial to maximizing the health of all workers.

Workplaces that encourage workers to maintain their capacity through physical activity and nutritious food can promote their workers' health (Chapter 3). When employees' capacity declines, the availability of assistive technologies and other reasonable accommodations can enable them to continue to work.

Another tool for maintaining the health, productivity and employability of older workers is to support workers before they are exhausted or lose motivation. Changing their tasks or the sequence of tasks, specifically, if these are mentally or physically exhausting over a long period, can help workers avoid illness and loss of motivation (*248*). Workers can perform a given job until they have reached their optimal productivity and then, before they lose this level of productivity, they can be moved to a new set of tasks that require a similar level of qualification or an increased level, depending on the individual's capacity (*258, 259*).

Create the conditions for volunteerism

The factors that influence volunteering are broad, but the desire to help, previous exposure to volunteering, having worked but being retired, becoming a caregiver, experiencing declines in health, or the death of a partner are important (*260–264*). However, older adults are most likely to volunteer because of their desire to help others and to stay active (*265, 266*).

Generativity – that is, the desire to work with the young and pass on knowledge – becomes more salient with age (*221, 263*). This report is unable to explore all the diverse ways that organizations can support older volunteers. However, research suggests a number of important considerations, including those described below.

- **Encourage people to have the self-confidence to volunteer**. Training is crucial in bolstering the confidence of older people and enabling them to become effective leaders. Older people may be concerned that if they volunteer they may become locked into large commitments of time and energy. At the same time, it can be costly for organizations to have a high turnover of volunteers. Providing clear information about an organization's requirements and ensuring that support is available are essential for helping volunteers make informed decisions.

- **Provide opportunities for organizations and volunteers to meet**. There are many ways to raise awareness about the availability and skills of older people and to create mechanisms for accessing their knowledge and skills, such as Thailand's "brain banks", which provide information about, and facilitate connections to, experienced, skilled retired workers for a range of organizations.

- **Ensure that the type and nature of the work provide satisfaction**. Ensuring personal satisfaction is essential to retaining volunteers. When volunteer workers were compared with a matched sample of paid employees performing identical tasks within the same organization, autonomy (that is, having choices and control over one's actions) and relatedness (that is, being able to develop and maintain secure and respectful relationships with others) were most positively related to volunteers' intentions to

remain with the organization, and this relationship is mediated by satisfaction with the task being done by the volunteer (*267*).

- **Ensure the "fit" between the motivations of the volunteer and the role**. Matching the motivations of potential volunteers with the messages used for recruitment has been shown to be important (*268*). Volunteers whose roles matched their motivations have been found to derive more satisfaction and more enjoyment from their service and to be more likely to intend to continue to volunteer (*268*). Matching volunteer opportunities to volunteers' motivations could thus increase satisfaction and lessen the rate of turnover in the volunteer labour force.

- **Provide compensation to encourage retention**. Although providing cash compensation is difficult for many organizations, turnover may be reduced by providing cash or in-kind compensation to meet the expenses of volunteers. The use of stipends has also been linked to the ability to involve diverse populations, increase retention and to ensure that the volunteers have the best possible experience (*269*).

- **Management matters**. The ways that volunteers are contacted, selected, trained and supervised influence recruitment and retention. For example, the most effective recruitment method is what is known as the personal ask (*264, 270*). Although older adults are less likely to be asked to volunteer, those who are asked agree to volunteer at rates five times higher than those who are not asked (*271*). The meaning attributed to the voluntary work, the support and guidance of staff, and relationships with other volunteers are all important to the quality of the volunteering experience (*221*). A study in England showed that the more appreciated the volunteers felt, the more satisfied they were with their lives in general (*272*).

Table 6.2. Examples of interventions that contribute to achieving the five abilities essential to *Healthy Ageing*, by sector

Abilities	Sector						
	Transport	Housing	Social protection and assistance	Urban development	Information and communication	Education and labour	Health and long-term care
Meet basic needs	- Ensure safe transport options for access to basic services, food and health-care services	- Provide access to adequate housing	- Implement social insurance to provide income security. - Provide assistance to families that care for older family members	- Ensure that structures and landscapes are accessible, safe and well designed	- Ensure that clear and accessible information is provided about the health and social services available for older people. - Ensure that emergency planning considers the needs of older people	- Provide retraining programmes adapted to older workers	- Ensure that an adequate range of healthcare and support services are available for promoting, maintaining and restoring capacity
Learn, grow and decide	- Ensure that front-line transportation operators are trained about the needs of older people and nondiscriminatory practices	- Ensure that older people have information about housing options	- Promote advance care planning	- Develop pedestrian infrastructure that uses principles of universal design. - Support the use of nonmotorized transport	- Provide educational programmes that introduce older people to new technologies that can help them combat loneliness and isolation	- Provide access to computers and the Internet at minimal cost (for example, in libraries or community centres). - Ensure that captioning is available for television broadcasts for people who are hearing impaired	Provide personal budgets
Be mobile	- Ensure that public transport is accessible to older people and people with disability. - Ensure that older people have priority seating	- Assist with home modifications	- Ensure that specialized transport options are available	- Ensure safe road conditions for driving and for pedestrians crossing streets. Provide priority parking for older people with disabilities. - Provide clean public toilets	- Ensure that information about transport options and timetables are available in accessible formats	- Ensure that workplaces are adapted to the needs of older people	- Provide early assessment of housing needs

Abilities	Sector						
	Transport	Housing	Social protection and assistance	Urban development	Information and communication	Education and labour	Health and long-term care
Build and maintain relationships	- Ensure that public transport provides sufficient stops and stations to allow older people to access senior centres, religious buildings and to visit their families	- Design housing that facilitates community integration. - Ensure that housing is not overcrowded	- Support voluntary organizations to facilitate older people's access to social activities	- Provide locations in the community where people can meet, such as community centres, senior centres, and public parks	- Provide accessible information on leisure and social activities	- Ensure that older workers have the opportunity to share their expertise with other workers	- Support older people to build and maintain their intrinsic capacity
Contribute	- Ensure that transportation is available to take people to work or volunteer opportunities	- Ensure that housing is located near services and opportunities for work or volunteering	- Provide unemployment insurance	- Facilitate safe walking for transport (for example, to get to work) and recreation	- Provide information on volunteer opportunities. - Implement communication campaigns to discourage ageism in the workplace by employers and younger employees	- Ensure that there are a range of opportunities for older workers. - Ensure that retirement is a choice and not mandatory. - Implement policies to prevent discrimination based on age	- Provide health insurance that includes coverage for catastrophic health expenditures

The way forward

Ensuring functional ability in older people is important in addressing population ageing. Relevant to all countries is the consideration of older people's abilities, which emphasizes personal and environmental resources as well as intrinsic capacity. Priorities for action will vary and countries will need to tailor actions to their specific contexts, but improving the fit between older people and their environments is universally achievable.

Placing an emphasis on maximizing functional ability supports governments, civil society and other partners in increasing their focus on results and impacts. Concentrating on abilities moves the focus from the inputs – for example, transportation – to outcomes – such as accessibility and mobility. In doing so, it focuses both on what is important to older people and the agendas of various sectors or agencies, which is a win–win approach. Also, this focus on functional ability moves beyond using only checklists, which have limitations because they do not consider the role of environments in nurturing capacity and fostering ability, they assume everybody will benefit equally from a particular resource, and they do not acknowledge that one factor might cancel out another, for example, making housing modifications may reduce the need for long-term care.

In times of heightened concerns over the implications of population ageing, increased national austerity and scarce aid dollars, the focus on abilities provides a way for all sectors at all levels of government to decide together how to most efficiently add health to years.

Each section of this chapter has provided options for actions that can be taken to enhance different domains of abilities. Table 6.2 illustrates the contributions that different sectors can make in enabling functional ability. The following three approaches are key to addressing these cross cutting issues, and are discussed in Chapter 7:

1. combating ageism;
2. enabling autonomy;
3. supporting *Healthy Ageing* in all policies and at all levels of government.

Engendering change requires collaborating across various levels of government and among government and nongovernmental actors, including, for example, academics and older people's organizations. Actions that can support intersectoral action on *Healthy Ageing* include (*273, 274*):

- raising awareness about *Healthy Ageing*;
- tailoring advocacy messages to particular sectors about how they can contribute to *Healthy Ageing*;
- drawing on previous successful experiences of intersectoral action;
- setting up organizational arrangements that promote ongoing collaboration to ensure *Healthy Ageing* across sectors;
- institutionalizing the goal of enhancing functional ability;
- measuring outcomes on ability and documenting specific measures or interventions that have been taken;
- addressing research gaps.

References

1. Attitudes about Aging: a global perspective.Washington (DC): Pew Research Center; 2014 (http://www.pewglobal.org/files/2014/01/Pew-Research-Center-Global-Aging-Report-FINAL-January-30-20141.pdf, accessed 10 July 2015).

2. Center for Excellence in Universal Design [website]. Dublin: National Disability Authority; 2012 (http://universaldesign.ie/, accessed 1 July 2015).

3. Global age-friendly cities: a guide. Geneva: World Health Organization; 2007 (http://www.who.int/ageing/publications/Global_age_friendly_cities_Guide_English.pdf, accessed 20 July 2015).

4. Safe streets for seniors. In: New York City Department of Transportation [website]. New York: City of New York; 2015 (http://www.nyc.gov/html/dot/html/pedestrians/safeseniors.shtml, accessed 1 July 2015).

5. Handi-Transit. In: City of Winnipeg [website]. Winnipeg: City of Winnipeg; 2015 (http://winnipegtransit.com/en/handi-transit/handi-transit, accessed 1 July 2015).

6. What is a men's shed? In: Australian Men's Shed Association [website]. Windale (NSW): Australian Men's Shed Association; 2015. (http://www.mensshed.org/what-is-a-men's-shed/.aspx, accessed 1 July 2015).

7. The universal declaration of human rights. New York: United Nations;1948(http://www.un.org/en/documents/udhr/, accessed 10 July 2015).

8. Naughton C, Drennan J, Treacy MP, Lafferty A, Lyons I, Phelan A, et al. Abuse and neglect of older people in Ireland. Report on the national study of elder abuse and neglect. Dublin: National Centre for the Protection of Older People; 2010. (http://www.ncpop.ie/userfiles/file/ncpop%20reports/Study%203%20Prevalence.pdf, accessed 20 July 2015.)

9. Wu L, Chen H, Hu Y, Xiang H, Yu X, Zhang T, et al. Prevalence and associated factors of elder mistreatment in a rural community in People's Republic of China: a cross-sectional study. PLoS One. 2012;7(3):e33857.doi: http://dx.doi.org/10.1371/journal.pone.0033857 PMID: 22448276

10. Shankar A, McMunn A, Banks J, Steptoe A. Loneliness, social isolation, and behavioral and biological health indicators in older adults. Health Psychol. 2011 Jul;30(4):377–85.doi: http://dx.doi.org/10.1037/a0022826 PMID: 21534675

11. Iliffe S, Kharicha K, Harari D, Swift C, Gillmann G, Stuck AE. Health risk appraisal in older people 2: the implications for clinicians and commissioners of social isolation risk in older people. Br J Gen Pract. 2007 Apr;57(537):277–82. PMID: 17394730

12. Commission on Social Determinants of Health. Closing the gap in a generation: health equity through action on social determinants of health. Final report of the Commission on Social Determinants of Health. Geneva: World Health Organization; 2008 (http://whqlibdoc.who.int/publications/2008/9789241563703_eng.pdf, accessed 10 July 2015).

13. Blazer DG, Sachs-Ericsson N, Hybels CF. Perception of unmet basic needs as a predictor of mortality among community-dwelling older adults. Am J Public Health. 2005 Feb;95(2):299–304.doi: http://dx.doi.org/10.2105/AJPH.2003.035576 PMID: 15671468

14. World Development Report 2000/2001: attacking poverty. New York: Oxford University Press; 2001 (https://openknowledge.worldbank.org/handle/10986/11856, accessed 20 July 2015).

15. Growing unequal? Income distribution and poverty in OECD countries. Paris: OECD Publishing; 2008 (http://www.keepeek.com/Digital-Asset-Management/oecd/social-issues-migration-health/growing-unequal_9789264044197-en#page1, accessed 20 July 2015).

16. Middleton S, Hancock R, Kellard K, Beckhelling J, Phung VH, Perren K. Measuring resources in later life: a review of the data. York, England: Joseph Rowntree Foundation; 2007. (http://www.jrf.org.uk/system/files/2001-measuring-resources-older-people.pdf, accessed 10 July 2015).

17. Zimmer Z, Das S. The poorest of the poor: composition and wealth of older person households in sub-Saharan Africa. Res Aging. 2014 May;36(3):271–96.doi: http://dx.doi.org/10.1177/0164027513484589 PMID: 25650994

18. World development report 2000/2001: attacking poverty. New York: Oxford University Press; 2001.(https://openknowledge.worldbank.org/handle/10986/11856, accessed 10 July 2015).

19. Rodrigues R, Huber M, Lamura G, editors. Facts and figures on healthy ageing and long-term care. Vienna: European Centre for Social Welfare Policy and Research; 2012.(http://www.euro.centre.org/data/LTC_Final.pdf, accessed 10 July 2015).

20. International covenant on economic, social and cultural rights. New York: United Nations; 1966 (http://www.ohchr.org/EN/ProfessionalInterest/Pages/CESCR.aspx, accessed 10 July 2015).

21. The right to adequate housing. Geneva: United Nations, Office of the High Commissioner for Human Rights; 2014 (Fact sheet No. 21/Rev. 1; http://www.ohchr.org/Documents/Publications/FS21_rev_1_Housing_en.pdf, accessed 20 July 2015).

22. Howden-Chapman P, Signal L, Crane J. Housing and health in older people: ageing in place. Soc Policy J NZ. 2010;13:14–30.

23. Thomson H, Thomas S, Sellstrom E, Petticrew M. Housing improvements for health and associated socio-economic outcomes. Cochrane Database Syst Rev. 2013;2:CD008657. PMID: 23450585

24. Healthy ageing: a challenge for Europe. Stockholm: Swedish National Institute for Public Health; 2006 (http://www.healthyageing.eu/sites/www.healthyageing.eu/files/resources/Healthy%20Ageing%20-%20A%20Challenge%20for%20Europe.pdf, accessed 10 July 2015).

25. Gibson M, Petticrew M, Bambra C, Sowden AJ, Wright KE, Whitehead M. Housing and health inequalities: a synthesis of systematic reviews of interventions aimed at different pathways linking housing and health. Health Place. 2011 Jan;17(1):175–84.doi: http://dx.doi.org/10.1016/j.healthplace.2010.09.011 PMID: 21159542

26. Beard JR, Cerdá M, Blaney S, Ahern J, Vlahov D, Galea S. Neighborhood characteristics and change in depressive symptoms among older residents of New York City. Am J Public Health. 2009 Jul;99(7):1308–14.doi: http://dx.doi.org/10.2105/AJPH.2007.125104 PMID: 19008519

27. Lipman B, Lubell J, Salomon E. Housing an aging population: are we prepared. Washington (DC): Center for Housing Policy; 2012. (http://www.nhc.org/media/files/AgingReport2012.pdf, accessed 10 July 2015).

28. Pope ND, Kang B. Residential relocation in later life: a comparison of proactive and reactive moves. J Hous Elder. 2010;24(2):193–207. doi: http://dx.doi.org/10.1080/02763891003757122

29. Dannefer D. Cumulative advantage/disadvantage and the life course: cross-fertilizing age and social science theory. J Gerontol B Psychol Sci Soc Sci. 2003 Nov;58(6):S327–37.doi: http://dx.doi.org/10.1093/geronb/58.6.S327 PMID: 14614120

30. James M, Graycar A, Mayhew P. A safe and secure environment for older Australians. Canberra: Australian Institute of Criminology; 2003. (http://www.aic.gov.au/media_library/publications/rpp/51/rpp051.pdf, accessed 10 July 2015).

31. Bachman R, Meloy ML. The epidemiology of violence against the elderly: implications for primary and secondary prevention. J Contemp Crim Justice. 2008;24(2):186–97. doi: http://dx.doi.org/10.1177/1043986208315478

32. Lachs MS, Williams CS, O'Brien S, Pillemer KA, Charlson ME. The mortality of elder mistreatment. JAMA. 1998 Aug 5;280(5):428–32.doi: http://dx.doi.org/10.1001/jama.280.5.428 PMID: 9701077

33. Hutton D. Older people in emergencies: considerations for action and policy development. Geneva: World Health Organization; 2008. (http://www.who.int/ageing/publications/Hutton_report_small.pdf?ua=1, accessed 10 July 2015).

34. Derges J, Clow A, Lynch R, Jain S, Phillips G, Petticrew M, et al. 'Well London' and the benefits of participation: results of a qualitative study nested in a cluster randomised trial. BMJ Open. 2014;4(4):e003596.doi: http://dx.doi.org/10.1136/bmjopen-2013-003596 PMID: 24694622

35. Guidelines for mainstreaming the needs of older persons in disaster situations. Washington (DC): Pan American Health Organization; 2012 (http://www.paho.org/disasters/index.php?option=com_docman&task=doc_download&gid=2000&Itemid=, accessed 20 July 2015).

36. Cooper K, Stewart K. Does money in adulthood affect adult outcomes? York, England: Joseph Rowntree Foundation; 2015. (http://www.jrf.org.uk/sites/files/jrf/money-adult-outcomes-full.pdf, accessed 10 July 2015).

37. Beard JR, Tracy M, Vlahov D, Galea S. Trajectory and socioeconomic predictors of depression in a prospective study of residents of New York City. Ann Epidemiol. 2008 Mar;18(3):235–43.doi: http://dx.doi.org/10.1016/j.annepidem.2007.10.004 PMID: 18083544

38. Gorman M. Age and security: how social pensions can deliver effective aid to poor older people and their families. London: HelpAge International (http://www.globalaging.org/pension/world/2004/security.pdf, accessed 20 July 2015).

39. Soares S, Osorio RG, Soares FV, Medeiros M, Zepeda E. Conditional cash transfers in Brazil, Chile and Mexico: impacts upon inequality. Estudios económicos. 2009;(1):207–24. (http://core.ac.uk/download/pdf/6327963.pdf, accessed 14 August 2015).

40. McKinnon R. Tax-financed old-age pensions in lower-income countries. Developments and trends: supporting dynamic social security. Geneva: International Social Security Association; 2007:31–7. (https://www.issa.int/html/pdf/publ/2DT07.pdf, accessed 10 July 2015).

41. Asher M. The future of old age income security. New York: International Longevity Centre Global Alliance; 2013 (Revised version of Robert Butler Memorial Speech, delivered at the International Centre Global Alliance Symposium on The Future of Ageing, Singapore, 21 June 2013; http://www.ilc-alliance.org/images/uploads/publication-pdfs/The_future_of_old_age_income_security_Oct_2013_1.pdf, accessed 20 July 2015).

42. Duflo E. Grandmothers and granddaughters: old age pension and intra-household allocation in South Africa. Cambridge (MA): National Bureau of Economic Research; 2000. (http://economics.mit.edu/files/732, accessed 10 July 2015).

43. World development report 2011: conflict, security, and development. Washington (DC): World Bank; 2011. doi: http://dx.doi.org/10.1596/978-0-8213-8439-8

44. Shin E, Do YK. Basic old-age pension and financial wellbeing of older adults in South Korea. Ageing Soc. 2015;35:1055–74. doi: http://dx.doi.org/10.1017/S0144686X14000051

45. Bussolo M, Koettl J, Sinnott E. Golden aging: prospects for healthy, active, and prosperous aging in Europe and Central Asia. Washington (DC): World Bank; 2015. (https://openknowledge.worldbank.org/handle/10986/22018, accessed 10 July 2015).

46. Why social pensions are needed now. London: HelpAge International; 2006 (http://www.helpage.org/silo/files/why-social-pensions-are-needed-now.pdf; accessed 20 July 2015).

47. Sadana R, Foebel AD, Williams AN, Beard JR. Population ageing, longevity, and the diverse contexts of the oldest old. Public Policy Aging Rep. 2013;23(2):18–25. doi: http://dx.doi.org/10.1093/ppar/23.2.18

48. Social protection floor. In: Social Protection Floor Initiative [website]. Geneva: Social Protection Floor Initiative; 2014 (http://www.socialprotectionfloor-gateway.org/4.htm, accessed 7 July 2015).

49. Maclean R, Wilson D, editors. International handbook of education for the changing world of work. Dordrecht, Netherlands: Springer; 2009. doi: http://dx.doi.org/10.1007/978-1-4020-5281-1

50. Asher M. Pension plans, provident fund schemes and retirement policies: India's social security reform imperative. ASCI J Manag. 2010;39(1):1–18. (http://journal.asci.org.in/Vol.39(2009-10)/39_1_Mukul%20G%20Asher.pdf, accessed 14 August 2015).

51. Wagner SL, Shubair MM, Michalos AC. Surveying older adults' opinions on housing: recommendations for policy. Soc Indic Res. 2010;99(3):405–12. doi: http://dx.doi.org/10.1007/s11205-010-9588-5

52. Braubach M, Power A. Housing conditions and risk: reporting on a European study of housing quality and risk of accidents for older people. J Hous Elder. 2011;25(3):288–305. doi: http://dx.doi.org/10.1080/02763893.2011.595615

53. Hui ECM, Wong FKW, Chung KW, Lau KY. Housing affordability, preferences and expectations of elderly with government intervention. Habitat Int. 2014;43:11–21. doi: http://dx.doi.org/10.1016/j.habitatint.2014.01.010

54. Wiles JL, Leibing A, Guberman N, Reeve J, Allen RES. The meaning of "aging in place" to older people. Gerontologist. 2012 Jun;52(3):357–66.doi: http://dx.doi.org/10.1093/geront/gnr098 PMID: 21983126

55. van der Pas S, Ramklass S, O'Leary B, Andersen S, Keating N, Cassim B. Features of home and neighbourhood and the live-ability of older South Africans. Eur J Ageing. 2015;30 May:1–13. doi: http://dx.doi.org/10.1007/s10433-015-0343-2

56. Keating N, Eales J, Phillips JE. Age-friendly rural communities: conceptualizing 'best-fit'. Can J Aging. 2013 Dec;32(4):319–32.doi: http://dx.doi.org/10.1017/S0714980813000408 PMID: 24128863

57. Convention on the rights of persons with disabilities and optional protocol. New York: United Nations; 2006 (http://www.un.org/disabilities/documents/convention/convoptprot-e.pdf, accessed 10 July 2015).

58. The National Evaluation of Partnerships for Older People Projects. executive summary. Canterbury (England): Personal Social Services Research Unit; 2013 (http://www.pssru.ac.uk/pdf/rs053.pdf, accessed 10 July 2015).

59. Wahl HW, Iwarsson S, Oswald F. Aging well and the environment: toward an integrative model and research agenda for the future. Gerontologist. 2012 Jun;52(3):306–16.doi: http://dx.doi.org/10.1093/geront/gnr154 PMID: 22419248

60. Nygren C, Oswald F, Iwarsson S, Fänge A, Sixsmith J, Schilling O, et al. Relationships between objective and perceived housing in very old age. Gerontologist. 2007 Feb;47(1):85–95.doi: http://dx.doi.org/10.1093/geront/47.1.85 PMID: 17327544

61. Tanner B, Tilse C, de Jonge D. Restoring and sustaining home: the impact of home modifications on the meaning of home for older people. J Hous Elder. 2008;22(3):195–215. doi: http://dx.doi.org/10.1080/02763890802232048

62. Perry TE, Andersen TC, Kaplan DB. Relocation remembered: perspectives on senior transitions in the living environment. Gerontologist. 2014 Feb;54(1):75–81.doi: http://dx.doi.org/10.1093/geront/gnt070 PMID: 23840021

63. McClure R, Turner C, Peel N, Spinks A, Eakin E, Hughes K. Population-based interventions for the prevention of fall-related injuries in older people. Cochrane Database Syst Rev. 2005; (1):CD004441. PMID: 15674948

64. Perracini M, Clemson L, Tiedmann A, Kalula S, Scott V, Sherrington C. Falls in older adults: current evidence, gaps and priorities. Gerontologist. 2016. (In press.).

65. Ytterstad B. The Harstad injury prevention study: community based prevention of fall-fractures in the elderly evaluated by means of a hospital based injury recording system in Norway. J Epidemiol Community Health. 1996 Oct;50(5):551–8.doi: http://dx.doi.org/10.1136/jech.50.5.551 PMID: 8944864

66. Zijlstra GA, van Haastregt JC, van Rossum E, van Eijk JT, Yardley L, Kempen GI. Interventions to reduce fear of falling in community-living older people: a systematic review. J Am Geriatr Soc. 2007 Apr;55(4):603–15.doi: http://dx.doi.org/10.1111/j.1532-5415.2007.01148.x PMID: 17397441

67. Lindqvist K, Timpka T, Schelp L. Evaluation of an inter-organizational prevention program against injuries among the elderly in a WHO Safe Community. Public Health. 2001 Sep;115(5):308–16.doi: http://dx.doi.org/10.1016/S0033-3506(01)00468-1 PMID: 11593439

68. Poulstrup A, Jeune B. Prevention of fall injuries requiring hospital treatment among community-dwelling elderly. Eur J Public Health. 2000;10(1):45–50. doi: http://dx.doi.org/10.1093/eurpub/10.1.45

69. Duff JM. Reducing the number of environmental hazards in the homes of community dwelling elderly: a comparison of approaches to fall prevention via environmental assessment and modification [thesis]. Ann Arbor: New York University; 2010.

70. Svanström L, Ader M, Schelp L, Lindstrom A. Preventing femoral fractures among elderly: the community safety approach. Saf Sci. 1996;21(3):239–46. doi: http://dx.doi.org/10.1016/0925-7535(95)00067-4

71. Kempton A, Van Beurden E, Sladden T, Garner E, Beard J. Older people can stay on their feet: final results of a community-based falls prevention programme. Health Promot Int. 2000;15(1):27–33. doi: http://dx.doi.org/10.1093/heapro/15.1.27

72. Fänge A, Iwarsson S. Changes in ADL dependence and aspects of usability following housing adaptation–a longitudinal perspective. Am J Occup Ther. 2005 May-Jun;59(3):296–304.doi: http://dx.doi.org/10.5014/ajot.59.3.296 PMID: 15969277

73. Heywood F. Money well spent: the effectiveness and value of housing adaptations. Bristol: Policy Press; 2001 (http://www.jrf.org.uk/system/files/jr100-effectiveness-housing-adaptations.pdf, accessed 10 July 2015).

74. The MetLife Study of Elder Financial Abuse. Crimes of occasion, desperation, and predation against America's elders. New York: MetLife Mature Market Institute; 2011 (https://www.metlife.com/assets/cao/mmi/publications/studies/2011/mmi-elder-financial-abuse.pdf, accessed 20 July 2015).

75. Wagner SL, Shubair MM, Michalos AC. Surveying older adults' opinions on housing: recommendations for policy. Soc Indic Res. 2010;99(3):405–12.

76. Help at home. My aged care [website]. Canberra: Australian Government, Department of Social Services; 2015. (http://www.myagedcare.gov.au/#!/help-home, accessed 27 July 2015).

77. Ageing in the twenty-first century a celebration and a challenge. New York: United Nations Population Fund; 2012 (http://www.unfpa.org/publications/ageing-twenty-first-century, accessed 10 July 2015).

78. Care & Repair England. In: Care & Repair England [website]. Nottingham (England): Care & Repair England. 2014 (http://careandrepair-england.org.uk/?page_id=30, accessed 10 July 2015).

79. Morris ME, Adair B, Miller K, Ozanne E, Hansen R, Pearce A, et al. Smarthome technologies to assist older people to live well at home. J Aging Sci. 2013;1(1):1–9. (http://www.esciencecentral.org/journals/smart-home-technologies-to-assist-older-people-to-live-well-at-home-jasc.1000101.pdf, accessed 10 July 2015).

80. World report on disability. Geneva: World Health Organization; 2011 (http://www.who.int/disabilities/world_report/2011/en/, accessed 10 July 2015).

81. Lansley P, McCreadie C, Tinker A. Can adapting the homes of older people and providing assistive technology pay its way? Age Ageing. 2004 Nov;33(6):571–6.doi: http://dx.doi.org/10.1093/ageing/afh190 PMID: 15347537

82. Mitchell OS, Piggott J. Unlocking housing equity in Japan. J Jpn Int Econ. 2004;18(4):466–505. doi: http://dx.doi.org/10.1016/j.jjie.2004.03.003

83. Rosenfeld O. Social and affordable housing finance – current trends and challenges in countries with mature social housing sector. Geneva: United Nations Economic Commission for Europe; 2014 (http://www.unece.org/fileadmin/DAM/hlm/prgm/hmm/social%20housing/geneva2014/1.05.rosenfeld.pdf, accessed 10 July 2015).

84. Ageing in cities. Paris: OECD Publishing; 2015. doi: http://dx.doi.org/10.1787/9789264231160-en

85. Beaulieu M, Dubé M, Bergeron C, Cousineau M-M. Are elderly men worried about crime? J Aging Stud. 2007;21(4):336–46. doi: http://dx.doi.org/10.1016/j.jaging.2007.05.001

86. Global population ageing: peril or promise. Geneva: World Economic Forum; 2011 (http://www3.weforum.org/docs/WEF_GAC_GlobalPopulationAgeing_Report_2012.pdf, accessed 20 July 2015).

87. James M, Graycar A. Preventing crime against older Australians. Canberra: Australian Institute of Criminology; 2000. (http://www.aic.gov.au/media_library/publications/rpp/32/rpp032.pdf, accessed 10 July 2015).

88. Pillemer KA, Burnes D, Riffin C, Lachs MS. Elder abuse. Gerontologist. 2016. Forthcoming. PMID: 3342992

89. Lachs M, Berman J. Under the radar: New York State elder abuse prevalence study. New York: Lifespan of Greater Rochester, Inc., Weill Cornell Medical Center of Cornell University, and New York City Department for the Aging; 2011.

90. Peterson JC, Burnes DP, Caccamise PL, Mason A, Henderson CR Jr, Wells MT, et al. Financial exploitation of older adults: a population-based prevalence study. J Gen Intern Med. 2014 Dec;29(12):1615–23.doi: http://dx.doi.org/10.1007/s11606-014-2946-2 PMID: 25103121

91. Kwok JST, Fritsch P, Raza A, Newport M. Loving the older people in times of cholera: preliminary findings from a study to analyse care and outcomes for cholera patients treated by Médecins Sans Frontières Operational Centre Amsterdam in Haiti and Zimbabwe 2008–12. London: Médecins Sans Frontières; 2012.

92. Guidance note on disability and emergency risk management for health. Geneva: World Health Organization; 2013 (http://apps.who.int/iris/bitstream/10665/90369/1/9789241506243_eng.pdf, accessed 20 July 2015).

93. Disabilities among refugees and conflict-affected populations: resource kit for fieldworkers. New York: Women's Commission for Refugee Women and Children; 2008 (https://womensrefugeecommission.org/resources/document/609-disabilities-among-refugees-and-conflict-affected-populations?catid=232, accessed 20 July 2015).

94. Duggan S, Deeny P, Spelman R, Vitale CT. Perceptions of older people on disaster response and preparedness. Int J Older People Nurs. 2010 Mar;5(1):71–6.doi: http://dx.doi.org/10.1111/j.1748-3743.2009.00203.x PMID: 20925760

95. Powell S, Plouffe L, Gorr P. When ageing and disasters collide: lessons from 16 international case studies. Radiat Prot Dosimetry. 2009 Jun;134(3-4):202–6.doi: http://dx.doi.org/10.1093/rpd/ncp082 PMID: 19435731

96. Fitzgerald KG. Evaluation of the preparedness of Massachusetts nursing homes to respond to catastrophic natural or human-made disasters. In: British Society of Gerontology [website]. York (England): British Society of Gerontology; 2008 (abstract; http://www.britishgerontology.org/DB/gr-editions-2/generations-review/evaluation-of-the-preparedness-of-massachusetts-nu.html, accessed 20 July 2015).

97. Kim HJ, Fritsch P. Older people in humanitarian contexts: the impact of disaster on older people and the means of addressing their needs. Gerontologist. 2016. (In press).

98. Boulton-Lewis GM. Education and learning for the elderly: why, how, what. Educ Gerontol. 2010;36(3):213–28. doi: http://dx.doi.org/10.1080/03601270903182877

99. Stephens C, Breheny M, Mansvelt J. Healthy ageing from the perspective of older people: a capability approach to resilience. Psychol Health. 2015;30(6):715–31. PMID: 24678916

100. Carstensen LL, Hartel CR, editors. When I'm 64. Washington (DC): National Academies Press; 2006. (http://www.nap.edu/openbook.php?record_id=11474&page=R1, accessed 10 July 2015).

101. Aspin DN, Chapman J, Evans K, Bagnall R. Second International handbook of lifelong learning. Dodrecht, Netherlands: Springer; 2012. doi: http://dx.doi.org/10.1007/978-94-007-2360-3

102. The lifelong learning needs of older people in Ireland: a discussion paper. Dublin: AONTAS, The National Adult Learning Organisation; 2007 (http://www.aontas.com/download/pdf/olderpeopleresearch_ppr_2007.pdf, accessed 10 July 2015).

103. Jeong H, Kim HS. Aging and text comprehension: interpretation and domain knowledge advantage. Educ Gerontol. 2009;35(10):906–28. doi: http://dx.doi.org/10.1080/03601270902834601

104. McNair S. Demography and lifelong learning: IFLL thematic paper No. 1. Leicester, England: National Institute of Adult Continuing Education; 2009.

105. Welford C, Murphy K, Wallace M, Casey D. A concept analysis of autonomy for older people in residential care. J Clin Nurs. 2010 May;19(9-10):1226–35.doi: http://dx.doi.org/10.1111/j.1365-2702.2009.03185.x PMID: 20345826

106. Lindberg C, Fagerström C, Sivberg B, Willman A. Concept analysis: patient autonomy in a caring context. J Adv Nurs. 2014 Oct;70(10):2208–21.doi: http://dx.doi.org/10.1111/jan.12412 PMID: 25209751

107. Laal M. Lifelong learning: what does it mean? Procedia Soc Behav Sci. 2011;28(0):470–4. doi: http://dx.doi.org/10.1016/j.sbspro.2011.11.090

108. Laal M. Barriers to lifelong learning. Procedia Soc Behav Sci. 2011;28(0):612–5. doi: http://dx.doi.org/10.1016/j.sbspro.2011.11.116

109. Rahhal TA, Hasher L, Colcombe SJ. Instructional manipulations and age differences in memory: now you see them, now you don't. Psychol Aging. 2001;16(4):697–706. doi: http://dx.doi.org/10.1037/0882-7974.16.4.697

110. Hess TM, Auman C, Colcombe SJ, Rahhal TA. The impact of stereotype threat on age differences in memory performance. J Gerontol B Psychol Sci Soc Sci. 2003 Jan;58(1):3–11.doi: http://dx.doi.org/10.1093/geronb/58.1.P3 PMID: 12496296

111. Kronfol NSA, Rizk A. Ageing in the Arab region: trends, implications and policy options. Beirut: Economic and Social Commission for Western Asia; 2013. (http://www.escwa.un.org/divisions/div_editor/Download.asp?table_name=divisions_other&field_name=ID&FileID=1588, accessed 10 July 2015).

112. Kothari B, Bandyopadhyay T. Same language subtitling of Bollywood film songs on TV: effects on literacy. Inf Technol Int Dev. 2014;10(4):31–47. (http://itidjournal.org/index.php/itid/article/view/1307, accessed 14 August 2015).

113. Vassilev I, Rogers A, Sanders C, Kennedy A, Blickem C, Protheroe J, et al. Social networks, social capital and chronic illness self-management: a realist review. Chronic Illn. 2011 Mar;7(1):60–86.doi: http://dx.doi.org/10.1177/1742395310383338 PMID: 20921033

114. Jacobson TA, Thomas DM, Morton FJ, Offutt G, Shevlin J, Ray S. Use of a low-literacy patient education tool to enhance pneumococcal vaccination rates. A randomized controlled trial. JAMA. 1999 Aug 18;282(7):646–50.doi: http://dx.doi.org/10.1001/jama.282.7.646 PMID: 10517717

115. Rogers A, Vassilev I, Sanders C, Kirk S, Chew-Graham C, Kennedy A, et al. Social networks, work and network-based resources for the management of long-term conditions: a framework and study protocol for developing self-care support. Implement Sci. 2011;6(1):56.doi: http://dx.doi.org/10.1186/1748-5908-6-56 PMID: 21619695

116. Wurzer B, Waters DL, Hale LA, Leon de la Barra S. Long-term participation in peer-led fall prevention classes predicts lower fall incidence. Arch Phys Med Rehabil. 2014 Jun;95(6):1060–6.doi: http://dx.doi.org/10.1016/j.apmr.2014.01.018 PMID: 24508186

117. Guo PJ, Reinecke K. Demographic differences in how students navigate through MOOCs. In: Proceedings of the first ACM conference on Learning @ scale conference. New York: Association of Computing Machinery; 2014. 21–30.

118. Löckenhoff CE, Carstensen LL. Socioemotional selectivity theory, aging, and health: the increasingly delicate balance between regulating emotions and making tough choices. J Pers. 2004 Dec;72(6):1395–424.doi: http://dx.doi.org/10.1111/j.1467-6494.2004.00301.x PMID: 15509287

119. McCormack B. Autonomy and the relationship between nurses and older people. Ageing Soc. 2001;21(4):417–46. doi: http://dx.doi.org/10.1017/S0144686X01008303

120. Boyle G. Facilitating choice and control for older people in long-term care. Health Soc Care Community. 2004 May;12(3):212–20.doi: http://dx.doi.org/10.1111/j.1365-2524.2004.00490.x PMID: 19777711

121. Ottmann G, Allen J, Feldman P. A systematic narrative review of consumer-directed care for older people: implications for model development. Health Soc Care Community. 2013 Nov;21(6):563–81. PMID: 23465034

122. Cui D, Wang P, Wang Q. A three-pronged approach to the care of elders with Alzheimer's Disease. Ageing Int. 2010;35(2):142–52. doi: http://dx.doi.org/10.1007/s12126-010-9058-z

123. Willis M, Dalziel R. LinkAge Plus: Capacity building – enabling and empowering older people as independent and active citizens. London: Department for Work and Pensions; 2009 (Research report No. 571; http://webarchive.nationalarchives.gov.uk/+/http://research.dwp.gov.uk/asd/asd5/rports2009-2010/rrep571.pdf, accessed 10 July 2015).

124. Evaluation on the model of inter-generational self-help club [website]. Vientiane (Vietnam); ISMS; 2014 (http://isms.org.vn/, accessed 10 July 2015) (in Vietnamese).

125. [Final evaluation of the project promotion the rights of the disadvantaged older people in Vietnam]. Vientiane (Vietnam): ISMS; 2014 (in Vietnamese).

126. Beales S. Empowerment and older people: enhancing capabilities in an ageing world. Expert Group Meeting on "Promoting people's empowerment in achieving poverty eradication, social integration and productive and decent work for all". New York: United Nations; 2012. (http://www.un.org/esa/socdev/egms/docs/2012/SylviaBeales.pdf, accessed 10 July 2015).

127. Crawford JO, Graveling RA, Cowie HA, Dixon K. The health safety and health promotion needs of older workers. Occup Med (Lond). 2010 May;60(3):184–92.doi: http://dx.doi.org/10.1093/occmed/kqq028 PMID: 20423949

128. Hamilton S, Tew J, Szymczynska P, Clewett N, Manthorpe J, Larsen J, et al. Power, choice and control: how do personal budgets affect experiences of people with mental health problems and their relationships with social workers and other practitioners? Br J Soc Work. 2015;23(April). doi: http://dx.doi.org/10.1093/bjsw/bcv023

129. Advance care planning. London: Royal College of Physicians; 2009 (National Guideline No. 12; (https://www.rcplondon.ac.uk/sites/default/files/documents/acp_web_final_21.01.09.pdf, accessed 10 July 2015).

130. Aw D, Hayhoe B, Smajdor A, Bowker LK, Conroy SP, Myint PK. Advance care planning and the older patient. QJM. 2012 Mar;105(3):225–30.doi: http://dx.doi.org/10.1093/qjmed/hcr209 PMID: 22075012

131. Billings JA. The need for safeguards in advance care planning. J Gen Intern Med. 2012 May;27(5):595–600.doi: http://dx.doi.org/10.1007/s11606-011-1976-2 PMID: 22237664

132. Detering KM, Hancock AD, Reade MC, Silvester W. The impact of advance care planning on end of life care in elderly patients: randomised controlled trial. BMJ. 2010;340 Mar 23 1:c1345. doi: http://dx.doi.org/http://dx.doi.org/10.1136/bmj.c1345 PMID:20332506doi: http://dx.doi.org/10.1136/bmj.c1345

133. Morrison RS, Chichin E, Carter J, Burack O, Lantz M, Meier DE. The effect of a social work intervention to enhance advance care planning documentation in the nursing home. J Am Geriatr Soc. 2005 Feb;53(2):290–4.doi: http://dx.doi.org/10.1111/j.1532-5415.2005.53116.x PMID: 15673354

134. Satariano WA, Guralnik JM, Jackson RJ, Marottoli RA, Phelan EA, Prohaska TR. Mobility and aging: new directions for public health action. Am J Public Health. 2012 Aug;102(8):1508–15.doi: http://dx.doi.org/10.2105/AJPH.2011.300631 PMID: 22698013

135. Ross LA, Schmidt EL, Ball K. Interventions to maintain mobility: What works? Accid Anal Prev. 2013 Dec;61:167–96.doi: http://dx.doi.org/10.1016/j.aap.2012.09.027 PMID: 23083492

136. Yeom HA, Keller C, Fleury J. Interventions for promoting mobility in community-dwelling older adults. J Am Acad Nurse Pract. 2009 Feb;21(2):95–100.doi: http://dx.doi.org/10.1111/j.1745-7599.2008.00390.x PMID: 19228247

137. Yeom HA, Fleury J, Keller C. Risk factors for mobility limitation in community-dwelling older adults: a social ecological perspective. Geriatr Nurs. 2008 Mar-Apr;29(2):133–40.doi: http://dx.doi.org/10.1016/j.gerinurse.2007.07.002 PMID: 18394514

138. Webber SC, Porter MM, Menec VH. Mobility in older adults: a comprehensive framework. Gerontologist. 2010 Aug;50(4):443–50.doi: http://dx.doi.org/10.1093/geront/gnq013 PMID: 20145017

139. Shumway-Cook A, Ciol MA, Yorkston KM, Hoffman JM, Chan L. Mobility limitations in the Medicare population: prevalence and sociodemographic and clinical correlates. J Am Geriatr Soc. 2005 Jul;53(7):1217–21.doi: http://dx.doi.org/10.1111/j.1532-5415.2005.53372.x PMID: 16108942

140. Nordbakke S, Schwanen T. Well-being and mobility: a theoretical framework and literature review focusing on older people. Mobilities. 2014;9(1):104–29. doi: http://dx.doi.org/10.1080/17450101.2013.784542

141. Mezuk B, Rebok GW. Social integration and social support among older adults following driving cessation. J Gerontol B Psychol Sci Soc Sci. 2008 Sep;63(5):S298–303.doi: http://dx.doi.org/10.1093/geronb.63.5.S298 PMID: 18818450

142. Yen IH, Fandel Flood J, Thompson H, Anderson LA, Wong G. How design of places promotes or inhibits mobility of older adults: realist synthesis of 20 years of research. J Aging Health. 2014 Dec;26(8):1340–72.doi: http://dx.doi.org/10.1177/0898264314527610 PMID: 24788714

143. Shumway-Cook A, Patla AE, Stewart A, Ferrucci L, Ciol MA, Guralnik JM. Environmental demands associated with community mobility in older adults with and without mobility disabilities. Phys Ther. 2002 Jul;82(7):670–81. PMID: 12088464

144. Cress ME, Orini S, Kinsler L. Living environment and mobility of older adults. Gerontology. 2011;57(3):287–94.doi: http://dx.doi.org/10.1159/000322195 PMID: 20980733

145. A guide for population-based approaches to increasing levels of physical activity: implementation of the WHO global strategy on diet, physical activity and health. Geneva: World Health Organization; 2007 (http://www.who.int/dietphysicalactivity/physical-activity-promotion-2007.pdf, accessed 20 July 2015).

146. Frank LD, Schmid TL, Sallis JF, Chapman J, Saelens BE. Linking objectively measured physical activity with objectively measured urban form: findings from SMARTRAQ. Am J Prev Med. 2005 Feb;28(2) Suppl 2:117–25.doi: http://dx.doi.org/10.1016/j.amepre.2004.11.001 PMID: 15694519

147. Chad KE, Reeder BA, Harrison EL, Ashworth NL, Sheppard SM, Schultz SL, et al. Profile of physical activity levels in community-dwelling older adults. Med Sci Sports Exerc. 2005 Oct;37(10):1774–84.doi: http://dx.doi.org/10.1249/01.mss.0000181303.51937.9c PMID: 16260980

148. Prohaska T, Belansky E, Belza B, Buchner D, Marshall V, McTigue K, et al. Physical activity, public health, and aging: critical issues and research priorities. J Gerontol B Psychol Sci Soc Sci. 2006 Sep;61(5):S267–73.doi: http://dx.doi.org/10.1093/geronb/61.5.S267 PMID: 16960240

149. Giles-Corti B, Donovan RJ. Relative influences of individual, social environmental, and physical environmental correlates of walking. Am J Public Health. 2003 Sep;93(9):1583–9.doi: http://dx.doi.org/10.2105/AJPH.93.9.1583 PMID: 12948984

150. Anderson LA, Slonim A, Yen IH, Jones DL, Allen P, Hunter RH, et al. Developing a framework and priorities to promote mobility among older adults. Health Educ Behav. 2014 Oct;41(1) Suppl:10S–8S.doi: http://dx.doi.org/10.1177/1090198114537492 PMID: 25274706

151. Booth ML, Owen N, Bauman A, Clavisi O, Leslie E. Social-cognitive and perceived environment influences associated with physical activity in older Australians. Prev Med. 2000 Jul;31(1):15–22.doi: http://dx.doi.org/10.1177/1090198114537492 PMID: 10896840

152. Wilcox S, Bopp M, Oberrecht L, Kammermann SK, McElmurray CT. Psychosocial and perceived environmental correlates of physical activity in rural and older african american and white women. J Gerontol B Psychol Sci Soc Sci. 2003 Nov;58(6):329–37.doi: http://dx.doi.org/10.1093/geronb/58.6.P329 PMID: 14614117

153. Bauman A, Singh M, Buchner D, Merom D, Bull F. Physical activity in older adults. Gerontologist. 2016. (In press).

154. Marottoli RA, Allore H, Araujo KLB, Iannone LP, Acampora D, Gottschalk M, et al. A randomized trial of a physical conditioning program to enhance the driving performance of older persons. J Gen Intern Med. 2007 May;22(5):590–7.doi: http://dx.doi.org/10.1007/s11606-007-0134-3 PMID: 17443366

155. Marmeleira JF, Godinho MB, Fernandes OM. The effects of an exercise program on several abilities associated with driving performance in older adults. Accid Anal Prev. 2009 Jan;41(1):90–7.doi: http://dx.doi.org/10.1016/j.aap.2008.09.008 PMID: 19114142

156. Garin N, Olaya B, Miret M, Ayuso-Mateos JL, Power M, Bucciarelli P, et al. Built environment and elderly population health: a comprehensive literature review. Clin Pract Epidemiol Ment Health. 2014;10(1):103–15.doi: http://dx.doi.org/10.2174/1745017901410010103 PMID: 25356084

157. Prince MJ, Wu F, Guo Y, Gutierrez Robledo LM, O'Donnell M, Sullivan R, et al. The burden of disease in older people and implications for health policy and practice. Lancet. 2015 Feb 7;385(9967):549–62.doi: http://dx.doi.org/10.1016/S0140-6736(14)61347-7 PMID: 25468153

158. Ackerman ML, Edwards JD, Ross LA, Ball KK, Lunsman M. Examination of cognitive and instrumental functional performance as indicators for driving cessation risk across 3 years. Gerontologist. 2008 Dec;48(6):802–10.doi: http://dx.doi.org/10.1093/geront/48.6.802 PMID: 19139253

159. Ball K, Edwards JD, Ross LA. The impact of speed of processing training on cognitive and everyday functions. J Gerontol B Psychol Sci Soc Sci. 2007 Jun;62(Spec. No. 1):19–31. PMID:17565162doi: http://dx.doi.org/10.1093/geronb/62.special_issue_1.19

160. Lane A, Green E, Dickerson AE, Davis ES, Rolland B, Stohler JT. Driver rehabilitation programs: defining program models, services, and expertise. Occup Ther Health Care. 2014 Apr;28(2):177–87. PMID: 24754768

161. Li G, Braver ER, Chen LH. Fragility versus excessive crash involvement as determinants of high death rates per vehicle-mile of travel among older drivers. Accid Anal Prev. 2003 Mar;35(2):227–35.doi: http://dx.doi.org/10.1016/S0001-4575(01)00107-5 PMID: 12504143

162. Löfqvist C, Nygren C, Széman Z, Iwarsson S. Assistive devices among very old people in five European countries. Scand J Occup Ther. 2005 Dec;12(4):181–92.doi: http://dx.doi.org/10.1080/11038120500210652 PMID: 16457091

163. Rosso AL, Auchincloss AH, Michael YL. The urban built environment and mobility in older adults: a comprehensive review. J Aging Res. 2011;2011:816106. doi: http://dx.doi.org/10.4061/2011/816106

164. Joint position paper on the provision of mobility devices in less-resourced settings. Geneva: World Health Organization; 2011 (http://whqlibdoc.who.int/publications/2011/9789241502887_eng.pdf?ua=1, accessed 20 July 2015).

165. World report on disability. Geneva: World Health Organization; 2011 (http://whqlibdoc.who.int/publications/2011/9789240685215_eng.pdf?ua=1, accessed 20 July 2015).

166. Proposed conceptual framework: universal design. In: Global Universal Design Commission [website]. Syracuse (NY): Global Universal Design Commission; 2015 (http://www.globaluniversaldesign.org/node/11, accessed 1 July 2015.)

167. About UD. The Center for Universal Design, College of Design, North Carolina State University [website]. Raleigh (NC): North Carolina State University; 2008. (http://www.ncsu.edu/ncsu/design/cud/about_ud/about_ud.htm, accessed 10 July 2015).

168. Norway: Oslo's Common Principles of Universal Design 2014. In: World Health Organization, Age-friendly World [website]. Geneva: World Health Organization; 2015 (http://agefriendlyworld.org/en/the-common-principles-of-universal-design-city-of-oslo-2014/, accessed 3 July 2015).

169. Accessibility in the built environment. In: Building and Construction Authority [website]. Singapore: Singapore Government; 2014 (http://www.bca.gov.sg/barrierfree/barrierfree_buildings.html, accessed 1 July 2015).

170. Kegler MC, Escoffery C, Alcantara I, Ballard D, Glanz K. A qualitative examination of home and neighborhood environments for obesity prevention in rural adults. Int J Behav Nutr Phys Act. 2008;5(1):65.doi: http://dx.doi.org/10.1186/1479-5868-5-65 PMID: 19077210

171. Li F, Fisher J, Brownson RC. A multilevel analysis of change in neighborhood walking activity in older adults. J Aging Phys Act. 2005 Apr;13(2):145–59. PMID: 15995261

172. Rantakokko M, Törmäkangas T, Rantanen T, Haak M, Iwarsson S. Environmental barriers, person-environment fit and mortality among community-dwelling very old people. BMC Public Health. 2013;13(1):783.doi: http://dx.doi.org/10.1186/1471-2458-13-783 PMID: 23981906

173. Hong SI, Morrow-Howell N. Health outcomes of Experience Corps: a high-commitment volunteer program. Soc Sci Med. 2010 Jul;71(2):414–20.doi: http://dx.doi.org/10.1016/j.socscimed.2010.04.009 PMID: 20510493

174. Fried LP, Carlson MC, Freedman M, Frick KD, Glass TA, Hill J, et al. A social model for health promotion for an aging population: initial evidence on the Experience Corps model. J Urban Health. 2004 Mar;81(1):64–78.doi: http://dx.doi.org/10.1093/jurban/jth094 PMID: 15047786

175. Rebok GW, Carlson MC, Glass TA, McGill S, Hill J, Wasik BA, et al. Short-term impact of Experience Corps participation on children and schools: results from a pilot randomized trial. J Urban Health. 2004 Mar;81(1):79–93.doi: http://dx.doi.org/10.1093/jurban/jth095 PMID: 15047787

176. Fujiwara Y, Sakuma N, Ohba H, Nishi M, Lee S, Watanabe N, et al. REPRINTS: effects of an intergenerational health promotion program for older adults in Japan. J Intergener Relatsh. 2009;7(1):17–39. doi: http://dx.doi.org/10.1080/15350770802628901

177. Frick KD, Carlson MC, Glass TA, McGill S, Rebok GW, Simpson C, et al. Modeled cost-effectiveness of the Experience Corps Baltimore based on a pilot randomized trial. J Urban Health. 2004 Mar;81(1):106–17.doi: http://dx.doi.org/10.1093/jurban/jth097 PMID: 15047789

178. Carstensen LL. The influence of a sense of time on human development. Science. 2006 Jun 30;312(5782):1913–5.doi: http://dx.doi.org/10.1126/science.1127488 PMID: 16809530

179. Berkman LF, Glass T, Brissette I, Seeman TE. From social integration to health: Durkheim in the new millennium. Soc Sci Med. 2000 Sep;51(6):843–57.doi: http://dx.doi.org/10.1016/S0277-9536(00)00065-4 PMID: 10972429

180. Ramlagan S, Peltzer K, Phaswana-Mafuya N. Social capital and health among older adults in South Africa. BMC Geriatr. 2013;13(1):100.doi: http://dx.doi.org/10.1186/1471-2318-13-100 PMID: 24073666

181. Holt-Lunstad J, Smith TB, Layton JB. Social relationships and mortality risk: a meta-analytic review. PLoS Med. 2010 Jul;7(7):e1000316.doi: http://dx.doi.org/10.1371/journal.pmed.1000316 PMID: 20668659

182. Giles LC, Glonek GF, Luszcz MA, Andrews GR. Effect of social networks on 10 year survival in very old Australians: the Australian longitudinal study of aging. J Epidemiol Community Health. 2005 Jul;59(7):574–9.doi: http://dx.doi.org/10.1136/jech.2004.025429 PMID: 15965141

183. Mendes de Leon CF, Gold DT, Glass TA, Kaplan L, George LK. Disability as a function of social networks and support in elderly African Americans and Whites: the Duke EPESE 1986--1992. J Gerontol B Psychol Sci Soc Sci. 2001 May;56(3):S179–90.doi: http://dx.doi.org/10.1093/geronb/56.3.S179 PMID: 11316843

184. Mendes de Leon CF, Glass TA, Berkman LF. Social engagement and disability in a community population of older adults: the New Haven EPESE. Am J Epidemiol. 2003 Apr 1;157(7):633–42.doi: http://dx.doi.org/10.1093/aje/kwg028 PMID: 12672683

185. Cohen S. Psychosocial models of the role of social support in the etiology of physical disease. Health Psychol. 1988;7(3):269–97.doi: http://dx.doi.org/10.1037/0278-6133.7.3.269 PMID: 3289916

186. Nyqvist F, Forsman AK, Giuntoli G, Cattan M. Social capital as a resource for mental well-being in older people: a systematic review. Aging Ment Health. 2013;17(4):394–410.doi: http://dx.doi.org/10.1080/13607863.2012.742490 PMID: 23186534

187. Kawachi I, Subramanian S, Kim D, editors. Social capital and health. New York: Springer; 2008. doi: http://dx.doi.org/10.1007/978-0-387-71311-3

188. Silverstein M, Giarrusso R. Aging and family life: a decade review. J Marriage Fam. 2010 Oct;72(5):1039–58.doi: http://dx.doi.org/10.1111/j.1741-3737.2010.00749.x PMID: 22930600

189. Murayama H, Fujiwara Y, Kawachi I. Social capital and health: a review of prospective multilevel studies. J Epidemiol. 2012;22(3):179–87.doi: http://dx.doi.org/10.2188/jea.JE20110128 PMID: 22447212

190. Nyqvist F, Cattan M, Andersson L, Forsman AK, Gustafson Y. Social capital and loneliness among the very old living at home and in institutional settings: a comparative study. J Aging Health. 2013 Sep;25(6):1013–35.doi: http://dx.doi.org/10.1177/0898264313497508 PMID: 23988810

191. Litwin H, Stoeckel KJ, Roll A. Relationship status and depressive symptoms among older co-resident caregivers. Aging Ment Health. 2014 Mar;18(2):225–31.doi: http://dx.doi.org/10.1080/13607863.2013.837148 PMID: 24047262

192. Grandparents parenting. Charlottetown: Community legal information association; 2015 (http://www.cliapei.ca/sitefiles/File/publications/PLA17.pdf, accessed 27 July 2015).

193. De Jong Gierveld J, Keating N, Fast J. Determinants of loneliness among older adults in Canada. Can J Aging. 2015;34(2):125–36. doi: http://dx.doi.org/10.1017/S0714980815000070

194. de Jong Gierveld J, Keating N, Fast JE. Determinants of loneliness among older adults in Canada. Can J Aging. 2015 Jun;34(2):125–36.doi: http://dx.doi.org/10.1017/S0714980815000070 PMID: 25707297

195. Dickens AP, Richards SH, Greaves CJ, Campbell JL. Interventions targeting social isolation in older people: a systematic review. BMC Public Health. 2011;11(1):647.doi: http://dx.doi.org/10.1186/1471-2458-11-647 PMID: 21843337

196. Tilvis RS, Laitala V, Routasalo PE, Pitkälä KH. Suffering from loneliness indicates significant mortality risk of older people. J Aging Res. 2011; 2011:534781. PMID:21423600doi: http://dx.doi.org/10.4061/2011/534781

197. Cattan M, Hogg E, Hardill I. Improving quality of life in ageing populations: what can volunteering do? Maturitas. 2011 Dec;70(4):328–32.doi: http://dx.doi.org/10.1016/j.maturitas.2011.08.010 PMID: 21958942

198. Findlay RA. Interventions to reduce social isolation amongst older people: where is the evidence? Ageing Soc. 2003;23(05):647–58. doi: http://dx.doi.org/10.1017/S0144686X03001296

199. Health Quality Ontario. Social isolation in community-dwelling seniors: an evidence-based analysis. Ont Health Technol Assess Ser. 2008;8(5):1–49. PMID: 23074510

200. The telephone rings at 5 program. In: Ageing with pleasure [website]. Setúbal (Portugal): Envelhecer com praza; 2015 (http://en.envelhecer.org/index.php?/programs/in-domo-nostra/, accessed 1 July 2015).

201. Englehart T, Melo R, Ranville M. Ageing in place with age-friendly conference calls. In: 2nd International Conference on Age-friendly Cities [website]. Québec, Canada: 2nd International Conference on Age-friendly Cities; 2013 (http://www.afc2013.ca/docs/PrésentationsVADA/2C_TerryEnglehart.pdf, accessed 10 July 2015).

202. Senior center without walls. In: Senior Center without Walls; Episcopal Senior Communities [website]. Oakland (CA): Episcopal Senior Communities; 2015 (http://www.seniorcenterwithoutwalls.org/, accessed 1 July 2015).

203. Mick P, Kawachi I, Lin FR. The association between hearing loss and social isolation in older adults. Otolaryngol Head Neck Surg. 2014 Mar;150(3):378–84. PMID: 24384545

204. Cotten SR, Anderson W, McCullough B. The impact of ICT use on loneliness and contact with others among older adults. Gerontechnology (Valkenswaard). 2012;11(2):161. doi: http://dx.doi.org/10.4017/gt.2012.11.02.378.00

205. Heaven B, Brown LJ, White M, Errington L, Mathers JC, Moffatt S. Supporting well-being in retirement through meaningful social roles: systematic review of intervention studies. Milbank Q. 2013 Jun;91(2):222–87.doi: http://dx.doi.org/10.1111/milq.12013 PMID: 23758511

206. Haus MG. Bundesministerium für Familie, Senioren, Frauen und Jugend [website]. Berlin: Bundesministerium für Familie, Senioren, Frauen und Jugend; 2015. [Multigenerational centres]. (http://www.mehrgenerationenhaeuser.de, accessed 10 July 2015).

207. Forte D. Relationships. In: Cattan M, editor. Mental health and well being in later life. Maidenhead, England: University Press, McGraw-Hill Education; 2009:84–111. (http://www.mheducation.co.uk/9780335228928-emea-mental-health-and-well-being-in-later-life/, accessed 10 July 2015).

208. Le cyclopousse: un service de transport de proximité destiné aux seniors. [The "cyclopousse":a local transport service for older people.] In: AREFO [website]. Lyons: AREFO; 2015 (http://www.arefo.com/arefo-services/le-cyclopousse/, accessed 24 July 2015) (in French).

209. De Silva MJ, McKenzie K, Harpham T, Huttly SR. Social capital and mental illness: a systematic review. J Epidemiol Community Health. 2005 Aug;59(8):619–27.doi: http://dx.doi.org/10.1136/jech.2004.029678 PMID: 16020636

210. Leyden KM. Social capital and the built environment: the importance of walkable neighborhoods. Am J Public Health. 2003 Sep;93(9):1546–51.doi: http://dx.doi.org/10.2105/AJPH.93.9.1546 PMID: 12948978

211. Ysseldyk R, Haslam SA, Haslam C. Abide with me: religious group identification among older adults promotes health and well-being by maintaining multiple group memberships. Aging Ment Health. 2013;17(7):869–79.doi: http://dx.doi.org/10.1080/13607863.2013.799120 PMID: 23711247

212. Senior City courses and workshops.[Cours et ateliers de Cité Seniors.] In: Ville de Genève [website]. Geneva: Ville de Genève; 2015 (http://www.ville-geneve.ch/themes/social/seniors/cite-seniors/cours-ateliers/, accessed 1 July 2015).

213. Russell C, Campbell A, Hughes I. Ageing, social capital and the Internet: findings from an exploratory study of Australian 'silver surfers'. Australas J Ageing. 2008 Jun;27(2):78–82.doi: http://dx.doi.org/10.1111/j.1741-6612.2008.00284.x PMID: 18713197

214. Rosso AL, Taylor JA, Tabb LP, Michael YL. Mobility, disability, and social engagement in older adults. J Aging Health. 2013 Jun;25(4):617–37.doi: http://dx.doi.org/10.1177/0898264313482489 PMID: 23548944

215. Choi NG, Dinitto DM. Internet use among older adults: association with health needs, psychological capital, and social capital. J Med Internet Res. 2013;15(5):e97.doi: http://dx.doi.org/10.2196/jmir.2333 PMID: 23681083

216. Veerle M. Cooking, caring and volunteering: unpaid work around the world. Paris: OECD Publishing; 2011 (OECD social, employment and migration working papers No. 116; http://www.oecd.org/officialdocuments/publicdisplaydocumentpdf/?cote=DELSA/ELSA/WD/SEM(2011)1&doclanguage=en, accessed 25 July 2015).

217. Maimaris W, Hogan H, Lock K. The impact of working beyond traditional retirement ages on mental health: implications for public health and welfare policy. Public Health Rev. 2010;31(2):532–48 (http://www.publichealthreviews.eu/upload/pdf_files/8/PHR_32_2_Maimaris.pdf, accessed 10 July 2015).

218. Kajitani S. Working in old age and health outcomes in Japan. Japan World Econ. 2011;23(3):153–62. doi: http://dx.doi.org/10.1016/j.japwor.2011.06.001

219. Calvo E, Haverstick K, Sass SA. Gradual retirement, sense of control, and retirees' happiness. Res Aging. 2009;31(1):112–35. doi: http://dx.doi.org/10.1177/0164027508324704

220. Aleksandrowicz P, Fasang A, Schömann K, Staudinger UM. Die Bedeutung der Arbeit beim vorzeitigen Ausscheiden aus dem Arbeitsleben. [The meaning of work at early retirement]. Z Gerontol Geriatr. 2010 Oct;43(5):324–9. PMID:19806292 (in German). doi: http://dx.doi.org/10.1007/s00391-009-0068-y

221. Decent work. In: International Labour Organization [website]. Geneva: International Labour Organization; 2015 (http://www.ilo.org/global/topics/decent-work/lang--en/index.htm, accessed 24 July 2015).

222. Thoits PA, Hewitt LN. Volunteer work and well-being. J Health Soc Behav. 2001 Jun;42(2):115–31.doi: http://dx.doi.org/10.2307/3090173 PMID: 11467248

223. Hao Y. Productive activities and psychological well-being among older adults. J Gerontol B Psychol Sci Soc Sci. 2008 Mar;63(2):S64–72.doi: http://dx.doi.org/10.1093/geronb/63.2.S64 PMID: 18441271

224. Greenfield EA. Felt obligation to help others as a protective factor against losses in psychological well-being following functional decline in middle and later life. J Gerontol B Psychol Sci Soc Sci. 2009 Nov;64(6):723–32.doi: http://dx.doi.org/10.1093/geronb/gbp074 PMID: 19825942

225. Brown SL, Brown RM, House JS, Smith DM. Coping with spousal loss: potential buffering effects of self-reported helping behavior. Pers Soc Psychol Bull. 2008 Jun;34(6):849–61.doi: http://dx.doi.org/10.1177/0146167208314972 PMID: 18344495

226. Piliavin JA, Siegl E. Health benefits of volunteering in the Wisconsin longitudinal study. J Health Soc Behav. 2007 Dec;48(4):450–64.doi: http://dx.doi.org/10.1177/002214650704800408 PMID: 18198690

227. Morrow-Howell N. Volunteering in later life: research frontiers. J Gerontol B Psychol Sci Soc Sci. 2010 Jul;65(4):461–9.doi: http://dx.doi.org/10.1093/geronb/gbq024 PMID: 20400498

228. Morrow-Howell N. Civic service across the life course. Generations. 2007;30:37–42.

229. Luoh MC, Herzog AR. Individual consequences of volunteer and paid work in old age: health and mortality. J Health Soc Behav. 2002 Dec;43(4):490–509.doi: http://dx.doi.org/10.2307/3090239 PMID: 12664678

230. Kumar S, Calvo R, Avendano M, Sivaramakrishnan K, Berkman LF. Social support, volunteering and health around the world: cross-national evidence from 139 countries. Soc Sci Med. 2012 Mar;74(5):696–706.doi: http://dx.doi.org/http://dx.doi.org/10.1016/j.socscimed.2011.11.017 PMID: 22305947

231. Burr JA, Tavares J, Mutchler JE. Volunteering and hypertension risk in later life. J Aging Health. 2011 Feb;23(1):24–51.doi: http://dx.doi.org/10.1177/0898264310388272 PMID: 20971920

232. Fried LP, Carlson MC, Freedman M, Frick KD, Glass TA, Hill J, et al. A social model for health promotion for an aging population: initial evidence on the Experience Corps model. J Urban Health. 2004 Mar;81(1):64–78.doi: http://dx.doi.org/10.1093/jurban/jth094 PMID: 15047786

233. Carlson MC, Helms MJ, Steffens DC, Burke JR, Potter GG, Plassman BL. Midlife activity predicts risk of dementia in older male twin pairs. Alzheimers Dement. 2008 Sep;4(5):324–31.doi: http://dx.doi.org/10.1016/j.jalz.2008.07.002 PMID: 18790459

234. McDonnall MC. The effect of productive activities on depressive symptoms among older adults with dual sensory loss. Res Aging. 2011 May;33(3):234–55.doi: http://dx.doi.org/10.1177/0164027511399106 PMID: 21686087

235. Kim J, Pai M. Volunteering and trajectories of depression. J Aging Health. 2010 Feb;22(1):84–105.doi: http://dx.doi.org/10.1177/0898264309351310 PMID: 19920207

236. Kahana E, Bhatta T, Lovegreen LD, Kahana B, Midlarsky E. Altruism, helping, and volunteering: pathways to well-being in late life. J Aging Health. 2013 Feb;25(1):159–87.doi: http://dx.doi.org/10.1177/0898264312469665 PMID: 23324536

237. Baker L, Cahalin L, Gerst K, Burr J. Productive activities and subjective well-being among older adults: the influence of number of activities and time commitment. Soc Indic Res. 2005;73(3):431–58. doi: http://dx.doi.org/10.1007/s11205-005-0805-6

238. Cattan M, Hogg E, Hardill I. Improving quality of life in ageing populations: what can volunteering do? Maturitas. 2011 Dec;70(4):328–32.doi: http://dx.doi.org/10.1016/j.maturitas.2011.08.010 PMID: 21958942

239. Bowen C, Staudinger UM. Images of aging in the workplace moderate age differences in promotion orientation. Gerontologist. 2010;50:79.

240. Burtless G. The impact of population aging and delayed retirement on workforce productivity. Chestnut Hill (MA): Center for Retirement Research at Boston College; 2013 (http://crr.bc.edu/working-papers/the-impact-of-population-aging-and-delayed-retirement-on-workforce-productivity/, accessed 10 July 2015).

241. Macarthur Foundation Research Network on an Aging Society. Facts and fictions about an aging America. Contexts. 2009;8(4):16–21. doi: http://dx.doi.org/10.1525/ctx.2009.8.4.16

242. Wacker RR, Roberto KA. Aging social policies: an international perspective. Thousand Oaks (CA): Sage Publications; 2011. (https://us.sagepub.com/en-us/nam/aging-social-policies/book229325, accessed 10 July 2015).

243. Allan LJ, Johnson JA. Undergraduate attitudes toward the elderly: the role of knowledge, contact and aging anxiety. Educ Gerontol. 2008;35(1):1–14. doi: http://dx.doi.org/http://dx.doi.org/10.1080/03601270802299780

244. Malinen S, Johnston L. Workplace ageism: discovering hidden bias. Exp Aging Res. 2013;39(4):445–65.doi: http://dx.doi.org/http://dx.doi.org/10.1080/0361073X.2013.808111 PMID: 23875840

245. Ragan AM, Bowen AM. Improving attitudes regarding the elderly population: the effects of information and reinforcement for change. Gerontologist. 2001 Aug;41(4):511–5.doi: http://dx.doi.org/http://dx.doi.org/10.1093/geront/41.4.511 PMID: 11490049

246. European Union. Council directive 2000/78/EC of 27 November 2000 establishing a general framework for equal treatment in employment and occupation. Brussels: Council of the European Union; 2000 (http://eur-lex.europa.eu/legal-content/EN/TXT/?uri=CELEX:32000L0078, accessed 10 July 2015).

247. Sonnet A, Olsen H, Manfredi T. Towards more inclusive ageing and employment policies: the lessons from France, the Netherlands, Norway and Switzerland. Economist. 2014;162(4):315–39. doi: http://dx.doi.org/http://dx.doi.org/10.1007/s10645-014-9240-x

248. Staudinger U, Finkelstein R, Calvo E, Sivaramakrishnan K. Ageing, work, and health. Gerontologist. 2016. (In press).

249. OECD employment outlook 2013. Paris: OECD Publishing; 2013 doi: http://dx.doi.org/http://dx.doi.org/10.1787/empl_outlook-2013-en doi: http://dx.doi.org/10.1787/empl_outlook-2013-en

250. Promoting longer working lives through pension reforms. First part: flexibility in retirement age provision. Brussels: European Commission, Social Protection Committee; 2007 (http://ec.europa.eu/social/BlobServlet?docId=745&langId=en, accessed 20 July 2015).

251. The SunAmerica Retirement Re-Set Study: redefining retirement post recession. Los Angeles: SunAmerica Financial Group; 2011 (http://www.agewave.com/research/retirementresetreport.pdf, accessed 4 June 2015).

252. Fairlie RW. Kauffman Index of Entrepreneurial Activity 1996–2012. Kansas City (MO): Ewing Marion Kauffman Foundation; 2013 (http://www.kauffman.org/~/media/kauffman_org/research%20reports%20and%20covers/2013/04/kiea_2013_report.pdf, accessed 10 July 2015).

253. Sundén A. The Swedish experience with pension reform. Oxf Rev Econ Policy. 2006;22(1):133–48. doi: http://dx.doi.org/10.1093/oxrep/grj009

254. Naegele GWA. A guide to good practice in age management. Luxembourg: European Foundation for the Improvement of Living and Working Conditions; 2006 (http://www.ageingatwork.eu/resources/a-guide-to-good-practice-in-age-management.pdf, accessed 10 July 2015).

255. Heckman JJ. Policies to foster human capital. Res Econ. 2000;54(1):3–56.

256. Pavlova M, Maclean R. Reskilling for all? The changing role of TVET in the ageing societies of developing countries. In: Karmel T, Maclean R, editors. Technical and vocational education and training in an ageing society: expert meeting proceedings. Adelaide: National Centre for Vocational Education Research; 2007:2401–15.

257. Munnell AH, Sass SA. Working longer: the solution to the retirement income challenge. Washington (DC): Brookings Institution Press; 2008 (http://www.brookings.edu/research/books/2008/workinglonger, accessed 10 July 2015).

258. Staudinger UM, Bowen CE. A systemic approach to aging in the work context. Zeitschrift für Arbeitsmarktforschung. 2011;44(4):295–306.

259. Bowen C, Staudinger UM. Age moderates the relationship between job satisfaction and performance. Gerontologist. 2012;52:2–3.

260. Tang F, Choi E, Morrow-Howell N. Organizational support and volunteering benefits for older adults. Gerontologist. 2010 Oct;50(5):603–12.doi: http://dx.doi.org/10.1093/geront/gnq020 PMID: 20211944

261. Tang F. What resources are needed for volunteerism? A life course perspective. J Appl Gerontol. 2006;25:375–90. doi: http://dx.doi.org/10.1177/0733464806292858

262. Hank K, Erlinghagen M. Dynamics of volunteering in older Europeans. Gerontologist. 2010 Apr;50(2):170–8.doi: http://dx.doi.org/10.1093/geront/gnp122 PMID: 19666783

263. Gray E, Khoo S-E, Reimondos A. Participation in different types of volunteering at young, middle and older adulthood. J Popul Res. 2012;29(4):373–98. doi: http://dx.doi.org/10.1007/s12546-012-9092-7

264. Butrica BA, Johnson RW, Zedlewski SR. Volunteer dynamics of older Americans. J Gerontol B Psychol Sci Soc Sci. 2009 Sep;64(5):644–55.doi: http://dx.doi.org/10.1093/geronb/gbn042 PMID: 19213847

265. Okun MA, Schultz A. Age and motives for volunteering: testing hypotheses derived from socioemotional selectivity theory. Psychol Aging. 2003 Jun;18(2):231–9.doi: http://dx.doi.org/10.1037/0882-7974.18.2.231 PMID: 12825773

266. Omoto AM, Snyder M, Martino SC. Volunteerism and the life course: investigating age-related agendas for action. Basic Appl Soc Psych. 2000;22:181–97. doi: http://dx.doi.org/10.1207/S15324834BASP2203_6

267. Boezeman EJ, Ellemers N. Intrinsic need satisfaction and the job attitudes of volunteers versus employees working in a charitable volunteer organization. J Occup Organ Psychol. 2009;82(4):897–914. doi: http://dx.doi.org/10.1348/096317908X383742

268. Clary EG, Snyder M, Ridge RD, Copeland J, Stukas AA, Haugen J, et al. Understanding and assessing the motivations of volunteers: a functional approach. J Pers Soc Psychol. 1998 Jun;74(6):1516–30.doi: http://dx.doi.org/10.1037/0022-3514.74.6.1516 PMID: 9654757

269. McBride ME, Huddleston CB, Balzer DT, Goel D, Gazit AZ. Hypoplastic left heart associated with scimitar syndrome. Pediatr Cardiol. 2009 Oct;30(7):1037–8.doi: http://dx.doi.org/10.1007/s00246-009-9479-1 PMID: 19495846

270. Musick MA, Wilson J. Volunteers: a social profile. Bloomington (IN): Indiana University Press; 2008 (http://www.iupress.indiana.edu/product_info.php?products_id=41769, accessed 10 July 2015).

271. America's senior volunteers. Washington (DC): Independent Sector; 2000 (https://www.independentsector.org/uploads/Resources/americas_senior_volunteers.pdf, accessed 10 July 2015).

272. McMunn A, Nazroo J, Wahrendorf M, Breeze E, Zaninotto P. Participation in socially-productive activities, reciprocity and wellbeing in later life: baseline results in England. Ageing Soc. 2009;29(05):765. doi: http://dx.doi.org/10.1017/S0144686X08008350

273. Closing the health equity gap: policy options and opportunities for action. Geneva: World Health Organization; 2013 (http://apps.who.int/iris/handle/10665/78335, accessed 20 July 2015).

274. Freiler A, Muntaner C, Shankardass K, Mah CL, Molnar A, Renahy E, et al. Glossary for the implementation of Health in All Policies (HiAP). J Epidemiol Community Health. 2013 Dec 1;67(12):1068–72.doi: http://dx.doi.org/10.1136/jech-2013-202731 PMID: 23986493

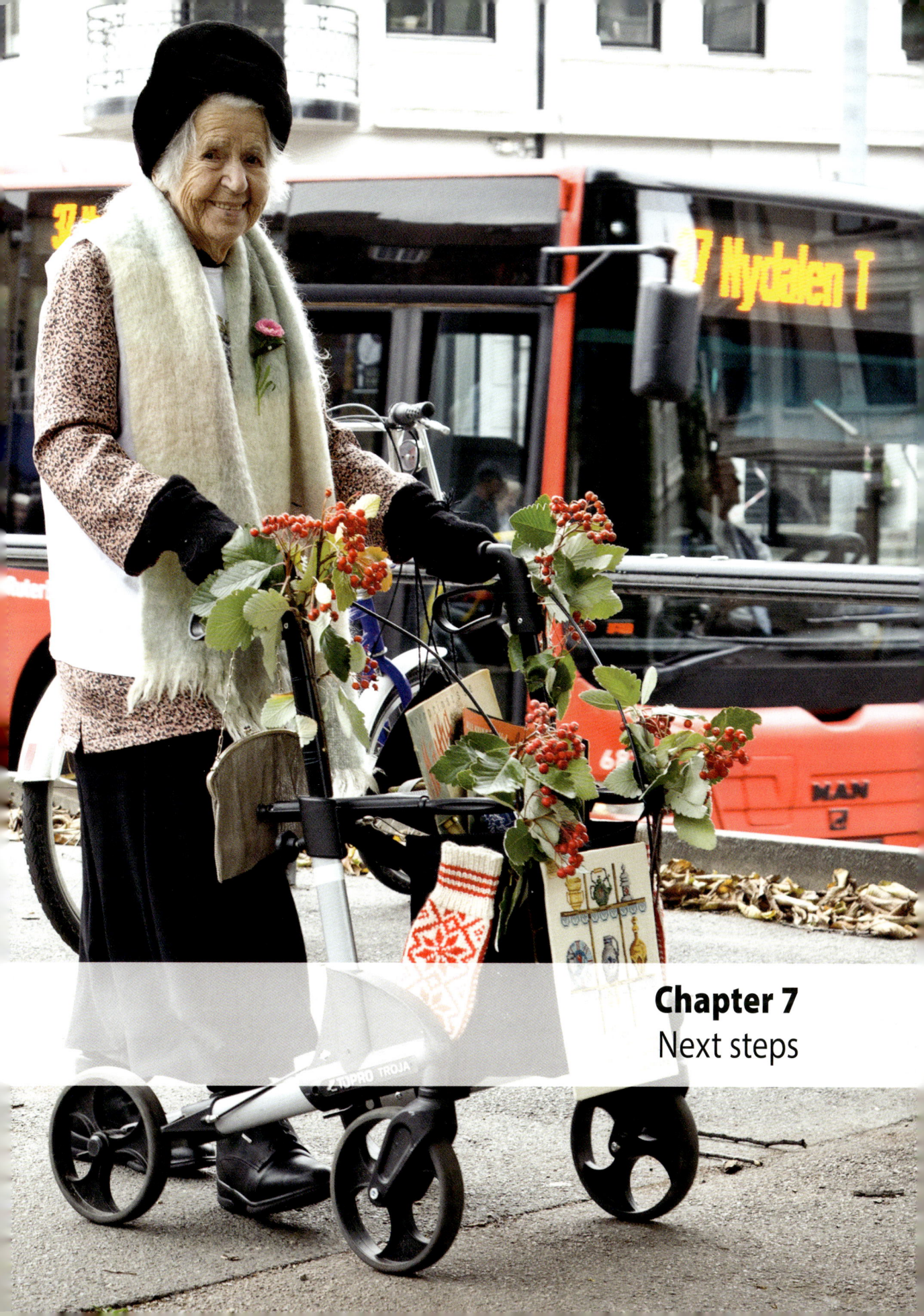

Chapter 7
Next steps

Ruth, 101, Norway

Ruth has been a regular participant in the Oslo "Walker Rally" . The annual event, organized by the City of Oslo in collaboration with non-government organizations and the Council for Senior Citizens, celebrates Healthy Ageing with a focus on accessibility, participation, volunteering and different generations working together.

Older people with walking sticks, walkers and wheelchairs take the centre stage with prizes awarded for the best decorated walker as well as the distance travelled.

"Staying active makes me forget about my back pains!" says Ruth who still lives at home at the age of 101 and praises her local day care centre for organising activities that help her stay active and socially connected.

7

Next steps

Introduction

Comprehensive public-health action on ageing is urgently needed. Although there are major knowledge gaps, we have sufficient evidence to act now, and there are things that every country can do, irrespective of their current situation or level of development.

The first step will be to focus on optimizing functional ability: the goal of *Healthy Ageing*. For individuals, this will require policies, systems and services that can optimize trajectories of ability across the life course. At a population level, strategies will need to look not just to raise overall levels of ability but also to narrow the distribution of ability by paying particular attention to those with the least resources or lowest level of functional ability.

Key opportunities for taking public-health action are outlined in Fig. 7.1, which builds on the public-health framework for *Healthy Ageing* described in Fig. 2.4. As described in Chapter 2, fostering the functional ability that enables well-being in older age requires strategies aimed at building and maintaining intrinsic capacity across the life course. But action will also be needed to enable older people to be and to do what they have reason to value, regardless of their level of capacity.

Chapters 4–6 have outlined many actions that can help achieve this. Choosing which of these are most appropriate or urgent, and how they are implemented, will vary according to the context. Although the health needs of older people are fairly consistent the world over, the preparedness to meet them varies among and within countries. One important consideration is a country's level of socioeconomic development. However, even among countries with similar resource levels there is great variation in how the needs of older people are currently met. For example, although many high-income countries provide universally affordable health care, the provision and financing of long-term care in these same settings varies considerably. In some it is sustainably financed through universal risk-pooling, but in others it remains the responsibility of individuals and their families, with the associated risks that have been highlighted in this report.

Thus, each country or region needs to assess its current situation and what is likely to work in its context before mapping the specific next steps that will be most appropriate.

Fig. 7.1. Opportunities for taking public-health action to ensure *Healthy Ageing*

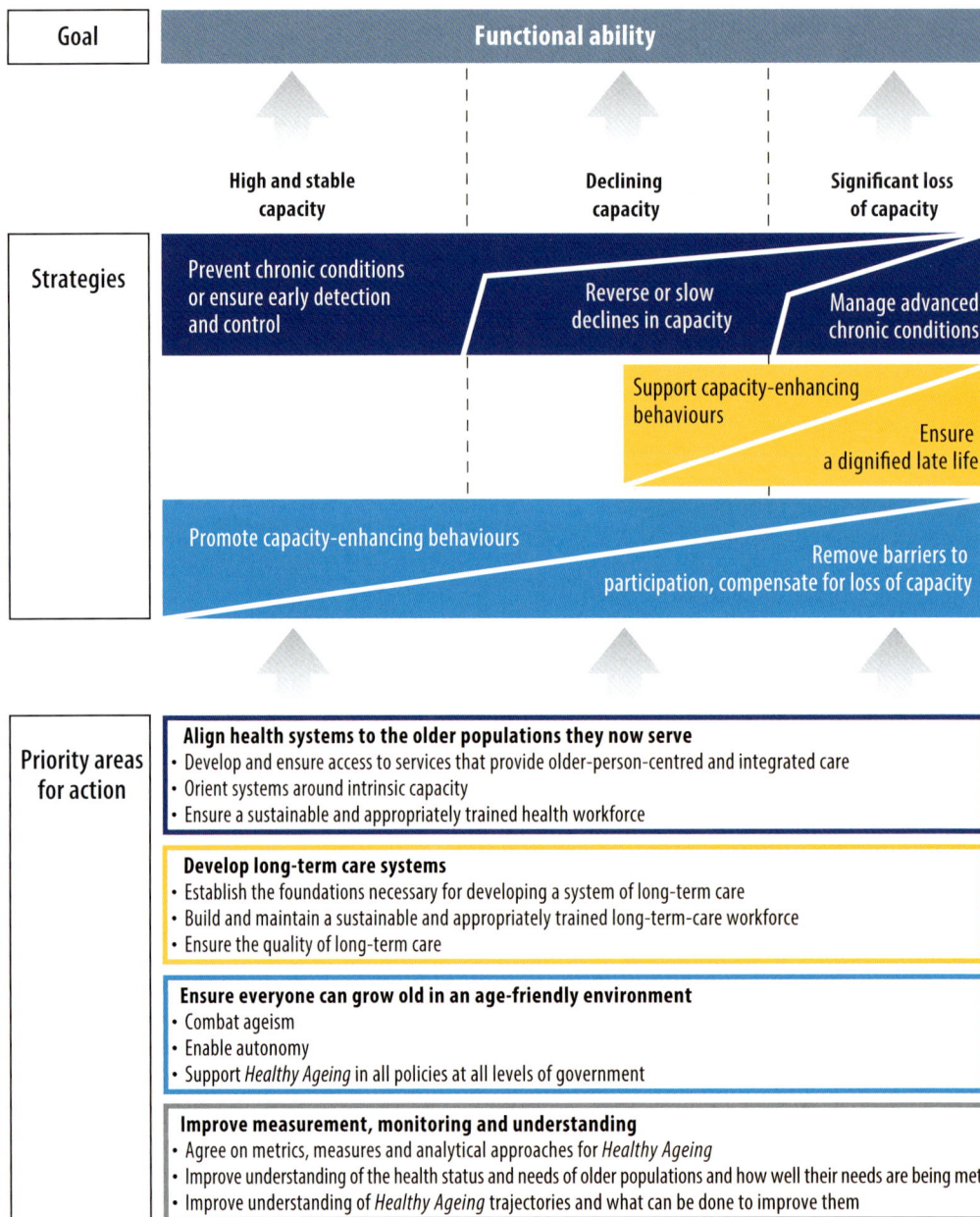

Goal	**Functional ability**

High and stable capacity | Declining capacity | Significant loss of capacity

Strategies

Prevent chronic conditions or ensure early detection and control

Reverse or slow declines in capacity

Manage advanced chronic conditions

Support capacity-enhancing behaviours

Ensure a dignified late life

Promote capacity-enhancing behaviours

Remove barriers to participation, compensate for loss of capacity

Priority areas for action

Align health systems to the older populations they now serve
- Develop and ensure access to services that provide older-person-centred and integrated care
- Orient systems around intrinsic capacity
- Ensure a sustainable and appropriately trained health workforce

Develop long-term care systems
- Establish the foundations necessary for developing a system of long-term care
- Build and maintain a sustainable and appropriately trained long-term-care workforce
- Ensure the quality of long-term care

Ensure everyone can grow old in an age-friendly environment
- Combat ageism
- Enable autonomy
- Support *Healthy Ageing* in all policies at all levels of government

Improve measurement, monitoring and understanding
- Agree on metrics, measures and analytical approaches for *Healthy Ageing*
- Improve understanding of the health status and needs of older populations and how well their needs are being met
- Improve understanding of *Healthy Ageing* trajectories and what can be done to improve them

However, four priority areas for action can be identified:

1. aligning health systems with the needs of the older populations they now serve;
2. developing systems for providing long-term care;
3. creating age-friendly environments;
4. improving measurement, monitoring and understanding.

The first three of these points mirror the focus of Chapters 4–6 of this report. The fourth priority reflects the stark gaps in knowledge that confront decision-makers and the urgent need to fill them.

Taking action in these four areas can help ensure that *Healthy Ageing* becomes a possibility for all older people, no matter what their level of capacity. But this will also require attention to the three different subpopulations of older people described in Chapter 2. For those with relatively high and stable capacity, the key objectives will be to breakdown the barriers that limit participation, to facilitate capacity-enhancing behaviours and self-care, and to prevent chronic conditions as well as to ensure their early detection and effective control. For those with declining capacity, the objectives extend to reversing declines, preventing further declines and enabling functional ability despite these decrements. For those with, or at high risk of, a significant loss of capacity, the objectives shift to a greater focus on enabling them to live with dignity and providing them with the health services to manage advanced chronic conditions. These subgroups are not rigid, nor do they cover the course of every older person's life. However, if the needs of these subgroups are addressed, most older people will find their functional ability enhanced.

Some of the key areas for action for achieving these outcomes are described in more detail below. Shortly after the release of this report, WHO will be working with its Member States to develop a global strategy and action plan on ageing and health. The strategy will draw on this report and other sources to identify global priorities for action and to identify the groups responsible for their implementation.

How action might be financed will vary among settings. Some may be financed by adapting current services to the changing demographic and epidemiological contexts. However, ensuring access to universal coverage for health care and long-term care is still a distant ambition in many countries. In these settings, concrete steps need to be taken and investments made to ensure that all older people have access to needed services – prevention, health promotion, treatment, rehabilitation and long-term care – without the risk of the associated financial hardship that may affect them or their families. Where this cannot be achieved immediately for the whole population, the initial target should be those with the greatest needs and with the least resources to meet their needs. Where countries are limited by resource constraints, some of the key areas for action, particularly those requiring technical assistance and capacity-building, can be included within the framework of international cooperation.

Key areas for action on *Healthy Ageing*

Align health systems to the needs of the older populations they now serve

As people age, their health-care needs tend to become more chronic and complex. Responding to these needs requires integrated care built around a common goal of optimizing trajectories of functional ability, with a specific focus on maximizing intrinsic capacity. Yet many existing services were designed to cure acute conditions or symptoms; health issues are often managed in a disconnected and fragmented manner; and coordination is frequently lacking across care providers, settings and time.

Transforming health systems from these outdated approaches requires action on several fronts. The following three approaches are crucial if alignment is to be achieved:

1. develop and ensure access to services that provide older-person-centred care;
2. orient systems around intrinsic capacity;
3. ensure a sustainable and appropriately trained workforce.

Develop and ensure access to services that provide older-person-centred and integrated care

The best way to reorient health systems towards achieving the goal of optimizing functional ability is by placing older people at the centre of service delivery. Practically, this means that systems are organized around older people's needs and preferences, and that services are age-friendly and coordinate closely with the older person and, when agreed and appropriate, with family and community members. Although the mix of strategies may vary, integration is crucial both among levels and across services, as well as between health care and long-term care services (Box 7.1). Key actions to take to achieve older-person-centred and integrated care include:

- ensuring that all older people are given a comprehensive assessment and have a single service-wide care plan that looks to optimize their capacity;
- developing services that are situated as close as possible to where older people live, including delivering services in their homes and providing community-based care;
- creating service structures that foster care by multidisciplinary teams;
- supporting older people to self-manage by providing peer support, training, information and advice;
- ensuring the availability of the medical products, vaccines and technologies that are necessary to optimize their capacity.

Orient systems around intrinsic capacity

If a health system is truly aligned with the needs of older populations, all its components will have a primary focus on intrinsic capacity. This orientation requires a significant transformation of the current systems that underpin service delivery. This might include changing the health and administrative information that the systems collect, the things they report, the way performance is monitored, the financing mechanisms and the incentives that are put in place, the training they offer and the behaviours they reward. Several actions are likely to assist this transformation:

- adapting information systems to collect, analyse and report data on intrinsic capacity;
- adapting performance monitoring, rewards and financing mechanisms to encourage care that optimizes capacity;

Box 7.1. Teams supporting ageing in place in Singapore

The Alexandra Health System in Singapore uses a comprehensive ageing-in-place programme to reduce avoidable hospital admissions and to improve the quality of life of older people. Older people who have a high utilization of hospital services (including care in the emergency department) receive home visits from a community nurse to review their needs and determine which of them may be unmet, develop a care plan and coordinate necessary follow-up (1).

Depending on a person's needs, follow-up visits might be conducted by nurses, physiotherapists, pharmacists, dietitians, occupational therapists or other community partners. For example, community nurses might teach an older person how to use a blood glucose monitoring kit; physiotherapists might teach simple strengthening exercises to foster independence; and pharmacists might review medications. The frequency of visits depends on a person's needs.

Through this approach, the health system has reduced hospital admissions by 67% and optimized the use of hospital resources.

- creating clinical guidelines to optimize trajectories of intrinsic capacity and updating existing guidelines so that their impact on capacity is clear.

Ensure a sustainable and appropriately trained health workforce

Ensuring a sustainable and appropriately trained health workforce for the 21st century will require careful consideration of the human resources that will be needed to deliver older-person-centred and integrated care. It will be important to ensure that service providers have basic gerontological and geriatric skills, as well as the more general competencies needed to work in integrated systems, including communication, teamwork, ICT and other technologies. But strategies should not be limited to current delineations of the workforce. Key actions that might be taken include:

- providing basic training about geriatric and gerontological issues during preservice training and in continuing professional development courses for all health professionals;
- including core geriatric and gerontological competencies in all health curricula;
- ensuring that the supply of geriatricians meets population need, and encouraging the development of geriatric units for the management of complex cases;
- considering the need for new workforce cadres (such as care coordinators and self-management counsellors) and extending the roles of existing staff, such as community health workers, to coordinate the health care of older people at the community level.

Develop systems for providing long-term care

In the 21st century, no country can afford not to have an integrated system of long-term care. In high-income countries, the challenges to achieving such a system are likely to revolve around the need to improve the quality of long-term care, develop financially sustainable ways to provide it to all who need it, and to better integrate it with health systems.

In low- and middle-income countries, the challenge may be to build a system where one does not already exist. In these settings, the responsibility for long-term care has often been left entirely to families. Socioeconomic development, population ageing and the changing roles of women mean that this practice is no longer sustainable or equitable.

Regardless of the setting, comprehensive systems of long-term care will be essential to meet the needs of older people, reduce inappropriate dependence on acute health services, help families avoid catastrophic care expenditures, and free women to play broader social roles. The central goal of these systems should be to maintain a level of functional ability in older people who have or who are at high risk of significant losses of capacity, and to ensure that this care is consistent with their basic rights, fundamental freedoms and human dignity. This includes acknowledging their continuing aspirations to well-being and respect.

Only governments can create and oversee these systems. But that does not mean long-term care is solely the responsibility of governments. Although the appropriate system for each country or setting will be different, it must be based on an explicit partnership with families, communities, other care providers and the private sector. The role of government (often implemented through ministries of health) will be to steward this partnership, train and support caregivers, ensure that integration occurs across various services (including the health sector), ensure the quality of services and directly provide services to those most in need (either because of their low intrinsic capacity or their socioeconomic status). These goals are achievable even for countries that are the most resource-constrained. Indeed, in these settings innovative action is already taking place (Box 7.2).

Box 7.2.   AgeWell: community based peer-to-peer support in Cape Town, South Africa

Older people can be an ageing community's greatest resource, drawing on their own experiences to identify and respond to issues faced by other older people. This is the premise of AgeWell, a pilot project to develop community-based peer-to-peer support in Cape Town, South Africa.

To improve the health and well-being of older people in Khayelitsha – South Africa's largest township and one of the poorest areas of Cape Town – 28 older community members were trained as peer supporters. Working in pairs, they made home visits to 211 older people in their community. The visits aimed to foster companionship and social support, and generate a sense of community; they were also used to identify health and social needs. Where needs were identified, older people were referred to health-care providers or social services.

Referrals were generated using a smartphone loaded with a screening instrument that included basic questions in addition to the observations made by the peer supporters during the home visit. The peer supporters became an important link between peers and community services.

A study assessed the benefits of this pilot project, and found that there were multiple benefits.

Older people who received home visits showed significant improvements. There was a 60% improvement in scores on measures of well-being; mean scores of satisfaction with social support improved by 50% over the study period. Peer supporters also reported their own health benefits while participating in the programme, including improved flexibility, agility, stamina, better sleep and decreased stress levels.

Older people's ability to meet their basic needs was enhanced. Peer supporters had greater financial security because they were paid a salary comparable to government-employed community health workers for 20 hours per week. Facilitating older people's access to community-based health and social services enabled them to meet their basic needs for health and social care. Referrals from AgeWell were credited with an increase in the use of clinic services, from 30 older clients to 200 during the study period.

Peer supporters' abilities to learn, grow and make decisions were enhanced through the training offered to them. They demonstrated improved self-esteem and self-efficacy, and a renewed sense of purpose and hope that were attributed to the training. They also described feeling a sense of empowerment and excitement about learning to use technology, such as smartphones and social media.

Older people's abilities to build and maintain relationships were strengthened, both for the peer supporters and the clients whom they visited. Membership in the local senior club tripled due to increased participation by AgeWell clients. Peer supporters reported feeling more connected to one another and their community, and that they had created stronger bonds with their neighbours, friends and other community members. They reported no longer feeling "isolated" and "alone" and saw their fellow peer supporters as "family" and clients as "friends".

The programme also enhanced older people's ability to contribute to their communities. Findings from focus groups of peer supporters demonstrated that the programme afforded a level of empowerment that stemmed from learning new skills and helping others. Becoming economically active again was described by many as "life-changing".

Source: M Besser and S Rohde; World Health Organization, Kobe Centre; Case study in South Africa: AgeWell, a peer-support service in a community setting to improve well-being and health among older persons living in a peri-urban township of Cape Town; 2015; unpublished data.

Three approaches will be crucial to realizing an accessible system of long-term care:
1. establish the foundations necessary for a system of long-term care;
2. build and maintain a sustainable and appropriately trained workforce;
3. ensure the quality of long-term care.

Establish the foundations necessary for developing a system of long-term care

Building an integrated system of long-term care that is oriented around enabling older people's ability requires a governance structure that can guide and oversee the system's development and clearly assign responsibility for progress.

Designing the system to fit the social, cultural and economic environments will be helped by a transparent process that draws on the knowledge and experience of older people, caregivers and researchers, considers current approaches, and assesses their strengths and weaknesses. This process can help define the key services and roles that are required, the barriers that may exist, who is best placed to deliver services, and who might best fill other roles, such as training and accreditation. A key focus should be on developing the system in ways that help older people to age in a place that is right for them and to maintain connections with their community and social networks. Ensuring access to this care, while reducing the risk that recipients or their caregivers incur financial hardship, will require adequate resources and a commitment to prioritizing support for those with the greatest health and financial needs.

Key actions that might be taken include:

- recognizing long-term care as an important public good;
- assigning clear responsibility for the development of a system of long-term care and planning how this will be achieved;
- creating equitable and sustainable mechanisms for financing care;
- defining the roles of government and developing the services that will be necessary to fulfil them.

Build and maintain a sustainable and appropriately trained long-term-care workforce

As with health systems, it will be crucial to develop a sustainable and appropriately trained workforce to provide long-term care. Many of the actions outlined in relation to health systems, will also be relevant for paid long-term caregivers. However, the field of long-term care has traditionally been undervalued. A crucial strategy for ensuring a sustainable workforce in the future will be to provide paid caregivers with the status and recognition that their contributions deserve.

Furthermore, unlike the health system, the majority of caregivers in the long-term-care system are currently family members, volunteers, members of community organizations, or paid but untrained workers. Most of them are women. Providing the training that allows them to do their job well, while relieving them of the stress that arises from being insufficiently informed about how to cope with challenging situations, will be central to building a long-term-care system. Providing concrete support to family caregivers by offering respite care or cash payments may also ease their load. It will be important also to look at how the responsibility for caregiving can be shared more equitably between the sexes and generations.

Exciting opportunities are arising in low- and middle-income countries from the empowerment of older volunteers in the form of older people's associations or organizations that advocate for the rights of older people and provide the care and support they may need. These concepts may be transferable to higher-income settings.

Key actions that can help build and maintain a sustainable and appropriately trained long-term-care workforce include:

- improving their salaries and working conditions and creating career pathways to allow them to advance to positions of increased responsibility and remuneration;
- enacting legislation supporting flexible working arrangements or leaves of absence for family caregivers;
- establishing support mechanisms for caregivers, such as offering respite care and accessible training or information resources;
- raising awareness of the value and rewards of caregiving, and combating social norms and roles that prevent men and young people from acting as caregivers;
- supporting community initiatives that bring older people together to act as a resource for caregiving and other community-development activities.

Ensure the quality of long-term care

The first step in ensuring the quality of long-term care is to orient services towards the goal of optimizing functional ability. This requires systems and caregivers to look at how they can optimize both the older person's trajectory of capacity, and compensate for a loss of capacity, by providing the care and transforming environments that help the older person to maintain functional ability at a level that ensures well-being. Coordination both across the system of long-term care and with health services will be essential if this is to be achieved. Quality-management systems can help maintain this coordinated focus on ability.

Key actions that can help achieve this include:

▪ developing and disseminating care protocols or guidelines that address key issues;
▪ establishing accreditation mechanisms for services and professional caregivers;
▪ establishing formal mechanisms for care coordination (including between long-term care and health-care services);
▪ establishing quality-management systems to help ensure that the focus on optimizing functional ability is maintained.

Creating age-friendly environments

Physical and social environments are powerful influences on *Healthy Ageing*. They shape trajectories of capacity and can extend what a person is able to do (their functional ability). Age-friendly environments allow older people to be and to do what they have reason to value by enabling them to maximize both their capacity and their ability.

Creating environments that are truly age-friendly requires action in many sectors – health, long-term care, transport, housing, labour, social protection, information and communication – by many actors – government, service providers, civil society, older people and their organizations, families and friends. It also requires action at multiple levels of government. Aiming towards the shared goal of optimizing functional ability allows these different stakeholders to work within their core areas but in a focused way that complements what is being done by others.

Opportunities for action on specific abilities have been given in Chapter 6. The following key approaches are relevant for each of these abilities and to all stakeholders:

1. combat ageism;
2. enable autonomy;
3. support *Healthy Ageing* in all policies at all levels of government.

Combat ageism

Age-based stereotypes influence behaviours, policy development and even research. Addressing these must lie at the core of any public-health response to population ageing. Although this will be challenging, experiences combating other widespread forms of discrimination, such as sexism and racism, show that attitudes and norms can be changed. There are also concrete examples of how this might be done for ageism (Box 7.3).

Tackling ageism will require building and embedding in the thinking of all generations, a new understanding of ageing. As this report emphasizes, this cannot be based on outdated conceptualizations of older people as burdens or on unrealistic assumptions that older people today have somehow avoided the health challenges of their parents and grandparents. Rather, it demands an acceptance of the wide diversity of the experience of older age, acknowledgement of the inequities that often underlie it, and an openness to asking how things might be done better.

Actions that may help tackle ageism include:
▪ undertaking communication campaigns to increase knowledge about and understanding of ageing among the media, general public, policy-makers, employers and service providers;
▪ legislating against age-based discrimination;

Box 7.3.   Say No to Ageism in Ireland

Ireland has run an ongoing campaign against ageism based on the wealth of evidence that negative stereotyping and discrimination against older people is pervasive and damaging. Say No to Ageism Week occurred annually from 2004 to 2012 to promote awareness and stimulate action against ageism. Developed by the Equality Authority and the Health Service Executive, with the support of the Office for Older People and older people's organizations, Say No to Ageism Week comprised two complementary strands: a public information campaign using advertising, radio, social media and posters; and the implementation of a series of sector-based actions designed to enhance the provision of age-friendly services.

Over the years, sectors that have participated included health, transportation, insurance, hospitality, sports and leisure. Actions taken by participating sectors have included holding focus groups with older adults to learn about the barriers they faced in using fitness facilities; providing age-awareness training for all frontline customer-facing staff of Dublin Bus; providing free transport to Say No to Ageism events; making improvements to information and signs to ensure they used more-age-friendly messages, including replacing the word "elderly" with "older people"; and showcasing older employees in marketing materials to emphasize the inclusiveness of Irish industries.

A review of the Say No to Ageism initiative was conducted in 2008 and highlighted the strong commitment, engagement and working relationships among partners and sectoral stakeholders as being key to the campaign's success.

Although information campaigns that raise awareness and stimulate debate about ageism among the general public are important in their own right, one of the strengths of the Irish initiative has been to underpin this awareness-raising with practical sector-based initiatives that provided tailored training with the aim of effecting positive changes in behaviours and the provision of services (2).

- ensuring that a balanced view of ageing is presented in the media, for example by minimizing sensationalist reporting of crimes against older people.

Enable autonomy

Older people have a right to make choices and take control over a range of issues including where they live, the relationships they have, what they wear, how they spend their time and whether they undergo a treatment or not. The possibilities for choice and control are shaped by many factors including the intrinsic capacity of the older person, the environments they inhabit, the personal and financial resources they can draw on, and the opportunities available to them. Together these determine the autonomy of older people, which has been shown to have a powerful influence on their dignity, integrity, freedom and independence, and has been repeatedly identified as a core component of their general well-being.

One key approach to enabling autonomy will be to maximize intrinsic capacity, and this is largely covered in the key areas for action by the health sector outlined above. But autonomy can also be enhanced regardless of an older person's level of capacity. This may be accomplished by changing the environments they inhabit or providing assistive devices that help them manage limitations in capacity. It may also arise by protecting their rights and strengthening their resilience and ability to control or change their environments. Autonomy is also heavily dependent on an older person's basic needs being met.

Actions that will be important in enabling autonomy include:

- legislating to protect the rights of older people (for example, by protecting them from elder abuse), supporting older people in becoming aware of and enjoying their rights, and creating mechanisms that can be used to address breaches of their rights, including in emergency situations;
- providing services that facilitate functioning, such as assistive technologies, and community-based or home-based services;
- providing mechanisms for advance care planning and supported decision-making that enable older people to retain the maxi-

mum level of control over their lives despite a significant loss of capacity;

- creating accessible opportunities for life-long learning and growth.

Support *Healthy Ageing* in all policies at all levels of government

In a rapidly increasing number of countries, more than 1 in 5 of the population are older than 60 years. There will be few policies or services that do not affect them in some way. If the goals of *Healthy Ageing* are to be achieved, all sectors need to consider their contribution to and impact on *Healthy Ageing*.

National, regional, state or municipal ageing strategies and action plans can help to guide this intersectoral response, and ensure a coordinated approach that spans multiple sectors and levels of government (Box 7.4). These will need to establish clear commitments to goals and clear lines of responsibility, have adequate budgets, and specify mechanisms for coordination, monitoring, evaluating and reporting across sectors.

Collecting and using age-disaggregated information about older people's abilities will also be important. This can facilitate reviews of the effectiveness of, and gaps in, existing policies, systems and services. Furthermore, mech-

Box 7.4. Live and age together (Vivre et vieillir ensemble): intersectoral action in Quebec

In 2011 the Secretariat aux aînés, a provincial agency for older adults, part of the government of Quebec, announced its first ageing policy aimed at fostering an inclusive and comprehensive approach to supporting older adults: Vivre et vieillir ensemble. At its core is collaboration across sectors and levels of government to enable older people to age in their homes and communities.

Intergovernmental – horizontal collaboration: this involves agencies and departments at the same level of government collaborating across missions and jurisdictions. For example:

- three province-level departments have collaborated to improve the quality of services, training and compensation for caregivers in order to improve the availability of support for older adults living at home;
- to improve the quality of life of older adults, two provincial bodies joined forces in 2010 (in the Programme d'infrastructures Quebec-Municipalites – Municipalite amie des aînés) to provide financial support for small infrastructure and facilities projects, such as renovating municipal buildings or enhancing recreational facilities to reflect the needs and expectations of older people (for example, by constructing accessible toilets or building walking paths).

Intergovernmental – vertical collaboration: this involves collaboration among the provincial level (Quebec), regional level and municipal (local) levels of government to achieve shared goals. In an effort to increase older people's use of public transit, two provincial bodies and one regional body, including county municipalities, partnered to review and modify public transportation plans to ensure that older adults had access to transport.

Collaboration between government and the private sector: this involves collaboration among the government, and local and provincial nongovernmental organizations and community-based organizations, private industry and academia. In Montreal, an action-based research project has been established between academia and the research division of the police department to develop and implement a police intervention to counter elder abuse; it comprises prevention, detection, first-line intervention, follow-up and investigation. This model emphasizes an intersectoral response to elder abuse that includes the police, a victim's assistance centre, community-based organizations, public health and social services, the public curator and the courts.

Collaboration between families, governments and the private sector: another example of collaboration between older people and their families that relates to enhancing long-term care. Family members caring for an older relative receive from the government both a tax credit as well as financial assistance for engaging caregivers and trained health-care professionals to come into the home to provide part-time care.

anisms to consult and involve older people or older people's organizations in the development and evaluation of policies can help ensure their relevance to local populations.

There are many areas for action, but opportunities include:

- establishing policies and programmes that expand housing options for older adults and assist with home modifications that enable older people to age in a place that is right for them;
- introducing measures to ensure that older people are protected from poverty, for example through social protection schemes;
- providing opportunities for social participation and for having meaningful social roles, specifically by targeting the processes that marginalize and isolate older people;
- removing barriers, setting accessibility standards and ensuring compliance in buildings, in transport, and in ICT;
- considering town-planning and land-use decisions and their impact on older people's safety and mobility;
- promoting age-diversity and inclusion in working environments.

Improve measurement, monitoring and understanding

Making progress on *Healthy Ageing* will require a far better understanding of age-related issues and trends. Many basic questions remain to be answered.

- What are the current patterns of *Healthy Ageing* and are they changing over time?
- What are the determinants of *Healthy Ageing*? Are inequalities increasing or narrowing?
- Which interventions work to foster *Healthy Ageing*? In which population subgroups do they work? What is the appropriate timing and sequencing of these interventions to maintain and increase intrinsic capacity and functional ability?

- What are the needs for health care and long-term care among older people, and how well are these being met?
- What are the real economic contributions made by older people and the true costs and benefits of fostering *Healthy Ageing*?

As a first step towards answering these, older people must be included in vital statistics and general population surveys, and analyses of these information resources should be disaggregated by age and sex. Appropriate measures of *Healthy Ageing* and its determinants and distributions will also need to be included in these studies.

But research will also need to be encouraged in a range of specific fields related to ageing and health, and this will require agreement on key concepts and how they can be measured. Approaches such as multicountry and multidisciplinary studies should be encouraged because they can be representative of a population's diversity and investigate the determinants of *Healthy Ageing* and the distinct context of older adults. So, too, should the involvement and contributions of older people. This may lead to more relevant and more innovative results (Box 7.5).

Finally, as new knowledge on ageing and health is generated, global and local mechanisms will be needed to ensure its rapid translation into clinical practice, population-based public-health interventions and health and social policies.

Key approaches include the following:
1. agree on metrics, measures and analytical approaches for *Healthy Ageing*;
2. improve understanding of the health status and needs of older populations and how well their needs are being met;
3. increase understanding of *Healthy Ageing* trajectories and what can be done to improve them.

Agree on metrics, measures and analytical approaches for *Healthy Ageing*

The current metrics and methods used in the field of ageing are limited, preventing a sound under-

Box 7.5. Research with, not just for, older people

The Manchester Institute for Collaborative Research on Ageing in England has undertaken a study on age-friendly cities that draws on the views, concerns and expertise of older residents (3). Working with targeted groups in three neighbourhoods of south Manchester, three key characteristics shape this work:

- **participation** – older residents act as co-investigators at all stages of the process, including planning, design and implementation;
- **collaboration** – a range of partners, including local government, voluntary organizations and other nongovernmental organizations, act as advisers, contributing via focus groups, interviews and ongoing partnerships;
- **action** – recommendations have been generated for urban design, regeneration, community engagement and policy implementation. A new space has been opened for insights to be fed directly into ongoing programmes and initiatives in Manchester and beyond.

A diverse group of 18 adults aged between 58 and 74 years, were trained as co-investigators. Participatory sessions and reflection meetings ensured that participants were involved – and became familiar with – all aspects of the research process, including design. In total, 68 in-depth interviews were conducted with older residents, many of whom experienced multiple forms of social exclusion, health problems, social isolation and poverty.

Taken as a whole, this study represents a significant methodological step forward in developing new models for community engagement. Interventions such as those used in the study represent excellent sources of data, valuable exercises in community engagement for all participants, and cost-effective mechanisms for producing informed policy in times of austerity.

standing of key aspects of *Healthy Ageing*. Often, appropriate methods do not yet exist. Sometimes, comprehensive approaches are used in other fields but not adapted to older populations. Consensus is needed on which approaches are most appropriate. These will need to allow comparisons and possibly

the linkage of data collected in a range of countries, settings and sectors. Priorities for action include:

- developing and reaching consensus on metrics, measurement strategies, instruments, tests and biomarkers for key concepts related to *Healthy Ageing*, including for functional ability, intrinsic capacity, subjective well-being, health characteristics, personal characteristics, genetic inheritance, multimorbidity and the need for services and care;
- reaching consensus on approaches for assessing and interpreting trajectories of these metrics and measures during the life course. It will be important to demonstrate how the information generated can serve as inputs for policy, monitoring, evaluation, clinical or public-health decisions;
- developing and applying improved approaches for testing clinical interventions that take account of the different physiology of older people and multimorbidity.

Improve understanding of the health status and needs of older populations and how well their needs are being met

Although general population-based research and surveillance need to place a greater emphasis on older people, specific population-based research about older people is also required to identify levels and the distribution of functional ability and intrinsic capacity, how these change over time, health and care needs, and how well these are being met. This research might include:

- establishing regular population surveys of older people that can reflect in detail the functional ability; intrinsic capacity; specific health states; need for health care or long-term care or broader environmental changes, and whether these needs are being met;
- mapping trends in intrinsic capacity and functional ability in different birth cohorts and determining whether increasing life expectancy is associated with added years of health;

- identifying indicators and mechanisms for the continuous surveillance of *Healthy Ageing* trajectories.

Increase understanding of *Healthy Ageing* trajectories and what can be done to improve them

Fostering *Healthy Ageing* will require a much better understanding of common trajectories of intrinsic capacity and functional ability, their determinants and the effectiveness of interventions to modify them. Key actions to achieving this understanding include:

- identifying the range and types of trajectories of intrinsic capacity and functional ability, and their determinants in different populations;
- quantifying the impact of health care, long-term care and environmental interventions on trajectories of *Healthy Ageing*, and identifying the pathways through which they operate;
- better quantifying the economic contribution of older people and the costs of providing the services they require, and developing rigorous, valid and comparable ways of analysing returns on investments.

Conclusion

Comprehensive public-health action on ageing is urgently needed. Although there are major knowledge gaps, we have sufficient evidence to act now, and there is something that every country can do irrespective of its current situation or level of development.

The societal response to population ageing will require a transformation of health systems that moves away from disease-based curative models and towards the provision of older-person-centred and integrated care. It will require the development, sometimes from nothing, of comprehensive systems of long-term care. And it will require a coordinated response from many other sectors and multiple levels of government. It must be built on a fundamental shift in our understanding of ageing to one that takes account of the diversity of older populations and responds to the inequities that often underlie ageing. And it will need to draw on better ways of measuring and monitoring the health and functioning of older populations.

Although these actions will inevitably require resources, they are likely to be a sound investment in society's future: a future that gives older people the freedom to live lives that previous generations could never have imagined.

References

1. Alexandra Health System's Ageing-in-Place Programme – first Singapore public healthcare programme to win 2014 UN Public Service Award. Singapore: Khoo Teck Puat Hospital; 2014 (https://www.ktph.com.sg/uploads/1403773586Media%20Release%20-%20First%20Singapore%20Public%20Healthcare%20Programme%20to%20Win%202014%20UN%20Public%20Service%20Award.pdf, accessed 29 June 2015).
2. Say No to Ageism Week (Ireland). In: Equinet; European Network of Equality Bodies [website]. Brussels: Equinet Secretariat; 2015 (http://www.equineteurope.org/Say-No-To-Ageism-Week-Ireland, accessed 15 July 2015).
3. Buffel T, editor. Researching age-friendly communities: stories from older people as co-investigators. Manchester: University of Manchester Library; 2015. (http://www.socialsciences.manchester.ac.uk/medialibrary/brochures/Age-Friendly-Booklet.pdf, accessed 27 July 2015).

Glossary

Accessibility

describes the degree to which an environment, service or product allows access by as many people as possible

Active ageing

the process of optimizing opportunities for health, participation and security in order to enhance quality of life as people age

Activities of daily living (ADLs)

the basic activities necessary for daily life, such as bathing or showering, dressing, eating, getting in or out of bed or chairs, using the toilet, and getting around inside the home

Activity

the execution of a task or action by an individual

Advance directive (or living will)

a mechanism by which competent individuals express their wishes so that should circumstances arise in which they no longer are able to make decisions regarding medical treatment, their preferences are respected; advance directives are made by writing living wills or granting power of attorney to another individual

Age (chronological)

the time lived since birth

Age-friendly cities and communities

a city or community that fosters Healthy and Active Ageing

Age-friendly environments

environments (such as in the home or community) that foster Healthy and Active Ageing by building and maintaining intrinsic capacity across the life course and enabling greater functional ability in someone with a given level of capacity

Ageing

at a biological level, ageing results from the impact of the accumulation of a wide variety of molecular and cellular damage that occurs over time

Ageing in (the right) place

ageing in place is the ability to live in one's own home and community safely, independently and comfortably, regardless of age, income or level of capacity. Ageing in the right place extends this concept to the ability to live in the place with the closest fit with the person's needs and preferences – which may or may not be one's own home

Ageism

stereotyping and discrimination against individuals or groups on the basis of their age; ageism can take many forms, including prejudicial attitudes, discriminatory practices, or institutional policies and practices that perpetuate stereotypical beliefs

Assistive technologies (or assistive health technology)

any device designed, made or adapted to help a person perform a particular task; products may be generally available or specially designed for people with specific losses of capacity; assistive health technology is a subset of assistive technologies, the primary purpose of which is to maintain or improve an individual's functioning and well-being

Barriers

factors in a person's environment that limit functional ability through their absence or presence

Built environment

the buildings, roads, utilities, homes, fixtures, parks and all other human-made entities that form the physical characteristics of a community

Care dependence

this arises when functional ability has fallen to a point where an individual is no longer able to undertake the basic tasks that are necessary for daily life without assistance

Caregiver

a person who provides care and support to someone else; such support may include:

- helping with self-care, household tasks, mobility, social participation and meaningful activities;
- offering information, advice and emotional support, as well as engaging in advocacy, providing support for decision-making and peer support, and helping with advance care planning;
- offering respite services; and
- engaging in activities to foster intrinsic capacity

caregivers may include family members, friends, neighbours, volunteers, care workers and health professionals

Case management

a collaborative process of planning services to meet an individual's health needs through communication with the individual and their service providers and coordination of resources

Chronic condition

a disease, disorder, injury or trauma that is persistent or has long-lasting effects

Comprehensive geriatric assessment

a multidimensional assessment of an older person that includes medical, physical, cognitive, social and spiritual components; may also include the use of standardized assessment instruments and an interdisciplinary team to support the process

Disability

an umbrella term for impairments, activity limitations and participation restrictions, denoting the negative aspects of the interaction between an individual (with a health condition) and that individual's contextual factors (environmental and personal factors)

Elder abuse

a single or repeated act, or lack of appropriate action, occurring within any relationship where there is an expectation of trust that causes harm or distress to an older person

Environments

all the factors in the extrinsic world that form the context of an individual's life; these include home, communities and the broader society; within these environments are a range of factors, including the built environment, people and their relationships, attitudes and values, health and social policies, systems and services

Facilitators

factors in a person's environment that through their absence or presence improve functional ability; these include factors such as a physical environment that is accessible, the availability of relevant assistive technology, and positive attitudes towards older people, as well as services, systems and policies that aim to increase the involvement of all people with a health condition in all areas of life; the absence of a factor can also be a facilitator – for example, the absence of stigma or negative attitudes; facilitators can prevent an impairment or activity limitation from restricting participation because the actual performance of an action is enhanced despite a person's problem with capacity

Frailty (or frail older person)

extreme vulnerability to endogenous and exogenous stressors that exposes an individual to a higher risk of negative health-related outcomes

Functional ability

the health-related attributes that enable people to be and to do what they have reason to value; it is made up of the intrinsic capacity of the individual, relevant environmental characteristics and the interactions between the individual and these characteristics

Functioning

an umbrella term for body functions, body structures, activities and participation; it denotes the positive aspects of the interaction between an individual (with a health condition) and that individual's contextual factors (environmental and personal factors)

Geriatric syndromes

complex health states that tend to occur only later in life and that do not fall into discrete disease categories; they are often a consequence of multiple underlying factors and dysfunction in multiple organ systems

Geriatrics

the branch of medicine specializing in the health and illnesses of older age and their appropriate care and services

Gerontology

the study of the social, psychological and biological aspects of ageing

Health

a state of complete physical, mental and social well-being, and not merely the absence of disease or infirmity

Health characteristics

underlying age-related changes, health-related behaviours, physiological risk factors (for example, high blood pressure), diseases, injuries, changes to homeostasis, and broader geriatric syndromes; the interaction among these health characteristics will ultimately determine the intrinsic capacity of an individual

Health condition

an umbrella term for acute or chronic disease, disorder, injury or trauma

Health inequality

differences in health status occurring among individuals or groups or, more formally, the total inter-individual variation in health for a population, which often considers differences in socioeconomic status or other demographic characteristics

Health inequity

differences in health that are unnecessary, avoidable, unfair and unjust

Health promotion

the process of enabling people to increase control over and to improve their health

Healthy Ageing

the process of developing and maintaining the functional ability that enables well-being in older age

Home modifications

conversions or adaptations made to the permanent physical features of the home environment to improve safety, physical accessibility and comfort

Impairment

a loss or abnormality in body structure or physiological function (including mental functions); in this report, abnormality is used strictly to refer to a significant variation from established statistical norms (that is, deviation from a population mean within measured standard norms)

Informal care

unpaid care provided by a family member, friend, neighbour or volunteer

Institutional care setting

refers to institutions in which long-term care is provided; these may include community centres, assisted living facilities, nursing homes, hospitals and other health facilities; institutional care settings are not defined only by their size

Instrumental activities of daily living (IADLs)

activities that facilitate independent living, such as using the telephone, taking medications, managing money, shopping for groceries, preparing meals and using a map

Integrated health services

integrated health services are managed and delivered in a way that ensures people receive a continuum of services including health promotion, disease prevention, diagnosis, treatment, disease-management, rehabilitation and palliative care at different levels and sites within the health system, and that care is provided according to their needs throughout their life course

International Classification of Functioning, Disability and Health

a classification of health and health-related domains that describe body functions and structures, activities and participation; the domains are classified from different perspectives: body, individual and societal; because an individual's functioning and disability occur within a context, this classification includes a list of environmental factors

Intrinsic capacity

the composite of all the physical and mental capacities that an individual can draw on

Life-course approach

this considers the underlying biological, behavioural and psychosocial processes that operate across the life course, which are shaped by individual characteristics and by the environments in which we live

Life expectancy (at age 60)

the average number of years that a 60-year-old can expect to live if he or she is subject to the age-specific mortality rate during a given period

Life expectancy (at birth)

the average number of years that a newborn would be expected to live if he or she is subject to the age-specific mortality rate during a given period

Longevity

how long people live

Long-term care

the activities undertaken by others to ensure that people with a significant ongoing loss of intrinsic capacity can maintain a level of functional ability consistent with their basic rights, fundamental freedoms and human dignity

Mobility

moving by changing body position or location, or by transferring from one place to another; by carrying, moving or manipulating objects; by walking, running or climbing; and by using various forms of transportation

Multimorbidity

the co-occurrence of two or more chronic medical conditions in one person

Noncommunicable diseases

diseases that are not passed from person to person; the four main types of noncommunicable diseases are cardiovascular diseases (such as heart attacks and stroke), cancers, chronic respiratory diseases (such as chronic obstructive pulmonary disease and asthma) and diabetes

Old

a social construct that defines the norms, roles and responsibilities that are expected of an older person; it is frequently used in a pejorative sense

Older person

a person whose age has passed the median life expectancy at birth

Out-of-pocket expenditure

payments for goods or services that include (i) direct payments, such as payments for goods or services that are not covered by any form of insurance; (ii) cost sharing – that is a provision of health insurance or third-party payment that requires the individual who is covered to pay part of the cost of the health care received; and (iii) informal payments, such as unofficial payments for goods and services, that should be fully funded from pooled revenue

Participation

a person's involvement in a life situation; it represents the societal perspective of functioning

People-centred services

an approach to care that consciously adopts the perspectives of individuals, families and communities, and sees them as participants as well as beneficiaries of health care and long-term-care systems that respond to their needs and preferences in humane and holistic ways; ensuring that people-centred care is delivered requires that people have the education and support they need to make decisions and participate in their own care; it is organized around the health needs and expectations of people rather than diseases

Performance

what individuals do in their current environment, including their involvement in life situations

Person–environment fit

the relationship between individuals and their environments; the fit between people and their environments requires (i) consideration of the person (that is, an individual's health characteristics and capacity) and societal needs and resources, (ii) awareness that the relationship is dynamic and interactive, and (iii) attention to the changes that occur in people and places over time

Polypharmacy

the simultaneous administration of multiple medications to the same patient

Population ageing

a shift in the population structure whereby the proportion of people in older age groups increases

Reasonable accommodation

the necessary and appropriate modifications and adjustments that can be made without imposing a disproportionate or undue burden to ensure that older persons with reduced functional ability can enjoy and exercise all human rights and fundamental freedoms on an equal basis with others

Rehabilitation

a set of measures aimed at individuals who have experienced or are likely to experience disability to assist them in achieving and maintaining optimal functioning when interacting with their environments

Resilience

the ability to maintain or improve a level of functional ability in the face of adversity through resistance, recovery or adaptation

Risk factor

a risk factor is an attribute or exposure that is causally associated with an increased probability of a disease or injury

Self-care (or self-management)

activities carried out by individuals to promote, maintain, treat and care for themselves, as well as to engage in making decisions about their health

Social care (services)

assistance with the activities of daily living (such as personal care, maintaining the home)

Social network

an individual's web of kinship, friendship and community ties

Social protection

programmes to reduce deprivation that arises from conditions such as poverty, unemployment, old age and disability

Social security

includes all measures providing benefits, whether in cash or in kind, to secure social protection

Supported decision-making

refers to people receiving support to exercise their legal capacity; supported decision-making can take many forms, including the use of support networks, a personal ombudsperson, community services, peer support, a personal assistant and advance planning

Universal design

the design of environments, products and systems to be usable by all people to the greatest extent possible without the need for adaptation or specialized design

Well-being

a general term encompassing the total universe of human life domains, including physical, mental and social aspects, that make up what can be called a "good life"

Index

O

OECD *see* Organisation for Economic Co-operation and Development
old **229**
older person *see* elder or older person
online *see* Internet
oral and dental health 72
    India, priority 98
Organisation for Economic Co-operation and Development (OECD) 46, 67
    long-term care 129, 131, 132, 144
    mortalities 45, 46, 47
    women's financial security 162
    see also high-income countries
organizations and associations
    older peoples' 138, 146, 177–178
    for volunteers 193
osteoarthritis 50, 54, 57, 71
osteoporosis 53–54
out-of-pocket payments/expenditure 16, 92, 131, **230**
outpatient care, sources of payment for 92
outreach, community 98, 105, 106, 107, 176

P

Pakistan, dementia day care 141
palliative care 103, 142
participation 222
    creating opportunities 183–184
    right to 15
    see also collaboration
payments and expenditure (incl. cash)
    choice and control enabled by 178
    out-of-pocket 16, 92, 131, **230**
    for outpatient care, sources 92
peers 176–177
    peer-to-peer support 176
        South Africa 216
pensions 163–165, 191
    early retirement-incentivizing 191
    inequities 9
people *see* persons
performance **230**

persons/individual people
    environment and, fit between 30, **230**
    person-centred services and interventions 34–35, 100–105, 113, 214
        dementia 140
        long-term care 135, 139, 140, 144
    personal characteristics 29
    personal health budgets 178
    personal security *see* safety and security
Peru, caregivers and care arrangements 130
pharmacists, Australia 110
    see also medications and drugs
physical accessibility to or in home 166–167, 168
physical activity/exercise 70–71, 101, 106–107, 181
    built environment and 182
    home-based 106–107
    maintaining mobility by 180, 181
physical capacity across life course 7, 31
police, community, New Delhi 170
policies (government) 4–7, 220–221
    development 7–13
    equity-enhancing 35
    financial security 165
    Healthy Ageing 111–112, 168, 220–221
    housing 166–169
    long-term care 146–147
    working and volunteering 189, 190
Political declaration 4, 5, 7, 27
polypharmacy 62, 110, **230**
population ageing 43–49, **230**
    economic impact on health systems 95–98
    long-term care and 129
Portugal, Telephone Rings at 5 186
positive messaging 178
postmarketing surveillance 114
poverty
    long-term care reducing 147
    meeting basic needs in 162–163
presbycusis (hearing loss) 54, 55, 60, 93
presbyopia 54

sexuality 56

SHARE (Survey of Health, Ageing and Retirement in Europe) 53, 59, 68, 69

Singapore
    ageing in place 214
    dementia respite care 141
    supporting ageing in place 214
    universal design 183

skills and competencies (workforce) 94, 215
    long-term care 139
    multidisciplinary teams 108

skin functions and conditions 57

smart-home technology 168

social care/services/support 143, 146, 178, **231**
    Turkey 154

social changes, global dimensions 12–13

social isolation and loneliness 111, 161, 184–185, 186–187

social networks 184, 186, 188, **231**

social pensions 164

social protection 49, 163, 163–164, 194–195, **231**

social relationships *see* relationships

social roles 188

social security 163, 165, **231**

socioeconomic development 10, 12, 45, 48, 66–67, 211, 215
    see also high-income countries; low- and/or middle-income countries

South Africa
    community-based peer-to-peer support in Cape Town 217
    housing subsidies 169
    pensions 164

South and Central (Latin) America, financing long-term care 144–145

specialist health services 93, 102, 104, 107, 109

Sri Lanka, accessibility to buildings 184

stereotypes 10–11, 159, 175
    see also ageism; negative attitudes

stewardship of long-term care systems 135, 144, 149

stroke 6, 15, 30, 58, 61, 71

Study on global AGEing and adult health (SAGE) 6, 53, 54, 65, 66, 68, 71, 92

sub-Saharan Africa
    financial security 162
    health system use 90, 93
    long-term care financing 144–145
    population ageing 43

subsidies
    housing 167, 169
    wage 141–142

supply of long-term caregivers 136–138

supported decision-making 177, 219–220, **231**

Survey of Health, Ageing and Retirement in Europe (SHARE) 53, 59, 68, 69

sustainability 15, 114
    financing of long-term care 144–146
    health workforce 215, 217

Switzerland, Cité Seniors in Geneva 188

T

teams *see* multidisciplinary teams

technologies (incl. innovative technologies) 36, 147
    accessibility 110–111
    assistive *see* assistive (health) technologies
    information and communication (ICT) 108, 109–110, 173–174, 187, 188, 194–195, 215
    medical 110

Telephone Rings at 5 (Portugal) 186

Thailand
    "brain banks" 193
    care integration and coordination 97

Torbay Care Trust 95–96

training and education
    community, on disaster risk management 174
    older persons 167, 175, 176, 181, 194–195
      volunteer 193
    workforce (paid and unpaid) 94, 108, 109, 167, 215